Novel Medical and General Hebrew Terminology from the Middle Ages

Novel Medical and General Hebrew Terminology from the Middle Ages

VOLUME 5

By

Gerrit Bos

BRILL

LEIDEN | BOSTON

Cover illustration: *Sefer Ṣedah la-Oreḥim u-ve-Lashon ha-Noṣrim BY'ṬYQW* (*Viatico*). Anonymous adaptation of the Hebrew translation by Abraham ben Isaac of Ibn al-Jazzar's *Zād al-musāfir wa-qūt al-ḥādir*. Ms Berlin, Staatsbibliothek Preußischer Kulturbesitz, Or. fol. 1058, fol. 88[b], copied in the fifteenth century in an Italian script. © STAATSBIBLIOTHEK ZU BERLIN – Preußischer Kulturbesitz, Orientabteilung. See also: Moritz Steinschneider, *Verzeichnis der hebräischen Handschriften in Berlin*, 2 vols. (Repr., Hildesheim 1980), no. 113.

Library of Congress Cataloging-in-Publication Data

Names: Bos, Gerrit, 1948- author.
Title: Novel medical and general Hebrew terminology from the Middle Ages. Volume 5 / Gerrit Bos.
Description: Boston : Brill, 2021. | Includes bibliographical references and index.
Identifiers: LCCN 2021038591 (print) | LCCN 2021038592 (ebook) | ISBN 9789004472792 (hardback) | ISBN 9789004472808 (ebook)
Subjects: LCSH: Medicine–Terminology. | Hebrew language, Medieval–Glossaries, vocabularies, etc.
Classification: LCC R123 .B6683 2021 (print) | LCC R123 (ebook) | DDC 610.1/4–dc23/eng/20211004
LC record available at https://lccn.loc.gov/2021038591
LC ebook record available at https://lccn.loc.gov/2021038592

Typeface for the Latin, Greek, and Cyrillic scripts: "Brill". See and download: brill.com/brill-typeface.

ISBN 978-90-04-47279-2 (hardback)
ISBN 978-90-04-47280-8 (e-book)

Contents

Sigla and Abbreviations

Sigla

a — Arabic text

BCD — G. Bos, *A Concise Dictionary of Novel Medical and General Hebrew Terminolog from the Middle Ages* (Leiden 2019).

BDB — F. Brown, S.R. Driver, and C.A. Briggs, *A Hebrew and English Lexicon of the Old Testament*, with an appendix containing the Biblical Aramaic, based on the lexicon of William Gesenius as translated by Edward Robinson (Repr., Oxford 1978).

BM — Eliezer Ben-Yehuda, *Millon ha-Lashon ha-Ivrit: Thesaurus Totius Hebraitatis et Veteris et Recentioris* (Repr., 8 vols., Tel Aviv, 1948–1959).

BMC — Maimonides, *On Coitus*, ed. and trans. by G. Bos, with editions of Medieval Hebrew translations by G. Bos, Medieval Latin translations by Ch. Burnett, and a Slavonic translation by W.F. Ryan and M. Taube (Leiden 2018).

BMH — Maimonides, *On Hemorrhoids*, ed. and trans. by G. Bos, with critical editions of Medieval Hebrew translations by G. Bos and Medieval Latin translations by M.R. McVaugh (Provo, UT 2012).

BMHA — Maimonides, *Commentary on Hippocrates'* Aphorisms, ed. and trans. by G. Bos, with critical editions of Medieval Hebrew translations, 2 vols. (Leiden 2020).

BMMN — Maimonides, *Medical Aphorisms: Hebrew Translation by Nathan ha-Me'ati*, ed. by G. Bos (Leiden 2020).

BMMZ — Maimonides, *Medical Aphorisms: Hebrew Translation by Zeraḥyah ben Isaac ben She'altiel Ḥen*, ed. by G. Bos (Leiden 2020).

BMP — Maimonides, *On Poisons and the Protection against Lethal Drugs*, ed. and trans. by G. Bos, with critical editions of Medieval Hebrew translations by G. Bos and Medieval Latin translations by M.R. McVaugh (Provo, UT 2009).

BMR — Maimonides, *On the Regimen of Health*, ed. and trans. by G. Bos, with critical editions of Medieval Hebrew translations by G. Bos and Latin translations by M.R. McVaugh (Leiden 2019).

BMZ — G. Bos, G. Mensching, and J. Zwink (eds.), *Medical Glossaries in the Hebrew Tradition: Shem Tov ben Isaac:* Sefer Almansur, with a supplement on the Romance and Latin terminology (Leiden 2017).

D — R.P.A. Dozy, *Supplément aux dictionnaires arabes*, 2 vols. (Leiden 1927).

DCVB — A.M. Alcover Sureda and F. de Borja Moll, *Diccionari català-valencià-balear*, 2nd ed., 10 vols. (Palma de Mallorca 1980–1985).

DKT — P. de Koning, *Trois traités d'anatomie arabes*, ed. by F. Sezgin (Repr., Frankfurt am Main 1986).

DMLBS *Dictionary of Medieval Latin from British Sources*, ed. by R.E. Latham, D.R. Howlett, and R.K. Ashdowne, 3 vols. (London 1975–2013).

DN W. Daems, *Nomina Simplicium Medicinarum ex Synonymariis Medii Aevi Collecta: Semantische Untersuchungen zum Fachwortschatz hoch- und spätmittelalterlicher Drogenkunde*, = *Studies in Ancient Medicine*, vol. 6 (Leiden 1993).

DT *Dioscurides Triumphans: Ein anonymer arabischer Kommentar (Ende 12. Jahrh. n. Chr.) zur Materia medica*, arabischer Text nebst kommentierter deutscher Übersetzung, ed. by A. Dietrich, vol. 2 (Göttingen 1988).

DW *Pedanii Dioscuridis Anazarbei De Materia Medica Libri Quinque*, ed. by M. Wellmann (Repr., 5 pts. in 1 vol., Berlin 1958).

EM Abraham Even-Shoshan, *Ha-Millon he-Ḥadash* (Repr., 7 vols., Jerusalem 1983).

EP I. Efros, *Philosophical Terms in the Moreh Nebukim* (New York 1924).

FAL A. Fonahn, *Arabic and Latin Anatomical Terminology chiefly from the Middle Ages* (Kristiania 1922).

FEW W. von Wartburg, *Französisches Etymologisches Wörterbuch* (Bonn 1922–).

FL G.W. Freytag, *Lexicon Arabico-Latinum*, vols. 1–4 (Halis Saxonum 1830–1837).

FM J. Feliks, *Mar'ot ha-Mishnah, Seder Zera'im* (Jerusalem 1967).

HA J. Hyrtl, *Das arabische und hebräische in der Anatomie* (Repr., Schaan, Liechtenstein 1981).

HCD A. Heschel, *A Concise Dictionary of Hebrew Philosophical Terms: Mimeographed for Use in the Philosophy Classes of the Hebrew Union College-Jewish Institute of Religion* (Cicinnati 1941).

HM S. Heymans, *Ha-Millim ha-She'ulot mi-Yewanit u-mi-Latinit ba-Mishnah. Leksikon we-Torat Hegeh* (PhD diss., Tel Aviv 2013).

HU M. Steinschneider, *Die hebräischen Übersetzungen des Mittelalters und die Juden als Dolmetscher* (Repr., Graz 1956).

IBF Ibn al-Bayṭār, *Traité des simples*, trans. by L. Leclerc, 3 vols. (Paris 1877–1883).

IJZ Ibn al-Jazzār, *Zād al-musāfir wa-qūt al-ḥāḍir* (*Provisions for the Traveller and Nourishment for the Sedentary*)*: Book 7* (*7–30*), critical edition of the Arabic text with English translation and critical edition of Moses ibn Tibbon's Hebrew translation (*Ṣedat ha-Derakhim*), ed. and trans. by G. Bos (Leiden 2015).

ISW Ibn Sayyār al-Warrāq, *Kitāb al-Ṭabīkh*, ed. by K. Öhrnberg and S. Mroueh, = *Studia Orientalia*, vol. 60 (Helsinki 1987).

JD M. Jastrow, *A Dictionary of the Targumim, the Talmud Bavli and Yerushalmi, and the Midrashic Literature* (Repr., 2 vols., New York 1950).

KA A. Kohut, *Arukh shalem: Aruch Completum*, and S. Krauss, *Tosefet he-Arukh*. Additamenta. (Repr., 9 vols., Tel Aviv 1970).

KB L. Koehler and W. Baumgartner, *The Hebrew and Aramaic Lexicon of the Old Testament*, subsequently revised by W. Baumgartner and J.J. Stamm, with assistance from B. Hartmann, Z. Ben-Hayyim, E.Y. Kutscher, and Ph. Reymond, ed. and trans. under the supervision of M.E.J. Richardson, 5 vols. (Leiden 1994–2000).

KDS D. Kaufmann, *Die Sinne: Beiträge zur Geschichte der Physiologie und Psychologie im Mittelalter aus hebräischen und arabischen Quellen*, repr. in: idem, *Die Spuren al-Baṭaljûsi's (Budapest 1880)*, and *Studien über Salomon ibn Gabirol (Budapest 1899)*, and *Die Sinne (Budapest 1884)*, with an introduction by L. Jacobs (Farnborough 1972).

KG S. Krauss, *Griechische und Lateinische Lehnwörter im Talmud, Midrasch und Targum*, mit Bemerkungen von I. Löw, 2 vols. (Berlin 1898–1899).

KM F. Käs, *Die Mineralien in der arabischen Pharmakognosie: Eine Konkordanz zur mineralischen Materia medica der klassischen arabischen Heilmittelkunde nebst überlieferungsgeschichtlichen Studien*, 2 vols. = *Akademie der Wissenschaften und der Literatur Mainz: Veröffentlichungen der Orientalischen Kommission*, vol. 54 (Wiesbaden 2010).

KR O. Kahl, *The Sanskrit, Syrian, and Persian Sources in the* Comprehensive Book *of Rhazes* (Leiden 2015).

KTP J. Klatzkin, *Thesaurus Philosophicus linguae hebraicae et veteris et recentioris* (Repr., 4 pts. in 2 vols., New York 1968).

L Latin text

LA I. Löw, *Aramäische Pflanzennamen* (Leipzig 1881).

Lane E.W. Lane, *Arabic-English Lexicon*, 8 vols. (London 1863–1879).

LF I. Löw, *Die Flora der Juden*, 4 vols. (Repr., Hildesheim 1967).

Low A. Lowinger, 'Register of Hebrew and Aramaic Terms, translated and edited by S. Paley,' in: J. Preuss, *Biblisch-talmudische Medizin: Beiträge zur Geschichte der Heilkunde und der Kultur überhaupt* (Repr., New York 1971).

LS Ch.T. Lewis and Ch. Short, *A Latin Dictionary Founded on Andrews' Latin Dictionary*, revised, enlarged, and in great part rewritten (Oxford 1966).

LSG H.G. Liddell and R. Scott, *A Greek English Lexicon*, revised and augmented throughout by H.S. Jones, a.o., with a supplement (Repr., Oxford 1989).

LW J. Levy, *Wörterbuch über die Talmudim und Midraschim*, nebst Beiträgen von H. Leberecht Fleischer, 2nd ed., mit Nachträgen und Berichtigungen von L. Goldschmidt, 4 vols. (Berlin 1924).

M Maimonides, *Moses Maimonides' Glossary of Drug Names*, trans. and annotated by F. Rosner from M. Meyerhof's French edition (*Sharḥ asmāʾ al-ʿuqqār (L'explication des noms des drogues): Un glossaire de matière médicale composé par Maïmonide*) (Haifa 1995).

MD A.M. Masie, *Dictionary of Medicine and Allied Sciences: Latin-English-Hebrew*, ed. by S. Tchernichowsky (Jerusalem 1934).

MIG Marwān ibn Janāḥ, *On the Nomenclature of Medicinal Drugs* (*Kitāb al-Talkhīṣ*), edition, translation, and commentary with special reference to the Ibero-Romance terminology, ed. by G. Bos, F. Käs, M. Lübke, and G. Mensching, 2 vols. (Leiden 2020).

MM S. Muntner, *Mavo-le-Sefer Asaph ha-Rofe* (Jerusalem 1957).

MMT M. Meyerhof, ed., *The Book of the Ten Treatises on the Eye Asribed to Ḥunain ibn Isḥāq* (809–877 A.D.) (Cairo 1928), and: *Al-morchid fi'l kohhl ou le guide d'oculiste: Ouvrage inédit de l'oculiste arabe-espagnol Mohammad ibn Qassoûm ibn Aslam al-Ghâfiqî* (Barcelona 1933); repr. in: *Augenheilkunde im Islam: Texte, Studien und Übersetzungen*, vol. 2: *Werke von Ḥunain b. Ishaq und Muḥammad al-Ġāfiqī*, ed. by F. Sezgin, = *Veröffentlichungen des Institutes für Geschichte der Arabisch-Islamischen Wissenschaften*, Reihe B: *Nachdrucke, Abteilung Medizin*, vol. 3.2 (Frankfurt am Main 1986).

NA N. Nasrallah (trans.), *Annals of the Caliphs' Kitchens: Ibn Sayyār al-Warrāq's Tenth-Century Baghdadi Cookbook*, with introduction and glossary, = *Islamic History and Civilization*, vol. 70 (Leiden 2007).

ND J. Norri, *Dictionary of Medical Vocabulary in English, 1375–1550*, 2 vols. (London 2016).

NM 1 G. Bos, *Novel Medical and General Hebrew Terminology from the 13th Century: Translations by Hillel Ben Samuel of Verona, Moses Ben Samuel Ibn Tibbon, Shem Tov Ben Isaac of Tortosa, Zeraḥyah Ben Isaac Ben She'altiel Ḥen*, = *Journal of Semitic Studies*, suppl. 27 (Oxford 2011).

NM 2 G. Bos, *Novel Medical and General Hebrew Terminology from the 13th Century*, vol. 2, = *Journal of Semitic Studies*, suppl. 30 (Oxford 2013).

NM 3 G. Bos, *Novel Medical and General Hebrew Terminology: Hippocrates'* Aphorisms *in the Hebrew Tradition*, = *Journal of Semitic Studies*, suppl. 37 (Oxford 2016).

NM 4 G. Bos, *Novel Medical and General Hebrew Terminology from the 13th Century*, vol. 4 (Leiden 2018).

PESHAT *Premodern Philosophic and Scientific Hebrew Terminology in Context: An Online Thesaurus 'PESHAT in Context'*, ed. by R. Leicht and G. Veltri (https://peshat.gwiss.uni-hamburg.de).

RL Fr. Raynouard, *Lexique roman: Ou dictionnaire de la langue des troubadours comparée avec les autres langues de l'Europe latine*, 5 vols. (Heidelberg 1970).

ROT al-Rāzī, *On the Treatment of Small Children* (*De curis puerorum*)*: The Latin and Hebrew Translations*, ed. and trans. by G. Bos and M.R. McVaugh (Leiden 2015).

SCP F. Steingass, *A Comprehensive Persian-English Dictionary* (Repr., London 1984).

SD M. Sokoloff, *A Dictionary of Jewish Palestinian Aramaic of the Byzantine Period* (Ramat Gan 1990).

SDA M. Sokoloff, *A Dictionary of Jewish Babylonian Aramaic of the Talmudic and Geonic Periods* (Ramat Gan 2002).

ShMM A.O. Shemesh, *Ḥomre marpe ba-Sifrut ha-Yehudit: Medical Materials in Medieval and Modern Jewish Literature—Pharmacology, History, and Halakha* (Ramat Gan 2013).

SHS 1 G. Bos, M. Hussein, G. Mensching, and F. Savelsberg (eds.), *Medical Synonym Lists from Medieval Provence: Shem Tov Ben Isaac of Tortosa:* Sefer ha-Shimmush, *Book 29—Part 1: Edition and Commentary of List 1 (Hebrew-Arabic-Romance/Latin)* (Leiden 2011).

Sin G. Mensching, *La Sinonima delos nombres delas medeçinas griegos e latynos e arauigos* (Madrid 1994).

SM G.B. Sarfatti, *Munaḥei ha-Matematikah ba-Sifrut ha-Madda'it ha-'Ivrit shel Yemei ha-Benayyim: Mathematical Terminology in Hebrew Scientific Literature of the Middle Ages* (Jerusalem 1968).

SMK H. Shy, *Al-Muršid al-Kāfī: The Lexicon of Tanḥūm ben Yosef Hayerushalmi to Mishné tora of Maimonides with a Translation from Judaeo-Arabic into Hebrew and References* (Jerusalem 2005).

SN D. Sontheimer, 'Nachricht von einer arabisch-medicinischen Handschrift, vermutlich des Ibn-Dschezla,' in *Janus* 2 (1847): 246–272, Repr. in: *Beiträge zur Geschichte der arabisch-islamischen Medizin: Aufsätze*, vol. 1 (1819–1869), ed. by F. Sezgin, in collaboration with M. Amawi, D. Bischoff, and E. Neubauer (Frankfurt am Main 1987), 92–128.

SP W. Schmucker, *Die pflanzliche und mineralische Materia Medica im* Firdaus al-ḥikma *des 'Alī ibn Sahl Rabban Ṭabarī* (PhD diss., Bonn 1969).

SpLA M.S. Spink and G.L. Lewis (eds.), *Albucasis: On Surgery and Instruments*, a definitive edition of the Arabic text with English translation and commentary (London 1973).

StH M. Steinschneider, 'Heilmittelnamen der Araber,' *Wiener Zeitschrift für die Kunde des Morgenlandes* 11 (1897): 259–278; 313–330; 12 (1898): 1–20; 81–101; 201–229; 319–334; 13 (1899): 75–94.

UW M. Ullmann, *Wörterbuch zu den griechisch-arabischen Übersetzungen des neunten Jahrhunderts* (Wiesbaden 2002).

UWS 1 M. Ullmann, *Wörterbuch zu den griechisch-arabischen Übersetzungen des neunten Jahrhunderts*, suppl. 1: A-O (Wiesbaden 2006).

UWS 2 M. Ullmann, *Wörterbuch zu den griechisch-arabischen Übersetzungen des neunten Jahrhunderts*, suppl. 2: Π-Ω (Wiesbaden 2007).

VL	I.A. Vullers, *Lexicon Persico-Latinum Etymologicum*, 2 vols. (Repr., Graz 1962).
WKAS	*Wörterbuch der klassischen arabischen Sprache*, ed. by Deutsche Morgenländische Gesellschaft (Wiesbaden 1957–).

Abbreviations

abl.	ablative case
acc.	accusative case
Arab.	Arabic
Aram.	Aramaic
Bibl. Hebr.	Biblical Hebrew
Class. Lat.	Classical Latin
dat.	dative case
Engl.	English
esp.	especially
Ex	Exodus
Ez	Ezekiel
f.	female
Gen	Genesis
Ger.	German
Gr.	Greek
Hebr.	Hebrew
Inf.	infinitive
Ital.	Italian
Lat.	Latin
L.Lat.	Late Latin
M.Fr.	Middle French
M.Lat.	Middle Latin
Mod. Fr.	Modern French
Ms	manuscript
nom.	nominative case
O.Cat.	Old Catalan
O.Fr.	Old French
O.Occ.	Old Occitan
Part.	participle
Pass.	passive
Pers.	Persian
Plur.	plural

poss.	possibly
prob.	probably
re	as related to
Rom.	Romance
Sing.	singular
syn.	synonym
tb	Babylonian Talmud
trans.	translated (by)
var.	variant
vern.	vernacular

Introduction

The current volume is part of a wider project aiming at mapping the novel[1] Hebrew[2] technical medical and general terminology as it features in medieval Hebrew medical works translated both from the Arabic and Latin.[3] In this way I hope to facilitate the consultation of these and other medical works and the identification of anonymous medical material.

The main texts consulted are:

1. *Sefer Ṣedat ha-Derakhim*; i.e., Moses ben Samuel ben Judah ibn Tibbon's translation of Ibn al-Jazzār's *Zād al-musāfir wa-qūt al-ḥādir* (*Provisions for the Traveller and Nourishment for the Sedentary*), bks. 1–3.[4] The terms selected are derived from the forthcoming critical editions. The basic Hebrew manuscripts consulted for these editions are Ms London, British Library, Ar. Or. 26 (cat. Margoliouth 1024) (for bks. 1–2) and Oxford, Bodleian Library, Poc. 353, Uri Heb. 314 (for bk. 3). Significant variant readings featuring in other Mss have been mentioned as well.
2. *Sefer Ya'ir Netiv*; a translation made from Constantine the African's *Viaticum*.[5] It was done by an anonymous author living in the Midi who, after his conversion to Christianity, called himself Do'eg ha-Edomi.[6] Between

---

1 With 'novel' I mean those terms that do not feature in the current dictionaries of the Hebrew language at all, or that feature in these dictionaries but without proper explanation or in a later period. Occasionally, I include terms that have already been mentioned in the first four volumes dealing with novel Hebrew medical terminology in order to show the wider distribution of a certain term.

2 In addition to the Hebrew terms, the list below also includes loan words from Latin and Romance.

3 Earlier volumes published are: NM 1 = *Novel Medical and General Hebrew Terminology from the 13th Century: Translations by Hillel Ben Samuel of Verona, Moses Ben Samuel Ibn Tibbon, Shem Tov Ben Isaac of Tortosa, Zeraḥyah Ben Isaac Ben She'altiel Ḥen*, = Journal of Semitic Studies, suppl. 27 (Oxford, 2011); NM 2 = *Novel Medical and General Hebrew Terminology from the 13th Century*, vol. 2, = Journal of Semitic Studies, suppl. 30 (Oxford 2013); NM 3 = *Novel Medical and General Hebrew Terminology: Hippocrates'* Aphorisms *in the Hebrew Tradition*, = Journal of Semitic Studies, suppl. 37 (Oxford 2016); and NM 4 = *Novel Medical and General Hebrew Terminology from the 13th Century*, vol. 4 (Leiden 2019). The terms listed in these four volumes feature in an alphabetical arrangement in: BCD = *A Concise Dictionary of Novel Medical and General Hebrew Terminology from the Middle Ages* (Leiden 2020). Cf. also BMZ 7–8.

4 For this translation, possibly hailing from the year 1259, cf. the introduction to the forthcoming critical edition of bks. 1–2.

5 I.e., his Latin translation of Ibn al-Jazzār's *Zād al-musāfir wa-qūt al-ḥādir*. The Hebrew translator attributed the text to Isaac Israeli.

6 For this translation, completed between 1197 and 1199, cf. the introduction to the forth-

 | DOI:10.1163/9789004472808_002

1197 and 1199 he completed the translation of a corpus of twenty-four medical texts, both practical and theoretical, from Latin to Hebrew. These texts were the first complete Hebrew translations of works by non-Jewish authors on secular subjects. The terms selected from bks. 1–3 are derived from the forthcoming critical editions. The basic Ms is London, British Library, Add. 18969. In the case of corruptions, omissions, or variant readings, I consulted Ms Oxford, Bodleian Library, Can. Or. 26; Ms Moscow, Russian State Library, Guenzburg 1481; and Ms Parma, Bibliotheca Palatina, Cod. Parm. 2474. A small number of terms consists of loan words from the Latin that are part of the standard technical vocabulary employed by Do'eg ha-Edomi. The parallel Latin terms from Constantine the African's translation are derived from the forthcoming critical editions. The parallel Arabic terms from Ibn al-Jazzār's *Zād al-musāfir wa-qūt al-ḥāḍir* are derived from the critical editions mentioned before.

3. *Sefer Ṣedah la-Oreḥim*; an incomplete translation made from the original Arabic text of Ibn al-Jazzār's *Zād al-musāfir wa-qūt al-ḥādir*, bk. 1, prepared by the otherwise unknown Abraham ben Isaac.[7] The translation is characterised by a unique number of Byzantine Greek medical terms in Hebrew transcription. These terms concern *materia medica*,[8] medical instruments,[9] illnesses,[10] body parts,[11] and general conditions of the body. The use of these terms probably indicates that Abraham ben Isaac lived and worked in Southern Italy, a region where Byzantyne Greek was

coming critical edition of bks. 1–2; see also NM 3:3 and the recent article by G. Freudenthal, M.R. McVaugh, and K. Mesler, 'Twelfth-Century Latin Medicine in Hebrew Garb: Do'eg the Edomite as a Cultural Intermediary,' *Medieval Encounters* 26 (2020): 226–284.

7 For this translation, which has only been preserved for bks. 1 and 6, probably predated that by Moses ibn Tibbon from 1259; cf. the introduction to the forthcoming critical edition of bks. 1–2.

8 For instance ליפתוקריאה is Greek λεπτοκάρυον, plur. λεπτοκάρυα 'hazelnut'; קוריאה (read: קודיאה) is Greek κωδύα 'poppy capsule'. I thank Petros Boutros-Vallianatos for his help in identifying the Greek terms.

9 Cf. the term סיקיאה, i.e., σικύα 'cupping glass'; אופיזימא, also written as איפוז(י)מא, i.e., Greek ἀπόζεμα, featuring for Arabic مطبوخ 'decoction'; a pot for preparing remedies (Hebrew אילפס representing Arabic قدر برام 'pot from serpentine stone' (cf. D 1:77)) is identified as Greek לפודי, i.e., Byzantine Greek λοπάδι from Greek λοπάδιον or λοπάς 'frying pan.'

10 The illness called אלבריאה, i.e., الإبرية 'dandruff,' is followed by the Greek parallel פיטרדש, i.e., πιτυρίς; 'sleeplessness' is rendered as אגריפצאה, perhaps a corruption of Greek ἀγρυπνία.

11 Cf. the term מלינגיש, i.e., Greek μήνιγγα, Plur. μήνιγγες in Byzantine Greek for 'the temples of the head,' called الصدغان in Arabic and in Hebrew הצדעים.

still used as spoken language and such terms could consequently be useful for the reader for correctly identifying the Arabic medical technical terms. Another indication for such a south-Italian origin of Abraham ben Isaac's translation are several parallel terms of *materia medica* in Italian.[12] The terms quoted below are derived from the forthcoming edition. The translation is extant in two manuscripts: Ms Florence, Biblioteca Medicina Laurenziana, Plut. 88.37 and Ms Jerusalem, National Library of Israel, Fr. 95. The basic Ms consulted for the edition is the one in Florence. Some of the terms quoted only feature in the Jerusalem Ms and have been indicated as such.

4. *Sefer Ṣedah la-Oreḥim*, Adaptation; an incomplete latinizing adaptation of Abraham ben Isaac's translation of bk. 1, which is extant in two manuscripts: Ms Berlin, Staatsbibliothek Preußischer Kulturbesitz, Or. fol. 1058[13] and Ms Moscow, Russian State Library, Guenzburg 165. The anonymous adapter probably consulted the *Viaticum*, i.e., the Latin translation of Ibn al-Jazzār's *Zād al-musāfir wa-qūt al-ḥādir* by Constantine the African, as is indicated by terms only featuring in the adaptation and the *Viaticum*, an example is דרך אפכא (see below).
5. *Sefer Ṣedah la-Oreḥim*, Abbreviation; an abbreviation and adaptation of bk. 1, which is extant in Ms St. Petersburg, Institute of Oriental Studies of the Russian Academy, B 133.
6. *Ma'amar ba-haqazah*; an anonymous Hebrew translation of Abū Bakr Muḥammad ibn Zakariyā al-Rāzī's *K. fī al-faṣd*. The translation is extant in Ms Parma, Bibliotheca Palatina, Cod. Parm. 2283,4, fols. 91[a]–97[b] (cat. Richler 1535[14]). The Arabic text is extant in Ms Escorial 857.
7. *Treatise on Melancholy*; an anonymous translation of Isḥāq ibn ʿImrān's *Maqāla fī al-mālankhūliyā*, uniquely quoted in the anonymous *Pinkas shel Rofe*, Ms Berlin, Staatsbibliothek Preußischer Kulturbesitz, Or. fol. 3088, fols. 42[a]–61[a], and copied in the fourteenth/fifteenth century in a Sephardic script.[15] The Ms has a double foliation, in Hebrew and Western

12 Cf. קרדמומו, *cardamomo* ('cardamon'); קטוניי, i.e., Italian QṬWNYY (*cotogne*?); בינידיטא, i.e., Italian *benedetta*, which stands for Latin *benedicta*; זולאבי, i.e., Italian *giulebbe*, lit., 'rosewater' (FEW 19:59b).

13 Moritz Steinschneider only knew this adaptation and accordingly suggested that the translation was not done on the basis of the Arabic text, as alleged by the translator, but on the basis of the Latin translation (*Viaticum*); cf. HU 705.

14 Cf. B. Richler, *Hebrew Manuscripts in the Bibliotheca Palatina in Parma: Catalogue*. Palaeographical and codicological descriptions: M. Beit-Arié (Jerusalem 2001).

15 Cf. M. Steinschneider, *Verzeichniss der hebräischen Handschriften in Berlin* (Repr., 1 vol., Hildesheim 1980).

(Arabic) numerals. When referring to a folio from this text, the Hebrew number will come first, followed by the Western (Arabic) between brackets. The translation is incomplete as it only covers fols. 89^{b}–107^{a} of the Arabic text extant in Ms Munich, Bayerische Staatsbibliothek, or. 251, that was copied in the year 1757 and used by Garbers for his facsimile edition.[16] The last part of the Arabic text discussing the healing properties of whey in the case of melancholy (fols. 107^{a}–109^{a}), and providing a wide variety of recipes to treat melancholy (fols. 109^{a}–120^{b}) is missing. The translation suffers from many corruptions and/or mistakes, possibly hailing from the copyist(s). Some of the mistakes can also be explained from the fact that the translator had a defective copy of the Arabic text in front of him.[17] In addition, one gets the impression that the translator was not familiar with standard Hebrew technical (i.e., medical-philosophical) terminology as coined by the Tibbonides.[18] On occasion the translation deviates from the original Arabic text as the translator adds explanatory remarks. While discussing epilepsy, he states: ועוד[19] קוראין אותו גונון ר״ל מצד השדים (It [i.e., epilepsy] is also called 'possession' by demons) and then adds: ורב׳ סעדיה ז״ל פריש בשגעון גנון (and R. Sa'adya [Gaon], of blessed memory, explains [the Arabic term] *junūn* as [Hebrew] *shigga'on*). And when discussing the differrent kinds of food stuff proper for melancholy patients, the translator remarks regarding the different kinds of fish recommended by the author: אמר המעתיק: כל אלו הדגים שזכר בשער זה הם דגים קטנים וקלים ולא ראינו בארצנו מהם כי הרצאצי (الرضراضي) והסכרי (الصخري) הם דגים כאצבע ולא גדולים ואינם גדולים יותר ובקשטילה הוא אלראבי והוא דק אומרים לו שמרוק (Says the translator: All these fish that he mentioned in this chapter are small and light fish. I have not seen them in my country because fish that live amongst the rocks, [i.e., rockfish] are small as a finger, not larger. In

16 Ibn 'Imrān, *Maqāla fī l-Mālīḫūliyā* (*Abhandlung über die Melancholie*) *und Constantini Africani libri duo* De melancholia, ed. Garbers (Hamburg 1977).

17 This was already noted by Garbers for the Munich Ms that he emended on several occasions.

18 A few examples of such non-standard terms are: גימטרייה for Arabic حساب 'arithmetic;' חכמת התכנית for Arabic علم الهندسة 'geometry;' גְּמָר/גֶּמֶר for Arabic تمام 'perfection;' דְּמָמָה for Arabic سكات 'apoplexy;' טִמְטוּם for Arabic سدّ 'obstruction;' הכח האוחז for Arabic القوة الماسكة 'the retentive faculty;' הכח ההודף for Arabic القوة الدافعة 'the excretory faculty;' הנפש החיית for Arabic النفس الحيوانية 'the vital soul;' נפש חכמה ממללת and נפש ממללת for Arabic النفس الناطقة 'the rational soul;' רַעְיוֹן for Arabic فكر 'reflection, rational thought, reason;' and תַּעֲרֹבֶת for Arabic خلط 'bodily humor.'

19 ועוד קוראין אותו גונון: = ويسمونه الجنون a.

Castile[20] they are called 'LR'BY (*al-rāy?[21]). They are small and they are also called ŠMRWQ). Parallel terms featuring in Constantine the African's Latin translation *De melancholia* have been mentioned as well.

8. *Treatise on Surgery* by Guillaume de Congenis (active first half of the thirteenth century); a Hebrew-Latin translation by the otherwise unknown R. Isaiah, Ms Paris, BN, 1165, fols. 44ᵃ–60ᵇ.[22] The Ms was copied in a Mughrabi script in the sixteenth/seventeenth century and bears the title: זה ספר אחר משרורגיאה אשר חבר גיללם דקונגיינש והעתיקו ר׳ ישעיה מלשון נוצרי ללשון הקודש בע״ה ובישועתו (*Another Book on Surgery Composed by Guillaume de Congenis, Translated by R. Isaiah from Latin into Hebrew with God's Help*).[23] The text in question is a collection of de Congenis's teachings, sets of classroom notes, that were made by students who heard his lectures at Montpellier, c. 1220. De Congenis' notes are based on Roger Frugardi,[24] who wrote the first general surgical textbook in the 1190s. He explains what Roger had said, adds his own further contributions and sometimes challenges what Roger had said instead of agreeing with him. For instance, to treat inguinal hernia when a portion of the intestine passes through the inguinal canal and lodges in the scrotum, Roger basically proposes cutting open at the opening of the inguinal canal, pushing the intestine back out of the scrotum, removing the testicle, and tying the inguinal canal shut so that the intestine (supposedly) won't pass through into the scrotum again. But Guillaume (the magister) criticizes this treatment and says that cutting the testicle free would produce too much

20 The reference to Castile and the translator's familiarity with the dialect spoken there might point to the fact that he hailed from that region.

21 For the identification of this fish, see BMR 62, n. 63.

22 Cf. HU 801; H. Zotenberg (ed.), *Catalogues des manuscrits hébreux et samaritains de la Bibliothèque Impériale* (Paris 1866), 213. In the mid-thirteenth century, Guillaume de Congenis lectured at Montpellier on surgery outside the curriculum, cf. M.R. McVaugh, *The Rational Surgery of the Middle Ages* (Florence 2006), 232, and esp. idem, 'Medieval Paths to Surgical Practice: The Example of Montpellier' (forthcoming in *Micrologus*); see also G. Karpp and O. Riha, 'Aus der Geschichte der Rogerglossen: Ein bisher unbekanntes Wilhelm von Congenis-Fragment,' *Sudhoffs Archiv* 99, no. 1 (2015): 73–104. For the Latin source, cf. K. Sudhoff, 'Eine therapeutische Rogerglosse aus Montpellier,' in: idem, *Beiträge zur Geschichte der Chirurgie im Mittelalter: Graphische und textliche Untersuchungen in mittelalterlichen Handschriften*, vol. 2 (Leipzig 1918), 265–297. I thank my colleague and friend Michael R. McVaugh for referring me to the Latin source.

23 The following description of the text derives from a series of communications with Michael R. McVaugh.

24 Cf. fol. 52ᵃ: דע כי המשיחה האחרת אשר צותה השרורגיאה מן רוגייר מועלת לכל התחלואים המולידים בשר רע (Know that the other salve recommended in the [book on] surgery by Roger is good for all illnesses that produce bad flesh).

blood; instead, he recommends scarring the inguinal canal with caustics to shut it without any blood flow from the vessels there.[25]

The Hebrew text also has incorporated material that features as marginal glosses in the Latin text and that obviously hailed from another student of Guillaume who added his own notes in the margin, making this a kind of accumulation of de Congenis's teachings. The list contains several examples of Hebrew loan words from Romance and/or Latin from this hitherto unresearched text. In addition to novel Hebrew terms, I also listed some of the more common Romance/Latin terms. The Ms has a number of marginal glosses in the same script, both corrections and explanations. Thus the term תולעים (earthworms) is glossed as לומבריקש (earthworms) (see entry), and זאב (lupus) (see entry) as לופוש נקרא בהמון לופאט (lupus, commonly called LWP'Ṭ), and the illness called אל תיגע בי (*noli me tangere*, a facial ulcer) (see entry) was glossed as: ונקרא בהמון נומיטוק (commonly called NWMYṬWQ). An unusual magical procedure against scrofula is the following (fol. 53ᵃ): 'On Saint John's Eve, the patient should go, at midnight, to a well, and have a little bit of blood extracted from each spot affected by scrofula, and throw the blood into the well.'[26]

9. *Shinnui ha-Shemot ha-Niqra'im Synonimi* (*On the Different Names Called 'Synonyms'*); an anonymous list of medical synonyms[27] extant in Ms Florence, Bibliotheca Laurenziana, Or. 17, copied in Anagni in 1464 in an Italian script by Abraham ben Daniel the physician; the glossary (synonym list) features on fols. 68ᵃ–92ᵇ; part of the text cannot be read due to severe staining. Every folio consists of four columns of terms with explanations in a variety of languages, such as Arabic, Italian, Hebrew, Latin, and Greek. The list, beginning with the letter Alef and the entry אכליל אל מלך (melilot, *Melilotus officinalis* (L.) Pall.) und ending abruptly with תין (fig, *Ficus carica* L.), is actually an adaptation of the index in Ibn Sīnā's *K. al-Qānūn*, bk. 2, with many additional entries.[28] On several occasions, the author adds explanations and different interpretations (e.g., by

---

25 For the Latin text, cf. Sudhoff, *Therapeutische Rogerglosse*, 290, ll. 745–757. For Guillaume's criticism, cf. Guillaume de Congenis, *Treatise on Surgery*, fol. 57ᵇ: החכם מונע הוצאת הביצה והשיג רוגייר אשר צוה להוציאה. I thank Michael R. McVaugh for this explanation; cf. Sudhoff, ibid., n. 1: "Nota quod M⟨agister⟩ uituperat multum ac⟨torem⟩, quia precipit testiculum abstrahi et prohibet, ne fiat."

26 The story features ibid., 282–283, ll. 523–527, and is told in the name of a lady from Montpellier.

27 I use the term 'synonym' in line with its medieval sense, i.e., for parallel terms both in the same language and in different languages.

28 According to Steinschneider (HU 839), the list contains 1,749 entries. An edition of the list

the *Noṣrim* (Christians)) and refers to explicit sources (e.g., Ibn Sīnā, al-Zahrāwī, Ibn Māsawayh, or al-Rāzī).

Similar synonym lists consulted are: Ms Leiden, Universiteitsbibliotheek, Or. 4719 (SCAL 2,2) (entitled: *Shinnui Shemot ha-Niqra Ṣinonimas*);[29] Ms Munich, Bayerische Staatsbibliothek, Cod. hebr. 8 (entitled: *Shinnui ha-Shemot ha-Niqra'im Synonimis*); and [*Synonima*], Ms Vatican, Biblioteca Apostolica, ebr. 550.[30]

10. *Sefer ha-Shimmush*, bk. 29, list 1; i.e, the translation by Shem Tov ben Isaac of Tortosa of the first (of two) indexes featuring in *K. al-Taṣrīf li-man ʿajiza ʿan al-taʾlīf* (*The Arrangement of Medical Knowledge for One Who Is Not Able to Compile a Book for Himself*) by the Andalusian physician Abū l-Qāsim Khalaf ibn ʿAbbās al-Zahrāwī.[31] Shem Tov omitted the original Arabic, Syrian, Persian, and Ibero-Romance indexes in his translation and substituted them instead with two lists as follows. The first list starts with the Hebrew or Aramaic term, followed by the Arabic synonym, and then—in about seventy percent of the entries—by the vernacular term, which is usually Old Occitan, and/or by a Latin synonym. This list was intended to help the reader identify and clarify the Hebrew terminology used by the author in his translation of the *K. al-Taṣrīf*. The second list starts with the Old Occitan or Latin term followed by its Arabic synonym and, in some cases, with its Hebrew or Aramaic equivalent, and was intended to be used and consulted independently of the *Sefer ha-Shimmush*.[32] The references to the first list are derived from the edition.
11. Zeraḥyah ben Isaac ben She'altiel Ḥen, Hebrew translation of Maimonides' *Medical Aphorisms*: The terms are derived from the critical edition (BMMZ) and are additional to the terms published in NM 1:121–195.
12. Nathan ha-Me'ati, Hebrew translation of Maimonides' *Medical Aphorisms*: The terms are derived from the critical edition (BMMN) and are additional to the terms published in NM 2:21–94.

(supported by the DFG) by Gerrit Bos, Sebastian Lauschus, Guido Mensching, and Frank Savelsberg, is in progress.

29 Cf. M. Steinschneider, *Catalogus Codicum Hebraeorum Bibliothecae Academiae Lugduno-Batavae* (Repr., Osnabrück 1977), 315.

30 Cf. B. Richler, *Hebrew Manuscripts in the Vatican Library: Catalogue*, compiled by the staff of the Institute of Microfilmed Hebrew Manuscripts, Jewish National and University Library, Jerusalem, palaeographical and codicological descriptions: M. Beit-Arié, in collaboration with N. Pasternak (Vatican City 2008), 466. The list has a double enumeration which will be referred to in the entries.

31 For the edition of the glossary, cf. SHS 1.

32 Cf. SHS 1:1 ff.

13. Ms Cambridge, T-S K14.14. The text on the four folios dating from the middle of the fifteenth century contains a copy of Abraham Avigdor's Hebrew translation of Gerard de Solo's commentary on the *Liber*[33] *nonus ad Almansorem*.[34] The text contains a fragmentary discussion of different illnesses affecting the ears, throat, and uvula. Abraham Avigdor severely abbreviates the original text by omitting questions and commentaries by Gerard de Solo. But he adds material from different explicitly mentioned sources, from the works of Islamic physicians, namely al-Rāzī and Ibn Sīnā, and from the *Sefer Ṣedat ha-Derakhim*; i.e., the Hebrew translation (composed by Moses ibn Tibbon in 1259) of the medical compendium *Zād al-musāfir wa-qūt al-ḥādir*, composed by Ibn al-Jazzār (see above). Other sources not explicitly mentioned are medical works composed by contemporaries, such as the *Practica seu Lilium medicinae* by Bernard de Gordon (1303). The same subject is often introduced by a double title, one in Hebrew and one in Latin (in Hebrew transcription).
14. Ms Cambridge, T-S K14.48: The 88 fragments contain a substantial part of an unidentified medical work in Hebrew, organized in chapters with rubricated headings.

33 I.e., the ninth book of the Latin translation of the *Kitābu'l-manṣūrī fi'ṭ-ṭibb* by Abū Bakr Muḥammad ibn Zakariyyā al-Rāzī (Al-Rāzī, lat. Rhazes), that was known as *Liber ad Almansorem* and was prepared by Gerard de Cremona (1175). On Abraham Avigdor (1351–1402), the first Provençal Jew to state explicitly that he studied in Montpellier at its university, see J. Shatzmiller, *Jews, Medicine, and Medieval Society* (Berkeley-Los Angeles-London 1994): 29–30; and L. Ferre *Práctica de Johannes de Parma: Un tratado farmacologico en sus versiones hebreas y catalana* (Granada 2002): 18–20.

34 An edition of the four folios and a comparison with Abraham Avigdor's Hebrew translation of Gerard de Solo's *Liber Nonus* by Gerrit Bos, Sandra Hajek, and Guido Mensching is forthcoming in *Aleph: Historical Studies in Science & Judaism*.

List of Terms

א

אָב • אב טרם הבן · **(lit., the father before the son); the seed of the Levant nut [*Anamirta cocculus* (L.) Wight & Arn.]**: O.Occ. **peire enans fil(h)* or O.Cat. **paire enans fill* · Shem Tov ben Isaac, *Sefer ha-Shimmush*, bk. 29, list 1 (SHS 1:104 (Alef 18)): אב טרם הבן ב״ה מאהיזהרה וב״ל פאירי איגנס פיל או אנטיפטרי ולטי׳ אקולוש קונשיליש (*av ṭerem ha-ben*, Arab. *māhīzahra*,[1] vern. **peire enans fil(h)* or **paire enans fill* or [Lat.] *antipater* and Lat. *oculus consulis*). In the sense of 'the seed of the Levant nut,' Hebr. אב טרם הבן is a non-attested calque of Rom. **peire enans fil(h)* or **paire enans fill*.[2]

אֲבוּבָא (*Aram.*) **• אבובא דרעיא** · **European water plantain [*Alisma plantago-aquatica* L.]**: Arab: زمارة الراعي or مزمار الراعي (cf. StH 948; IBF 2126; DT 3:144 (505–506); LA 34, no. 2: אבוב רועה) · *Shinnui ha-Shemot ha-Niqra'im Synonimis*, Ms Munich, Bayerische Staatsbibliothek, Cod. hebr. 8, fol. 197ᵇ: זמארה אלרעי כלומר מזמר הרועה ובלשונינו אבובא דרעיא ([Arab.] *zammāra al-rāʿī*; i.e., [Hebr.] MZMR *ha-roʿeh*; and in our language [i.e., Aram.] *abbuba de-raʿya*). In the sense of 'European water plantain,' Aram. אבובא דרעיא features as אבוב רעיא in LA 34, no. 2; Löw (ibid.) also mentions the Hebrew equivalent אבוב רועה featuring in Rabbinic literature (cf. JD 3; FM 1: 'common knot-grass' [*Polygonum aviculare* L.] = Arab. عصى الراعي; cf. MIG 980). For Hebr. מזמר הרועה, see entry מזמר.

אֶבֶן • אבן ההר · **(lit., mountain stone); hematite**: Arab. حجر الطور (cf. القول في الأماطيطس وهو حجر الشادنج ... ويسمى بالعربيّة حجر الدم ويقال له حجر الطور وذلك أنّ معدنه بطور تابور من عمل طبرية ('Abhandlung über den Hämatit; das ist der Stein Šādanağ [...]: und auf Arabisch heißt er Blutstein. Man sagt auch Bergstein dazu, denn seine Grube befindet sich im Berge Tabor, der unter der Verwalting von Tiberias steht.'))[3] · *Shinnui ha-Shemot ha-Niqra'im Synonimis*, Ms Munich, Bayerische Staatsbibliothek, Cod. hebr. 8, fol. 198ᵃ: חגר אלדם הוא אבן הדם נקרא שאדנג[4] ונקראת אבן ההר ([Arab.] *ḥajar al-dam*; i.e., [Hebr.] *even ha-dam*, is [also] called *shādanaj* and [in Hebr.] *even ha-har*). Hebr. אבן ההר does not feature in the current dictionaries. For the Hebrew synonym אבן הדם, cf. BCD 15 (NM 2:27).

• אבן החלב · **milk stone**: Arab. حجر اللبن (cf. IBF 596, s.v. حجر لبني) (Gr. γαλακτίτης (cf. DW 5:132)) · *Shinnui ha-Shemot ha-Niqra'im Synonimis*, Ms Munich, Bayerische

---

1 *Māhīzahra*: The term is not Arabic but Persian; cf. VL 2:130 f.: "n.c. cortex radicis plantae valde niger, iecori piscis similis et pisces necans;" SCP 1147: "A poisonous yellow-flowering milk-grass which, thrown into water, intoxicates the fish and brings them to the surface." The Arabic equivalent is *māhīzahraj*; cf. SP 697.

2 According to Löw (LF 2:252), there are no Hebrew or Aramaic equivalents.

3 J. Schönfeld (ed. and trans.), *Über die Steine: Das 14. Kapitel aus dem* Kitāb al-Muršid *des Muḥammad Ibn Aḥmad at-Tamīmī, nach dem Pariser Manuskript herausgegeben, übersetzt und kommentiert* (Freiburg 1976), BXI, 1 (66).

4 שאדנג: emendation editor לאדנם Ms.

Staatsbibliothek, Cod. hebr. 8, fol. 198[b]: חגר אללבן הוא אבן החלב ([Arab.] *ḥajar al-laban*; i.e., [Hebr.] *even he-ḥalav*). Hebr. אבן החלב does not feature in the current dictionaries.

• **אבן משחזת** · **whetstone:** Arab. حجر المسن (cf. D 1:251) · *Shinnui ha-Shemot ha-Niqra'im Synonimis*, Ms Munich, Bayerische Staatsbibliothek, Cod. hebr. 8, fol. 198[b]: חגר אלמסן היא אבן המשחזת ([Arab.] *ḥajar al-misann*; i.e., [Hebr.] *even ha-mashḥezet*). Hebr. אבן משחזת features as משחזת in Rabbinic literature and modern Hebrew ethical literature (cf. JD 851; KT 2:307; BM 3367; EM 1075); and in medieval medical literature; cf. entry מַשְׁחֶזֶת.

• **אבן הספוג** · **sponge stone (i.e., stone found among sponges):** Arab. حجر الإسفنج (cf. IBF 511) (Gr. λίθοι οἱ ἐν τοῖς σπόγγοις (the stones in the sponges)) · *Shinnui ha-Shemot ha-Niqra'im Synonimis*, Ms Munich, Bayerische Staatsbibliothek, Cod. hebr. 8, fol. 198[b]: חגר אלאספנג היא אבן הספוג ([Arab.] *ḥajar al-isfanj*; i.e., [Hebr.] *even ha-sefog*). Hebr. אבן הספוג features in BM 32 as אבן ספוג and is explained by Ben-Yehuda as 'a stone that is as porous as a sponge and that is used for planing wood and the like.'

אַבְנִינוּת · **calcification:** Arab. تحجّر · Maimonides, *Medical Aphorisms* 23.89 · trans. Zeraḥyah Ḥen (BMMZ 229): הרופאים באמרם טחולים ירצו לומר במי שיקרה בטחולו קושי ואבנינות מבלתי מורסא (When speaking of 'spleen patients,' physicians mean those patients whose spleen is affected by induration and calcification without an inflammation). Hebr. אַבְנִינוּת does not feature in the current dictionaries. Nathan ha-Me'ati translates Arab. تحجّر as הִתְאַבְּנוּת (see entry).

[אבק] • *Pi'el* **אִבֵּק** · **to pulverize:** Arab. سحق · Ibn al-Jazzār, *Zād al-musāfir wa-qūt al-ḥādir* · trans. Abraham ben Isaac, *Sefer Ṣedah la-Oreḥim*, Adaptation; cf. bk. 1, ch. 1 (Ms Berlin, Staatsbibliothek Preußischer Kulturbesitz, Or. fol. 1058, fol. 89[a]): אחר כן שים עליו איפורבייו שחוק עם שמן לאורינו או שים עליו שרשי קנים שרופים או נשטרוצי מאובק ומעורב עם שמן או קח קצף הים הנקרא שפומא מרינה ואבקנה וערבנה עם אבק ניטרו ועם שמן שקדים מרים ושים עליו (Subsequently, it [i.e., the bald spot on the head] should be anointed with pulverized resin spurge together with bay laurel oil. Burnt reed roots, or pulverized garden cress mixed with oil may also be rubbed on it. Or take sepiolite, called *spuma marina*, pulverize it and mix it with pulverized natron and oil of bitter amonds and put it on [the spot]). In the sense of 'to pulverize,' Hebr. אִבֵּק features in BM 36 in a later attestation from the *Lev Aryeh*, a memory treatise composed by Judah Aryeh mi-Modena (Leon of Modena).[5] Moses ibn Tibbon and Abraham ben Isaac render Arab. سحق as שחק.

---

5 For this treatise, see G. Bos, 'Jewish Traditions on Strengthening Memory and Leone Modena's Evaluation,' *Jewish Studies Quarterly* 2, no. 1 (1995): 39–58.

• *Part. Pu'al* **מְאֻבָּק** · **pulverized**: Arab. مسحوق · Ibn al-Jazzār, *Zād al-musāfir wa-qūt al-ḥādir* · trans. Abraham ben Isaac, *Sefer Ṣedah la-Oreḥim*, Adaptation, bk. 1, ch. 1 (Ms Berlin, Staatsbibliothek Preußischer Kulturbesitz, Or. fol. 1058, fol. 89[a]): אחר כן שים עליו איפורבייו שחוק עם שמן לאורינו או שים עליו שרשי קנים שרופים או נשטרוצי מאובק ומעורב עם שמן או קח קצף הים הנקרא שפומא מרינה ואבקנה וערבנה עם אבק ניטרו ועם שמן שקדים מרים ושים עליו. Hebr. מְאֻבָּק features in Rabbinic literature in the sense of 'powdered' (cf. JD 8). Ben-Yehuda mentions the term in the sense of 'pulverized' in an attestation from the *Lev Aryeh*, mentioned in the previous entry. Do'eg ha-Edomi renders Lat. *in pulverem redactus* as שחוק לאבק. In the sense of 'pulverized' (for Lat. *pulverizatus*), Hebr. מְאֻבָּק also features in Bonfos Bonfil Astruc's translation of *On the Treatment of Small Children* attributed to al-Rāzī (Cf. ROT 45, l. 19). Moses ibn Tibbon and Abraham ben Isaac translate Arab. مسحوق as שחוק.

אָבָק · **powder**: Lat. *pulvis* (Arab. سفوف) · Constantinus Africanus, *Viaticum* · trans. Do'eg ha-Edomi, *Sefer Ya'ir Netiv*, bk. 1, ch. 23: אבק מועיל: טורביט שרפין עשב טיטימל קולוקונטידא[6] זרע שיקודא אפי אניש אשטיקדוש אקורי (A powder that is good: [Take] St. Thomas lidpod, sagapenum, resin spurge, colocynth pulp, Syrian rue seed, celery, anise, French lavender, sweet flag …). In the sense of 'powder,' Hebr. אָבָק features in BCD 15 (NM 4:11) in a later attestation from Moses ibn Tibbon's *Sefer Ṣedat ha-Derakhim*. Arab. سفوف is translated by Moses ibn Tibbon as קֶמַח (see entry).

• **אבק העופרת** · **(lit., lead powder); white lead**: Arab. اسفيداج · *Shinnui ha-Shemot ha-Niqra'im Synonimi*, Ms Florence, Bibliotheca Laurenziana, Or. 17, fol. 69[b]: אספידאג׳ ה׳ אבק העופרת ('SPYD'Ğ [i.e., Arab. *isfīdāj* (KM 241–246; SHS 1:98–99 (Aleph 10))]; i.e., white lead). Hebr. אבק העופרת is not attested for in the current dictionaries.

אֵבֶר • *Plur.* **אברים** • **האברים הרוחניים** · **the[7] spiritual members (organs)**: Lat. *membra spiritualia* · Guillaume de Congenis, *Treatise on Surgery* · trans. Isaiah, fol. 55[a]: ובזה ירחץ החבורים והזרועות וזה יקרר החום והאברים הרוחניים (With this [remedy] he should wash the joints and the arms [because] it cools the heat and the spiritual members). Hebr. האברים הרוחניים features in BCD 16 (NM 4:12–13) in an attestation from Estori ha-Parḥi's Hebrew translation of Armengaud Blaise's *Tabula Antidotarii*.

• **תרדמת האיברים** → תַּרְדֵּמָה.

אגריפא · **an ointment, supposedly used by Agrippa**: Lat. *agrippa* (DMLBS 73; ND 33–34) · Guillaume de Congenis, *Treatise on Surgery* · trans. Isaiah, fol. 44[a]: ומיום השלישי והלאה יאות למשוח המכה משמנינות חזיר או מאגריפא ופלומצולש גדולים מנוערת רחוצות במים וסחוטות יושמו עליו ויוקשרו (From the third day on one should rub the wound with fat from a pig or with an ointment [called] *agrippa*, and large feather pads

---

6 קולוקונטידא זרע שיקודא: emendation editor קולוקונטידא שיקודא זרע Mss.

7 'the spiritual members (organs): Lat. *membra spiritualia*': I.e., bodily members (organs) involved in breathing (and so in taking in air and spirit), namely the lungs, the trachea, and the epiglottis, cf. NM 4:11, n. 4.

made from chaff should be put and fastened on it once they have been washed and wrung out). Hebr. אגריפא is a non-attested loan word from Lat. *agrippa* (and var.).

אדומה → אֲדֻמָּה.

אֲדִיּוּת · I. **vaporous [substance] (h.l., type)**: Arab. بخارية · a) Maimonides, *Medical Aphorisms* 10.23 · trans. Nathan ha-Me'ati (BMMN 126): לפעמים יתהפך הדם כשיתעפש וישוב אדומיי או שחוריי ותהיה הקדחת ממין השלישית או ממין הרביעית ואין ביניהם הפרש אלא שאותה היא רעה ומגונה וזאת ההווה מהתהפכות הדם אינה מגונה כי החום כשיהיה יותר נוטה אל האידיות ופחות[8] מזיק ומצער המשוש[9] אז היא מעפוש שתי המרות (Sometimes [the quality of] the blood changes when it putrefies: it turns into yellow bile or black bile. In these cases, the fever is either tertian or quartan. The only difference between these cases is that in the first one the fever is malignant; but when it originates from the transformation of the blood, it is not malignant. For when the heat tends more toward the vaporous type and is less aggressive and harmful when one touches [the body], it[10] comes from [the transformation of] the blood, but when it is biting and smarting when one touches [the body], it comes from the putrefaction of [one of] the two biles). Hebr. אֲדִיּוּת features in BM 59 in the sense of 'evaporation' in a quotation of this particular aphorism; see also BCD 17 (NM 3:24) for אדיות in the sense of 'transudation' (for Arab. رشح). Zeraḥyah Ḥen translates Arab. بخارية as אדיית.

b) Ms Cambridge, T-S K14.14, fol. 2[b]: וירחיק היין וכו': הטעם כי היין רב האידיות (He [i.e., someone suffering from earache (tinnitus)] should abstain from wine etc.: The reason is that wine is very vaporous [i.e., its digestion produces many vapors]).

· II. (**אדיית**) · **smoky, gaseous [substance]**: Arab. دخانية · Maimonides, *Medical Aphorisms* 10.67 · trans. Zeraḥyah Ḥen (BMMZ 130): המילוי הנקרא תכמה אשר ישתנה המזון בו אל חימוץ לא יתחדש ממנו קדחת. אבל אפשר שיתחדש הקדחת בעבור המילוי ההוא אשר ישתנה בו המזון אל האדיית (No fever develops from an indigestion in which the food turns sour. But fever can occur from an indigestion in which the food becomes gaseous). Nathan ha-Me'ati translates Arab. دخانية as עֲשָׁנִיּוּת (see entry).

אֹדֶם • אודם אשר באחת קצוות העין · **(lit., redness in one of the corners of the eyes); hyposphagma (bloodshot eyes)**: Arab. طرفة (cf. MMT 195) · Ibn al-Jazzār, *Zād al-musāfir wa-qūt al-ḥādir* · trans. Moses ibn Tibbon, *Sefer Ṣedat ha-Derakhim*, bk. 2, ch. 3: השער השלישי באודם אשר באחת קצוות העין הנקרא בער' אלטרפא (Ch. 3: On hyposphagma [lit., redness in one of the corners of the eyes], called *ṭarfa*, or *ṭurfa* in Arabic). Hebr. אודם אשר באחת קצוות העין is not attested for in the current dictionaries. Do'eg ha-Edomi translates Lat. *sanguis in oculis* as דם העינים (see entry דָּם).

---

8 وأقلّ عادية وأذى :ופחות מזיק ומצער a.

9 המשוש: فهي من الدم. ومتى كانت لذاعة قارضة للمس add. a.

10 'it comes from [the transformation of] the blood, but when it is biting and smarting when one touches [the body]': add. according to a.

אֲדַמְדַּם • צמח אדמדם → צֶמַח.

אֲדֻמָּה • **האדומה השחרחורת** · **black bile:** Lat. *colera nigra* (Arab. المرّة السوداء) · Constantinus Africanus, *Viaticum* · trans. Do'eg ha-Edomi, *Sefer Ya'ir Netiv*, bk. 1, ch. 10: ואם הוא מן האדומה השחרחורת יהיה הכאב בצד השמאלי עם קרירות ותעורה (If it (i.e., the headache) originates from black bile, the pain is in the left side [of the head] and is accompanied by cold and sleeplessness). Hebr. אֲדֻמָּה only features in the current dictionaries in the sense of 'red bile'; cf. BM 54, s.v. אדומה; KTP 1:22. Abraham ben Isaac translates Arab. المرّة السوداء as מרירה השחורה and Moses ibn Tibbon as מרה שחורה.

אַדְמוּת · **reddening; redness:** Arab. احمرار · Ibn al-Jazzār, *Zād al-musāfir wa-qūt al-ḥādir* · trans. Abraham ben Isaac, *Sefer Ṣedah la-Oreḥim*, bk. 1, ch. 10 (Ms Jerusalem, National Library of Israel, Fr. 95, fol. 89[a]): אם יהיה מחמת ריבוי דם אז ירגיש החולה חמות בראשו וכובד במצחו ואדמות בגידי עיניו ובפנים ומילאוי הגידים בשתי הצדעין ואם יהיה מחמת מרירה האדומה אז ירגיש חמות חדה ויובש באפיו ובלשונו ונדידת שינה וצמאה (If [headache] originates from a surplus of blood, the patient feels heat in his head, heaviness in his forehead, reddening of the blood vessels of the eyes and face, and repletion of the veins of the temples. If it originates from yellow bile, he feels a sharp heat and dryness of his nostrils and his tongue and suffers from sleeplessness and thirst). Hebr. אַדְמוּת features in EM 20 in attestations from Rabbinic literature and in BM 70 in an attestation from Menahem Recanati's commentary on the Torah. Moses ibn Tibbon translates Arab. احمرار as אדמות as well.

אודם → אֹדֶם.

[אוה] • *Part. Pi'el* מְאַוֶּה · **whetting the appetite** · Ms Cambridge, T-S K14.48, P11 (recto): פלפל מאוה ומעכל המזון (Pepper whets the appetite and is good for digesting the food). Hebr. מְאַוֶּה is not attested for in this sense in the current dictionaries.

אִוּוּי · **desire:** Arab. شوق · Ibn al-Jazzār, *Zād al-musāfir wa-qūt al-ḥādir* · trans. Abraham ben Isaac, *Sefer Ṣedah la-Oreḥim*, bk. 1, ch. 20: החשק הוא מן החלאים הנולדים במוח הראש והוא רוב איווי עם הירהור ותאוה ועל זה יקרה לכל מי שיארע לו חולי זה מקצת מקראות הנפש המה נדידת השינה גם ההירהור (Lovesickness belongs to the diseases that originate in the brain. It is an excess of desire accompanied by brooding and longing. Therefore, it is followed by afflictions of the soul, which is to say sleeplessness and brooding). Hebr. אִוּוּי features in BM 93 with attestations from medieval liturgical literature only. Moses ibn Tibbon translates Arab. شوق as תשוקה. Do'eg ha-Edomi translates the parallel Latin term *concupiscentia* as חמדה.

אוזן → אֹזֶן.

אוֹחֵז (*Part.*) → אָחַז.

אֲוִיר • **האויר הבא על הנחירים** · **the inhaled air:**[11] Arab. الهواء المستنشق · Isḥāq ibn 'Imrān, *Treatise on Melancholy* · trans. Anonymous, fol. 51[a] (52[a]): זו היא הנהגתם מצד האויר

11 See also entry נְשִׁימָה: נשימת האויר על הנחירים והפה.

הבא על הנחירים (This is their regimen regarding the inhaled air). Hebr. האויר הבא על הנחירים does not feature in the current dictionaries.

• נְשִׁימָה → נשימת האויר על הנחירים והפה.

אוכל → אֹכֶל.

אוּמָה · **main lobe of the lung** · Guillaume de Congenis, *Treatise on Surgery* · trans. Isaiah, fol. 55b: אם תעשה מכה באומה או באונת הפולמון הדקה או בקצה תוכל לעזור לפי החכם (If the main lobe of a lung or one of the minor lobes is injured because of a blow [to the chest] affecting [the lobes] or part of it, it can be cured according to the learned Master). My translation of Hebr. אוּמָה as 'main lobe' follows that by Rabinowitz and Grossmann in their translation of Maimonides, *Mishneh Torah, Sefer ha-'Avodah, Hilkhot Shechitah*, bk. 7:3, 5.[12] Ben-Yehuda (BM 103) defines the term as 'that part of the lungs to which the lobes are attached' (חלק הריאה שאונות מחוברות אליו). Cf. the definition featuring in Tanḥum Yerushalmi, *Al-Murshid al-kafi*, 40–41, s.v. 'm: 'the *om* is the larger part of the lung from which the smaller *unnot* branch out.'[13] Sokoloff (SDA 90) translates the parallel Aramaic term אומא as '(small) lobe' and אונא as '(large) lobe' (see next entry). A variant reading of אומה, namely אוֹם, features in Maimonides, *Mishneh Torah, Sefer ha-'Avodah, Hilkhot Shechitah* 7:5: האום של ריאה שנמצאת סמוכה לדופן (When the main lobe of the lung is found adhering to the flank).

אוּנָה • האונה הדקה · **minor lobe of the lung** · Guillaume de Congenis, *Treatise on Surgery* · trans. Isaiah, fol. 55b: אם תעשה מכה באומה או באונת הפולמון הדקה או בקצה תוכל לעזור לפי החכם (If the main lobe of a lung or one of its minor lobes is injured because of a blow [to the chest] affecting [the lobes] or a part of it, it can be cured according to the learned Master). Hebr. האונה הדקה refers to the 'minor lobe of the lung.' The term אוּנָה on its own has the same meaning; cf. the translation by Rabinowitz and Grossmann of Maimonides, *Mishneh Torah, Sefer ha-'Avodah, Hilkhot Shechitah*, bk. 7:3; 8:1. Sokoloff (SDA 90) translates the parallel Aramaic term אונא as '(large) lobe.'

אונקלי · **uvula**: Arab. لهاة · Ibn al-Jazzār, *Zād al-musāfir wa-qūt al-ḥādir* · trans. Moses ibn Tibbon, *Sefer Ṣedat ha-Derakhim*, bk. 2, ch. 21: תאר שנון יטהר השנים ויסיר החפירות וייטיב הריח ויוריד הליחה ויועיל מן האונקלי הנופל אללהאת בערבי ומכאב הגרון ושאר כאיבי השנים והטוחנות והפה מנוסה (Recipe of a dentifrice that cleanses the teeth, removes holes, improves the smell of breath, brings down moistness, and which is beneficial for prolapse of the uvula, called in Arabic *lahāt*, for sore throat, and other aches of the teeth, the molars, and the mouth—it has been tested). Hebr. אונקלי is a non-attested loan word from Rom. *angle* or **auncle* ('angle') (FEW 24:571). Do'eg ha-Edomi renders the parallel Latin term *uvula* as אובילא.

12 See Maimonides, *The Code of Maimonides*, bk. 5: *The Book of Holiness*, ed. Nemoy, trans. Rabinowitz and Grossman (Repr., New Haven 1965), 288–289.

13 Tanḥum Yerushalmi, *Al-Murshid al-kafi*, ed. and trans. Shy (Jerusalem 2005).

אוסיא • **substance:** Gr. οὐσία (Arab. جوهر) · Ibn al-Jazzār, *Zād al-musāfir wa-qūt al-ḥādir* · trans. Abraham ben Isaac, *Sefer Ṣedah la-Oreḥim*, bk. 1, ch. 14: דע כי יושר הגירסא שיגרוס האדם ולא ישכח הוא יזכיר הדברים הטמונים בלב ודבר זה יוכיח שהאוסיא שלקצה מוח הראש ממול העורף אשר יקראו שמו הרופאים זכרון ובלשון ישמעאל אל דכר האוסיא דההיא פרה ורבה גם הקראסיס שוה (Know that a good memory means that one remembers and does not forget the things hidden in the heart and this indicates that the substance of the rear part of the brain—which the physicians call 'memory,' *al-dhikr* in Arabic—is healthy[14] and sound, and that its temperament is balanced[15]). Hebr. אוסיא is a non-attested loan translation of Gr. οὐσία. Moses ibn Tibbon translates the parallel Arabic term جوهر as עצם.

אוסף → אֹסֶף.

[אור] • *Hif'il* הֵאִיר • **to show:** Lat. *declaro* (Arab. أظهر) · Constantinus Africanus, *Viaticum* · trans. Do'eg ha-Edomi, *Sefer Ya'ir Netiv*, bk. 1, ch. 22: אמר גלינוס: זה החולי נקרא איפילימסיא הוא ליחה לחה אשר בסבתה בטני המוח או המדורים הם סגורים ולא[16] על נכון ומונעת הנפש להאיר פעולתה (Galen says: The disease called 'epilepsy' is a viscous humor that causes an incomplete obstruction of the ventricles of the brain. It prevents the soul from showing its actions). Hebr. הֵאִיר does not feature in this sense in the current dictionaries. Abraham ben Isaac and Moses ibn Tibbon translate Arab. أظهر as הראה.

אוֹר • *Plur.* **אורות** • **mallow** [***Malva sylvestris*** **L.**]: Lat. *malva* · *Shinnui ha-Shemot ha-Niqra'im Synonimi*, Ms Florence, Biblioteca Laurenziana, Or. 17, fol. 69[b]: אורות ה' מלבא ('WRWT; lit., 'lights;' i.e., mallow). Hebr. אורות does not feature in this sense in the current dictionaries.

אֹזֶן • **אוזן העכבר** • **(lit., mouse ear); a plant of uncertain identity, poss., madwort [*Asperugo procumbens* L.], or a species of forget-me-not (perhaps field forget-me-not [*Myosotis arvensis* (L.) Hill]), or lichwort [*Parietaria officinalis* L. or *Parietaria* lusitanica L.]**: Arab. أذن الفأر (cf. MIG 48) · *Shinnui ha-Shemot ha-Niqra'im Synonimi*, Ms Florence, Biblioteca Laurenziana, Or. 17, fol. 68[a]: אדן אלפאר ר"ל אוזן העכבר והוא עשב ונקרא בלשונם אאורקוליס מוריס ([Arab.] *udhun al-fa'r*, i.e., mouse ear, and that is an herb, and it is called *auriculares muris* in their language [i.e., Latin]). Hebr. אוזן העכבר is a non-attested loan translation of Arab. أذن الفأر.

• *Dual* **אזנים** • **הברה באזנים** → הֲבָרָה.

אָח • **המקור אשר בין האצבע הקטן לאחיהו** → מָקוֹר.

• *Plur.* **אחים** • **דם שני האחים** → דָּם.

אָחַז • *Part.* **אוֹחֵז** • **הכח האוחז** → כֹּחַ.

איורי → אִוּוּי.

אַיָּל • **לשון איל** → לָשׁוֹן.

---

14 'healthy and sound': Hebr. פרה ורבה; lit., 'is fertile and increases' (cf. Gen 1:22); om. a.
15 'balanced': سيالا ('fluid') a.
16 ולא על נכון: *non perfecte* L.

איסטניסות → אִסְטְנִיסוּת.

איפוזימא · **decoction**: Gr. ἀπόζεμα (cf. LSG 198) (Arab. مطبوخ) · Ibn al-Jazzār, *Zād al-musāfir wa-qūt al-ḥādir* · trans. Abraham ben Isaac, *Sefer Ṣedah la-Oreḥim*, bk. 1, ch. 10: ואם יבוא מחמת פלגמוני שיהיה בראש או מחמת נפילה או מכה אז ראוי להקיז מגיד אל קפיאל ויוציא מן הדם שני פעמים בכדי כחו אם לא יעכב שום עלילה להקיז ואחר כך ישלשלהו באיפוזימא שלתמררינדי (If [headache] originates from a tumor occurring in the head, or from a fall or blow, the [patient's] cephalic vein should be venesected. The blood should be extracted in two sessions, according to the strength [of the patient]. This can only be done if there are no obstacles that make a venesection impossible. After this, he should be purged with a decoction made from tamarinds ...). Hebr. איפוזימא is a non-attested loan word from Greek ἀπόζεμα. Moses ibn Tibbon translates Arab. مطبوخ as בשול.

איצטגנין • *Plur.* **איצטגנינים** · **astronomers** · Isḥāq ibn ʿImrān, *Treatise on Melancholy* · trans. Anonymous, fol. 44ª (45ª): והחוזים בעילות הגלגלים והכוכבים הם האיצטגנינים הנ׳ בלשון יון האסטרונומיאה[17] (Those who study the causes of the orbs and stars, i.e., those [who practice astronomy] that is called 'astronomia' [i.e., ἀστρονομία] in Greek).[18] For the use of the term איצטגנין[19], *Plur.* איצטגנינים, referring to both 'astrologers' and 'astronomers' in medieval literature, cf. Sela.[20]

אישטופאש · **tow**: Lat. *estupa*, Plur. acc. *estupas* (with prothetic -*e*) · Guillaume de Congenis, *Treatise on Surgery* · trans. Isaiah, fol. 44ª: כאשר שבירת העצם גדולה ונכרת באותות אז יאות לקחת אבק לבונה ולשים על האם קשה ואחר יושם עליו בגד טבול בלובן ביצה בין העצם והאם הקשה ואחר לפי כמות העצם יתכן לשום פלומצול מאישטופאש רחוצות במים לבדה (When the fracture of the bone [in the head] is large and can be diagnosed [i.e., recognized] from the symptoms, one should take incense powder and put this on the dura mater. Then, one should put a cloth dipped in egg white between the bone and the dura mater and then one can—according to the size of the bone—put a pledget on it that is made from tow and has been washed with water only). Hebr. אישטופאש is a non-attested loan word from Lat. *estupa*, Plur. acc. *estupas*. In addition to the Latin loan word, the Hebrew translator uses Hebr. נעורת.

אישפונגא • **אישפונגא מן הים** · **sponge**: Rom. *espunge marine* / Lat. *espongia marina*[21] (DMLBS 3521) · Guillaume de Congenis, *Treatise on Surgery* · trans. Isaiah, fol. 50ª: אישפונגא מן הים ג׳ דרכמונים (Three *dirhams* of sponge [as part of a compound good for

---

17 האסטרונומיאה: emendation editor המתרטֶומ׳נא Ms.

18 Cf. the Arabic text: والنظر في علل الفلك والكواكب وهو علم التنجيم المسمّى باليونانية الأسطرنوميا.

19 Variant readings: אצטגנין and אסטגנין, cf. JD 89; KG 2:119, 601; KA 1:166; 9:41; LW 1:118.

20 Sh. Sela, 'The Fuzzy Borders between Astronomy and Astrology in the Thought and Work of Three Twelfth-Century Jewish Intellectuals,' *Aleph* 1 (2001): 59–100. I thank Shlomo Sela for this reference and for correcting my original translation.

21 Lat. *espongia marina*, with prothetic -*e* and emendation of Heb. אשפונגא as: אשפונגיא.

treating cancer]). Lat./Rom.-Hebr. אישפונגא מן הים is a non-attested combined loan word and translation from Rom. *espunge marine* or Lat. *espongia marina*. In addition to אישפונגא מן הים, Isaiah renders the Romance-Latin term as אשפונגא מרינא (see entry אשפונגא).

אישרוף · **syrup**: Lat. *siropus* (Arab. شراب) · Constantinus Africanus, *Viaticum* · trans. Do'eg ha-Edomi, *Sefer Ya'ir Netiv*, bk. 1, ch. 16: ונתן לו לשתות מליקרט ארומטיק ואוקשימל עם אישרוף[22] העשוי מן קלמינט (We administer [the patient] a drink of fragrant hydromel as well as oxymel with a syrup prepared from mint). Hebr. אישרוף is a non-attested loan translation from O.Occ. *exirop* ('syrup'). The variant reading אישרוב (cf. Ms Oxford, Bodleian Library, Can. Or. 26) features in BCD 20 (NM 4:15) in a later attestation from Shem Tov ben Isaac's *Sefer ha-Shimmush*, bk. 27. Moses ibn Tibbon translates Arab. شراب as משקה, and Abraham ben Isaac as זולאבי (cf. entry below).

אֲכִילָה • *Plur.* **אכילות** · **foods; dishes**: Lat. *cibi* (Arab. أغذية) · Ibn al-*Jazzār, Zād al-musāfir wa-qūt al-ḥādir* · trans. Abraham ben Isaac, *Sefer Ṣedah la-Oreḥim*, Adaptation, bk. 1, ch. 2 (Ms Berlin, Staatsbibliothek Preußischer Kulturbesitz, Or. fol. 1058, fol. 90a): אם נראה שנפילת השיער תהא מחמת חסרון הפרנוס כאמור למעלה אז נצוה לחולה שיכנס במרחץ מזוג תדיר ונאכילהו אכילות קלות ומיושרות (If we see that the hair loss originates from a decrease of nourishment as stated above, we order the patient frequent visits to the bathhouse, moderately [heated], and administer him light and balanced foods). In the sense of 'food,' Hebr. אֲכִילָה features in the current dictionaries with attestations from the Bible and Rabbinic literature only (cf. BDB 38; JD 63; BM 206). Moses ibn Tibbon translates Arab. أغذية as מזונות. Do'eg ha-Edomi translates Lat. *cibi* as האכיל.

[אכל] • *Nif'al* **נֶאֱכַל** · **to vanish**: Arab. فني (Lat. *pereo*) · Ibn al-Jazzār, *Zād al-musāfir wa-qūt al-ḥādir* · trans. Abraham ben Isaac, *Sefer Ṣedah la-Oreḥim*, bk. 1, ch. 23: וירוצצו אותם וישימום עם השמן והמים ויבשלום באש רפה קלה עד שיאכל המים וישאר השמן (Crush these [ingredients], add them to the oil and the water, and cook this on a low fire until the water vanishes and only the oil remains). Hebr. נֶאֱכַל features in the current dictionaries in the sense of 'to be eaten, devoured, consumed, wasted, destroyed' (cf. BDB 37; BM 212–213). Moses ibn Tibbon translates Arab. فني as הלך. Do'eg ha-Edomi translates the parallel Latin term *pereo* as כלה.

• *Part. Nif'al* **נֶאֱכָל** · **affected by caries, corrosion**: Arab. مأكول · Ibn al-Jazzār, *Zād al-musāfir wa-qūt al-ḥādir* · trans. Moses ibn Tibbon, *Sefer Ṣedat ha-Derakhim*, bk. 2, ch. 19: ואם יבשל שמרי יין במי בוסר עד שישוב כדבש וישים ממנו על השן הנאכלת יעקר אותה ויקל עקירתה (If he cooks lees of wine with the juice of unripe grapes until it turns into a honey-like substance and puts this on the tooth affected by caries, he can pull it out easily). Hebr. נֶאֱכָל does not feature in this sense in the current dictionaries. In

22 אישרוף: אישרוב Ms Oxford, Bodleian Library, Can. Or. 26.

bk. 2, ch. 18, Moses ibn Tibbon uses the noun אִכּוּל in אכול השנים for Arab. تأكّل الأسنان (caries; corrosion of the teeth). Cf. BCD 21 (NM 4:15–16).

אֹכֶל • הבדלת האוכל והמשתה → הַבְדָּלָה.

אַל • אל תיגע בי ‧ **'touch me not' (i.e., a facial ulcer)**: Lat. *noli me tangere*[23] · Guillaume de Congenis, *Treatise on Surgery* · trans. Isaiah, fol. 50ª:[24] כנגד אל תיגע בי זהו נולימיטנגרי קח אבק שלגיימה דקה ושים עליו (Against 'touch me not' (*noli me tangere*): Take the fine powder of rock salt and put it on the spot). Hebr. אל תיגע בי is a non-attested loan translation of Lat. *noli me tangere.*

אֵם ‧ **uterus; womb**: Lat. *matrix* (Arab. رحم) · Constantinus Africanus, *Viaticum* · trans. Do'eg ha-Edomi, *Sefer Ya'ir Netiv*, bk. 1, ch. 18: ונאמר כי כל אחד ממיני החולי הזה נולד מחולי אחר או מצמח הנולד בקרב הוא דיאפרגמא או מחולי האיסטומכ׳ או מן האם (I say that every type of this illness [i.e., phrenitis] originates from another illness, either from an inflammation occurring in the diaphragm or from an illness of the stomach or from the uterus). In the sense of 'uterus,' Hebr. אֵם is attested for in Rabbinic literature (cf. JD 74, BM 261–262) and in medieval encyclopaedic literature, i.e., Gershon ben Solomon, *Sha'ar ha-Shamayim* and Me'ir Aldabi, *Shevilei Emunah* (cf. BM ibid.). Moses ibn Tibbon renders Arab. رحم as רחם.

• **האם הטובה** ‧ **pia mater**: Lat. *pia mater*: Guillaume de Congenis, *Treatise on Surgery* · trans. Isaiah, fol. 43ᵇ: אם האם הטובה מוכה לא יוכל להעזר כי המות ישיגנו ליום חמישי או לשביעי לגבורות אך מעט נצולים לג׳ ימים (When the pia mater is hit, the patient cannot be cured; he will die on the fifth or seventh day when he is strong, only a few live after three days). Hebr. האם הטובה features in BM 262 in a later attestation from Me'ir Aldabi, *Shevilei Emunah*, and in MD 571 (s.v. 'pia mater') referring to the *Sefer ha-Qanun.*

• **אם קשה** ‧ **dura mater**: Lat. *dura mater*: Guillaume de Congenis, *Treatise on Surgery* · trans. Isaiah, fol. 44ª: כאשר שבירת העצם גדולה ונכרת באותות אז יאות לקחת אבק לבונה ולשים על האם קשה ואחר יושם עליו בגד טבול בלובן ביצה בין העצם והאם הקשה ואחר לפי כמות העצם יתכן לשום פלומצול מאישטופאש רחוצות במים לבדה (When the fracture of the bone [in the head] is large and can be diagnosed [i.e., recognized] from the symptoms, one should take incense powder and put this on the dura mater. Then, one should put a cloth dipped in egg white between the bone and the dura mater and then one can—according to the size of the bone—put a pledget on it that is made from tow and has been washed with water only). Hebr. אם קשה is a non-attested loan translation from Lat. *dura mater.*

---

23 Cf. Th.C. Benedek, 'Historical Background of Discoid and SLE,' in *Dubois' Lupus Erythematosus and Related Syndromes*, 8th ed., eds. Wallace and Hahn (Philadelphia 2013): e1: 'Toward the end of the 12th century, Rogerius Frugardi, Salernitan surgeon, introduced the term *noli me tangere* (touch me not) to designate a facial ulcer.'

24 נולימיטנגרי: emendation editor נולימינטראגי Ms ונקרא בהמון נומיטוק Ms[1].

אמידום · **starch**: Lat. *amidum* (Arab. نشاستج) · Constantinus Africanus, *Viaticum* · trans. Do'eg ha-Edomi, *Sefer Ya'ir Netiv*, bk. 3, ch. 1: ונתן לו לאכול במדה מועטת מאיזה מרק או מזרע מילונש ואבטיחים או בשרם כתוש וכן אמידום דרגגן עם שמן שקדים מכל אלה יעשה מרק שינתן לו בצום או אמידום עם חלב ועם פניס ושמן שקדים (We let him eat a little bit of broth from melon seed, watermelon, or from its pulp. Similarly from starch, gum tragacanth with almond oil. The broth prepared from all these ingredients should be given to the patient on an empty stomach. [One can also make it from] starch with milk, sugar candy and almond oil). Hebr. אמידום is a non-attested loan word from Lat. *amidum*. Moses ibn Tibbon uses the same term to translate Arab. نشاستج.

אמצעי • **אֶמְצָעִי** • המקור האמצעי → מָקוֹר.

אנגילא · **eel**: Lat. *anguilla* · Guillaume de Congenis, *Treatise on Surgery* · trans. Isaiah, fol. 47b: לאדמימות העינים קח דג הנקרא אנגילא והוצא את דמו ויבש אותו הדם ושחוק עד אשר דק ומועבר בנפה ואחר יושם בעינים טוב הוא להם ומסיר הדם עד להפליא (For red eyes: Take the fish called 'eel;' extract its blood, dry and pound it until it is a fine substance, sieve it and then put it on the eyes; it is beneficial and removes the blood in an amazing way). Hebr. אנגילא is a non-attested loan word from Lat. *anguilla*.

אסטניסות • **אִסְטְנִיסוּת** • איסטניסות · **want of appetite**: Lat. *fastidium* · Constantinus Africanus, *Viaticum* · trans. Do'eg ha-Edomi, *Sefer Ya'ir Netiv*, bk. 3, ch. 6: אישרוף העשוי מפראשי זה יועיל אל השעול הקר מהלבנה ומרוח ומאיסטניסות ולכל חולי החזה לזקנים (A syrup made from white horehound that is beneficial for cold cough caused by phlegm, for winds, for want of appetite, and for any illness of the chest affecting old people). In the sense of 'want of appetite,' Hebr. אִסְטְנִיסוּת features in BCD 24 (NM 3:26) in a later attestation from Hillel ben Samuel's translation of Hippocrates' *Aphorisms* 4.17.

אסף • **אֹסֶף** • אוסף · **firmness; solidity**: Arab. اكتناز · Maimonides, *Medical Aphorisms* 16.36 · trans. Zeraḥyah Ḥen (BMMZ 168): ההרה כשחלבה יוצא משדיה העובר הוא חלוש ומפני חולשתו אינו מושך הדם וישוב אל השדים ויתילד החלב. ואם יהיה בשדים הרבה אוסף העובר הוא יותר בריא (If the milk of a pregnant woman flows [copiously], the fetus is weak. Because of its weakness, it does not attract the blood, which recedes to the breasts and milk is produced. If the breasts are firmer, the fetus is healthier). In the sense of 'firmness; solidity,' Hebr. אֹסֶף is a non-attested semantic borrowing from Arab. اكتناز. Nathan ha-Me'ati translates Arab. اكتناز as קבוץ חלקים.

אף • קנה האף → קָנֶה.

• *Dual* אַפַּיִם • שם באפיו → [שים].

אפושטוליקון · **apostolicon (an ointment)**: Lat. *apostolicon* (ND 58–59: 'Apostles' plaster or ointment') · Guillaume de Congenis, *Treatise on Surgery* · trans. Isaiah, fol. 44b: מגיד שאלו האבקים צריך לשים במקום אפושטוליקון (It tells us that these powders must be applied instead of apostolicon). Hebr. אפושטוליקון is a non-attested loan word from Lat. *apostolicon*.

אֲפִיסָה · **weakness**: Lat. *defectio* (Arab. ضعف) · Constantinus Africanus, *Viaticum* · trans. Do'eg ha-Edomi, *Sefer Ya'ir Netiv*, bk. 1, ch. 25: אך אפיסת הכח המניע הלאצרטוש

הם ברדונש הוא סבה להתחלת החרדה (But weakness of the faculty that moves the [muscles], i.e., [Romance] BRDWNŠ, causes the beginning of a tremor). In the sense of 'weakness,' Hebr. אֲפִיסָה is a non-attested semantic borrowing from Lat. *defectio*, which can mean both 'defect; weakness' and 'failure; omission.' For other names of illnesses coined with אֲפִיסָה, see BCD 25 (NM 3:27–28). Moses ibn Tibbon translates Arab. ضعف as חולשה, and Abraham ben Isaac as חלישות.

אֲפִיקוֹמָן · **dessert**: Arab. نُقْل · Ibn al-Jazzār, *Zād al-musāfir wa-qūt al-ḥāḍir* · trans. Moses ibn Tibbon, *Sefer Ṣedat ha-Derakhim*, bk. 1, ch. 19: ויהיה מזונו פיישאן הנקרא בערב׳ דראג׳ ותרנוגלים קטנים ומאכלים חמוצים עשויים בקני הלגלוגות ומי בוסר ומי חמיצות האתרוג ויקח אפיקומן רמונים חמוצים ממוצעים ושורבש ותפוחים (The [patient's] food should consist of francolins, called *durrāj* in Arabic, young chickens, and verjuice stews made from common purslane stalks, juice from unripe grapes, and citron pulp. As dessert, he should take sourish pomegranates, true service tree fruits, and apples). Hebr. אֲפִיקוֹמָן is not attested for in medieval medical literature. Abraham ben Isaac translates Arab. نُقْل as פַּרְפְּרָאוֹת (see entry פַּרְפֶּרֶת). Do'eg ha-Edomi translates Lat. *refocilandus est* (for Arab. يتّخذ من النقل) as יאות לחזקו.

אֵפְכָא (*Aram.*) • **דרך אפכא** → דֶּרֶךְ.

[אפס] • *Part. Nif'al* **נֶאֱפָס** • **נאפסת הרגשתו** · **losing one's sensory perceptions**: Arab. فقدان الحسّ · Ibn al-Jazzār, *Zād al-musāfir wa-qūt al-ḥāḍir* · trans. Abraham ben Isaac, *Sefer Ṣedah la-Oreḥim*, bk. 1, ch. 22: אך מקראות המאורעים לבעל חולי זה בכל עת שיבוא לו החולי נאפסת הרגשתו (The symptoms that affect someone suffering from this disease [i.e., epilepsy] in general are: loss of sensory perceptions …). Hebr. נֶאֱפָס only features in EM 102 in an attestation from medieval poetry, i.e., Samuel ha-Nagid, *Ben Mishlei*, and from modern literature. Moses ibn Tibbon translates Arab. فقدان الحسّ as העדר החוש. Do'eg ha-Edomi translates Lat. *sensus et uoluntarii motus fiunt ablatiua* as ההרגשות ותנועות החפץ כשלו.

אֶצְבַּע • **אצבע צפור** · **(lit., birds' finger); greater celandine [*Chelidonium majus* L.]**: Arab. إصبع أصفر (cf. al-Zahrāwī, *K. al-Taṣrīf* II 417, s.v. pl. أصابع صفر, who states that it is identical with الماميران (i.e., the greater celandine); see also MIG 1040) · *Shinnui ha-Shemot ha-Niqra'im Synonimi*, Ms Florence, Bibliotheca Laurenziana, Or. 17, fol. 68ᵃ: אצבע צפור הוא עשב ככף יד ונקרא צילידוניאה כפי זהוראוי (The greater celandine; i.e., a herb like a hand palm, and it is called [in Rom.] *celidonia* according to al-Zahrāwī). Hebr. אצבע צפור features in BM 366 as אצבעות כרכומיים (*digitalis purpurea*).

• **המקור אשר בין האצבע הקטן לאחיהו** → מָקוֹר.

• **המקור העומד בין האצבע הקטון לחבירו** → מָקוֹר.

• **העורק אשר בין האצבע הקטן וחברו** → עוֹרֵק.

• **צמח בצפורן האצבע** → צֶמַח.

• *Plur.* **אצבעות** • **אצבעות הרמוס** · **(lit., Hermes' fingers); autumn crocus [*Colchicum autumnale* L.]**: Arab. أصابع هرمس (Gr. ἑρμοδάκτυλος) (cf. M 276 (Meyerhof)) · *Shinnui* *ha-Shemot ha-Niqra'im Synonimis*, Ms Munich, Bayerische Staatsbibliothek, Cod. hebr. 8, fol. 193[b]: אצבעות הרמוס הוא פרח ארמודוטולי (Hermes' fingers; i.e., flowers [i.e., bulb] of [Rom.] *ermodactuli* [read: *ermodactili*; cf. BMZ 57 (Samekh 1)]). In the sense of 'autumn crocus,' Hebr. אצבעות הרמוס is a non-attested calque from Arab. أصابع هرمس.

אֲרֻבָּה • *Plur.* **ארובות** ‣ **catarrhs**: Lat. *cataractae* (Arab. نوازل) · Constantinus Africanus, *Viaticum* · trans. Do'eg ha-Edomi, *Sefer Ya'ir Netiv*, bk. 2, ch. 14: ולא ירגיל לישן מאד כי השינה פותחת הארובות (And he [i.e., someone suffering from a cold] should not sleep much because sleep opens the catarrhs [i.e., makes them flow]). Hebr. אֲרֻבָּה, *Plur.* ארובות, is not attested for in this sense in the current dictionaries. Moses ibn Tibbon translates Arab. نوازل as ירידות (cf. BCD 120 (NM 3:110)). Zeraḥyah Ḥen translates the Arabic synonym نزلات as נזילות in his translation of Maimonides, *Commentary on Hippocrates'* Aphorisms 7.38 (390) (BMHA 1:507–508; cf. BCD 172 (NM 3:152–153)). See also NM 2:116, 147 for a definition of Hebr. נזל, *Plur.* נזלים, by Nathan ha-Me'ati in his glossary to the *Sefer ha-Qanun*.

ארובה → אֲרֻבָּה.

ארוך → אָרֹךְ.

ארטיטיקא • **טפה ארטיטיקא** → טִפָּה.

אֲרִי • **ארי הארץ** ‣ **(lit., earth lion); February daphne [*Daphne mezereum* L.]**: Arab. أسد الأرض (cf. MIG 57) · Shem Tov ben Isaac, *Sefer ha-Shimmush*, bk. 29, list 1 (SHS 1:128 (Alef 53)): ארי הארץ ב"ה מאזריון וב"ל לוריולה (*ari ha-areṣ*; Arab. *māzaryūn*; vern. LWRY-WLH [i.e., Lat. or O.Occ. *laureola*]). In the sense of 'February daphne,' Hebr. ארי הארץ is a non-attested calque from Arab. أسد الأرض.

אָרֹךְ • **בארוכה** ‣ **for a long time**: Lat. *diu* · Constantinus Africanus, *Viaticum* · trans. Do'eg ha-Edomi, *Sefer Ya'ir Netiv*, bk. 2, ch. 7: ולא תתעכב בארוכה באוזן בפנים (And it [i.e., the remedy] should not stay inside the ear for a long time). In the sense of 'for a long time,' Hebr. בארוכה features as a modern term in EM 117 in attestations from Aḥad ha-Am and Samuel Joseph Agnon.

אַרְעָא (*Aram.*) • **חלבא דארעא** → חֶלְבָּא.

אֶרֶץ • **ארי הארץ** → אֲרִי.

אֵשׁ • **אש קרה** ‣ **cold fire (i.e., quicklime)** · Ibn al-Jazzār, *Zād al-musāfir wa-qūt al-ḥāḍir* · trans. Abraham ben Isaac, *Sefer Ṣedah la-Oreḥim*, bk. 1, ch. 1: הסיד החי המרוקח היא אש קרה (Quicklime, i.e., 'cold fire'). Hebr. אש קרה does not feature in the current dictionaries. See also entry סִיד: סיד מרוקח.

אֶשֶׁךְ • *Plur.* **אשכים** ‣ **castoreum (i.e., a medicament often defined as testicles of a water animal; in fact, it is an excretion derived from the scent glands of the Eurasian beaver [*Castor fiber* Linnaeus, 1758])**: Lat. *castoreum* (cf. DMLBS 388) · *Shinnui ha-Shemot ha-Niqra'im Synonimi*, Ms Florence, Bibliotheca Laurenziana, Or. 17, fol. 69[b]: אשכים ה' קסטורו (Testicles, that is [Rom.] QSṬWRW). Hebr. אשכים is not attested for in this sense in the current dictionaries, cf. BM 416.

אשפונגא • אשפונגא מרינא · **sponge**: Rom. *espunge marine* / Lat. *espongia marina*[25] (DMLBS 3521) · Guillaume de Congenis, *Treatise on Surgery* · trans. Isaiah, fol. 44[b]: האשפונגא מרינא אינה ראויה לשום בין העצם והאם הקשה בלא מחיצה (One should not put a sponge between the [fractured] bone and the dura mater without a partition). Hebr. אשפונגא מרינא is a non-attested loan word from Rom. *espunge marine* or Lat. *espongia marina*. In addition to אשפונגא מרינא, Isaiah translates Rom. *espunge marine*/Lat. *espongia marina* as אישפונגא מן הים (see entry אישפונגא).

אשפטולה · **spatula**: Lat. *espatula* (with prothetic -*e*) · Guillaume de Congenis, *Treatise on Surgery* · trans. Isaiah, fol. 49[a]: וזה מעשה המשיחה: קח השומן והרתיחנו באש ויסונן ובסנון יושם האבק הנזכר וינער יפה באשפטולה ויועיל גם כנגד כל סרטן ישן לפי החכם (This is the recipe of the salve:[26] Take the fat [of an old pig], boil it on a fire, filter it, put the mentioned powder into the filtrate, and stir it well with a spatula. According to the learned [Master, i.e., Guillaume de Congenis] it is also good for an inveterate cancer). Hebr. אשפטולה is a non-attested loan word from Lat. *espatula*.

אֶתְרוֹג • חומץ אתרוג → חֹמֶץ.

---

25 Lat. *espongia marina*, with emendation of Heb. אשפונגא as: אשפונגיא.

26 I.e., the one mentioned under the entry יָרֹק.

ב

בָּאְשָׁה[27] **• באשת הפה** · **bad breath**: Arab. بخر (cf. FL 1:90: *foetor oris*) · Ibn al-Jazzār, *Zād al-musāfir wa-qūt al-ḥādir* · trans. Moses ibn Tibbon, *Sefer Ṣedat ha-Derakhim*, bk. 2, ch. 23: ולו גם כן תאר גרגרים חברם לבאשת הפה המתהוה מן האצטו׳ וחוזק סרחון הפה יסירהו ויבריאהו (He [i.e., Ibn Māsawayh] also has a recipe for pills that he composed to stop and cure bad breath originating from the stomach and a very bad smell in the mouth). Hebr. באשת הפה features in BM 456 in an attestation from the Hebrew *Sefer ha-Qanun*.[28] In addition to באשת הפה, Moses ibn Tibbon translates Arab. بخر as ריח הפה (cf. BCD 261 (NM 4:195)).

בֶּגֶד · **pannus; ailment of the eyes; cataract?**: Lat. *pannus* (cf. DMLBS 2455: '(med. or anat.): a) membrane; b) false membrane, morbid formation; c) ([*pann*]*us oculorum* or ellipt.) pannus, ailment of the eyes, ? cataract; d) birthmark') · Guillaume de Congenis, *Treatise on Surgery* · trans. Isaiah, fol. 48ᵃ: וזאת האבק מסיר בגד הישן בעין אך לא יתמיד בה יותר מדאי (This powder removes inveterate pannus from the eyes, but one should not use it too frequently). In the sense of 'pannus' Hebr. בֶּגֶד is a non-attested semantic borrowing from Lat. *pannus*, which can also mean 'a piece of cloth.' In addition to בֶּגֶד, Isaiah translates Lat. *pannus* as דק (see entry).

בַּד[1] · **shoot; twig; branch**: Arab. غصن · Ibn al-Jazzār, *Zād al-musāfir wa-qūt al-ḥādir* · trans. Moses ibn Tibbon, *Sefer Ṣedat ha-Derakhim*, bk. 2, ch. 19: וממה שיועיל ג״כ מרקיקת הדם שישתה החולה פרח גפן ב׳ שקלים במים קרים בקר וערב או יקח בדי ורד רבים ויודקו ויעצור מימיהם ויתיך במיץ ההוא ב׳ שקלים סחיטת אפוקישטידוש וישתה אותו ([A remedy that is] also good against spitting of blood: Let the patient take in the morning and evening two *sheqels*[29] [Arab. *mithqāl*s] of grapevine blossom with cold water, or take a large quantity of rose shoots, pound them, extract their juice, dissolve two *sheqel*s of hypocist [*Cytinus hypocistis* (L.) L.] in it, and let the patient take it). In the sense of 'branch; shoot; twig,' Hebr. בַּד is only attested for in the Bible, as well as in Rabbinic and modern Hebrew literature (cf. KB 109; BM 460; JD 138; EM 134).

בַּד[2] **• בד בבד** · **one part of each**: Arab. من كلّ واحد جزء · Ibn al-Jazzār, *Zād al-musāfir wa-qūt al-ḥādir* · trans. Abraham ben Isaac, *Sefer Ṣedah la-Oreḥim*, bk. 1, ch. 17: מרקחת אחר להרדים ולישן בטוב: קח אופיו ובנג׳ וזרע יברוחין בד בבד כתוש הכל ונפה ולוש במים ושים בשמש ה׳ ימים וכשתצטרך לו תקח ממנו במעט מוך ומשח בו המצח וגם בין העינים (Another

27 Ben-Yehuda (BM 456) vowelizes the term באשה as בְּאָשָׁה.

28 '*Sefer ha-Qanun*': I.e., one of the translations of Ibn Sīnā's *K. al-Qānūn*, composed by Nathan ha-Me'ati, Zeraḥyah Ḥen, or Joshua Lorki. For an extensive discussion, see NM 4:3–4.

29 '*shekel*s [Arab. *mithqāl*s]': One *mithqāl* is 4.46 grams; cf. W. Hinz, *Islamische Maße und Gewichte umgerechnet ins metrische System*, photomechanischer Nachdruck mit Zusätzen und Berichtigungen, = *Handbuch der Orientalistik*, vol. 1, suppl. 1.1 (Leiden1970), 4–7.

remedy to fall asleep and sleep well: Take one part each of opium, henbane, and mandrake seeds. Pulverize all this, sieve it, knead it with water, and let it stand in the sun for five days. When you need it, take some of it in a piece of cotton and rub it on the forehead and between the eyes). Hebr. בד בבד is not attested for in medieval Hebrew medical literature. It features in the Bible in Ex 30:34: קח לך סמים נטף ושחלת וחלבנה ... בד בבד יהיה (Take the herbs stacte, onycha, and galbanum [...], let there be an equal part of each);[30] cf. BDB 94. Moses ibn Tibbon translates Arab. من كلّ واحد جزء as מ״א חלק.

[בדל] • *Part. Hifʿil* **מַבְדִּיל** • **הוולון המבדיל** → וולון.

בָּדַק • **בדק נקביו** · **to defecate**: Arab. تغوّط · Maimonides, *Medical Aphorisms* 24.20 · trans. Zeraḥyah Ḥen (BMMZ 235): מי שראה מי שיש בו חולי העין הנקרא רמד והוא בלתי מורגל לראות זה עיניו יתמלאו תחלה מליחות ואם יאריך לראותם גם הוא יחלה זה החולי. וכן כמו שאדם יראה אדם אחר ישתין או יבדוק נקביו או יגהק או יפהק[31] מיד[32] ירצה הוא לעשות כמוהו (If someone sees someone else suffering from the eye disease called 'ophthalmia' and he is not used to seeing such a thing, his eyes will initially fill with moisture, and if he looks for a long time, he will also suffer from this illness. Similarly, sometimes a person sees someone else urinating, or defecating, or yawning, or stretching[33] oneself, and this prompts him to do exactly the same thing). Hebr. בדק נקביו does not feature in the current dictionaries. A variant reading בדק עצמו (for Arab. تبرّز) features in BCD 30 (NM 1:79) in an attestation from Shem Tov ben Isaac, *Sefer ha-Shimmush*, bk. 30. Nathan ha-Me'ati translates Arab. تغوّط as יצא.

בַּהֶרֶת · **spot or opaque place on the eye; cataract; leucoma**: Lat. *macula* (DMLBS 2032) · Guillaume de Congenis, *Treatise on Surgery* · trans. Isaiah, fol. 48ª: דע כי זה האבק תועיל לדוק שבעין ולבהרת (Know that this powder is useful for pannus of the eyes and for a spot or opaque place on the eye [i.e., cataract; leucoma]). Hebr. בַּהֶרֶת features in the Bible and Rabbinic literature in the sense of 'brightness, bright spot, of eruption on the skin'; cf. BDB 97; JD 143; BM 475–476; Low XXXIX.

• **בהרת לבנה** · **leucoma**: Lat. *albugo* (DMLBS 76: 'white spot or film on eye, cataract;' Arab. بياض) · Constantinus Africanus, *Viaticum* · trans. Do'eg ha-Edomi, *Sefer Ya'ir Netiv*, bk. 2, ch. 2: ב׳ מאלבוגני הוא בהרת לבנה (Ch. 2: On *albugo*; i.e., leucoma). Hebr. בהרת לבנה features in Lev 13:4 in the sense of a 'white discoloration on the skin;' cf. KB 1:1112.

בּוֹל • **בול חתום** · **terra sigillata**: Arab. خواتيم البحيرة (cf. MIG 569) · Ibn al-Jazzār, *Zād al-musāfir wa-qūt al-ḥādir* · trans. Moses ibn Tibbon, *Sefer Ṣedat ha-Derakhim*, bk. 2, ch. 23: וזה תואר עוגות מחתימות נוטות אל הקביצות מעט חברם בן מאסויה לפתיחת העורקים

---

30 Trans. JPS.
31 יפהק: يتمطّى a.
32 מיד ירצה הוא فيدعوه ذلك a.
33 'stretching oneself': Trans. after a.

בחזה ובריאה ובקיעתם ולראשית התחדש הנגע ויפסיק רבוי יציאת דם הנדות ערובו: יקח בול חתום ג׳ דר׳ בול ארמיני ורדים (Recipe of pastilles composed by Ibn Māsawayh that close up [the wound], that are slighty astringent, and that are good against blood vessels in the chest and lungs that open and break, and against a beginning tumor and severe menstrual bleeding: Take three *dirhams* of terra sigillata, Armenian earth, roses …). Hebr. בול חתום is a non-attested combined term, consisting of O.Occ. *bol* (cf. SHS 1:239–240 (Ṭet 1)) and Hebr. חתום. In Shem Tov ben Isaac's *Sefer ha-Shimmush*, bk. 29, list 1, we find the Hebrew term טיט חתום for the Arabic variant طين مختوم (cf. SHS 1:239 (Ṭet 1)): טיט חתום ב״ה טין מכתום וב״ל בול שג׳ילאטום (see also entry טִיט).

בּוּעָה ‣ **hunchback:** Lat. *gibbositas* (DMLBS 1347: 'protuberance, swelling (on body);' ND 459, s.v. 'gibbosity': 'hump on back') (Arab. حدب) · Constantinus Africanus, *Viaticum* · trans. Do'eg ha-Edomi, *Sefer Ya'ir Netiv*, bk. 1, ch. 23: שמן אחר טוב לחולי קר ולבועה זה הוא גיבושיטט ([Recipe of] another oil beneficial for cold illnesses and hunchback; i.e., GYBWŠYṬṬ [Lat. *gibbositate*]). Hebr. בּוּעָה only features in the current dictionaries in the sense of 'swelling, abscess' (cf. JD 147, s.v. Aram. בועא, BM 489) and 'bulla or blister on the lung or outside the body' (Low XXXIX). Moses ibn Tibbon translates Arab. حدب as גבנות (cf. BCD 43 (NM 4:30)).

בורקיה ‣ **alkalinity:** Arab. بورقية · Isḥāq ibn 'Imrān, *Treatise on Melancholy* · trans. Anonymous, fol. 52ª (53ª): צריך להיות בהם בורקיה או מליחות ([The remedies] must have alkaline or salt [properties]). Hebr. בורקיה is a non-attested loan word from Arab. بورقية. The same Arabic term is translated as בורקיות by Nathan ha-Me'ati in his translation of Maimonides, *Medical Aphorisms* 21.59 (BMMN 203). Constantine the African translates Arab. بورقية as *salsa*. For the adj. בורקי 'alkaline,' featuring in the Hebrew translations of Maimonides, *Medical Aphorisms* 21.59, by both Nathan ha-Me'ati (BMMN 203) and Zeraḥyah Ḥen (BMMZ 201), see BCD 31 (NM 2:30).

בָּחוּר • **תרנגול בחור** → תַּרְנְגוֹל.

בְּטוּלִי ‣ **numb:** Arab. خدري (Gr. ναρκώδης) · Maimonides, *Medical Aphorisms* 6.60 · trans. Zeraḥyah Ḥen (BMMZ 68): ואם יהיה הכאב בקרום אשר תחת העור אשר יהיה נפשט עמו ויתחדש בעבורו כאב המשכי בטוליי (When the pain is in the membrane that lies under the skin and can be stripped off with it, it causes a tensive numb pain). Hebr. בְּטוּלִי is not attested for in the current dictionaries.

בֶּטֶן • **הפוך הבטן** → הִפּוּךְ.

• *Plur.* **בטנים** ‣ **ventricles:** a) Lat. *ventriculi* · Constantinus Africanus, *Viaticum* · trans. Do'eg ha-Edomi, *Sefer Ya'ir Netiv*, bk. 1, ch. 22: אמר גלינוס: זה החולי נקרא איפילימסיא הוא ליחה לחה אשר בסבתה בטני המוח או המדורים הם סגורים ולא[34] על נכון ומונעת הנפש להאיר פעולתה (Galen says: The disease called 'epilepsy' is a viscous humor that causes an

34 ולא על נכון: *non perfecte* L.

incomplete obstruction of the ventricles of the brain. It prevents the soul from showing its actions). In the sense of 'ventricle [of the brain],' Hebr. בֶּטֶן, *Plur.* בטנים, is a non-attested semantic borrowing from the Lat. *ventriculus* (cf. DMLBS 3977).

b) Arab. بطون · Ibn al-Jazzār, *Zād al-musāfir wa-qūt al-ḥādir* · trans. Moses ibn Tibbon, *Sefer Ṣedat ha-Derakhim*, bk. 1, ch. 22: ונאמר כי זה החולי הנקרא בלשון יונים אפילמסיא והוא הכפיה לחות נגר יסתום בטני המוח סתום חסר וימנע הנפש מהראות פעולותיה (I say that the disease that is called in Greek 'PYLMSY' [i.e., ἐπιληψία]; i.e., epilepsy, [originates] from a fluid, which incompletely obstructs the ventricles of the brain and prevents the soul from showing its actions). In the sense of 'ventricle [of the brain],' Hebr. בֶּטֶן, *Plur.* בטנים, is a non-attested semantic borrowing from Arab. بطون. Abraham ben Isaac translates Arab. بطون as חדרים (see entry חֶדֶר).

בָּטְנָה • *Plur.* **בטנים** · **pine cone(s)**: Lat. *pinea* · Constantinus Africanus, *Viaticum* · trans. Do'eg ha-Edomi, *Sefer Ya'ir Netiv*, bk. 3, ch. 6: ויאות גם כן לתת לו מרק חטה עם שמן שקד גם להאכילו בטנים תאנים שקדים וישתה מליקרט עם ארומטיקש ויאכל מרק זרעונים (One should also give him to eat broth prepared from wheat with almond oil, and pine cones, figs, and almonds. He should drink hydromel with spices and eat a broth prepared from chickpeas). In the sense of 'pine cone,' Hebr. בָּטְנָה is attested for in BCD 33 (NM 4:25–26) in a later attestation from Moses ibn Tibbon, *Sefer Ṣedat ha-Derakhim*, bk. 2, ch. 8.

בֵּיצָה • *Plur.* **ביצים • ביצי הפיל** · **marking nut (Ger. *Elefantenlaus*) (fruit of the marking nut tree [*Semecarpus anacardium* L.])**: Arab. بلاذر (cf. MIG 2[35]) · *Shinnui ha-Shemot ha-Niqra'im Synonimi*, Ms Florence, Bibliotheca Laurenziana, Or. 17, fol. 72ª: בלאדור הוא פרי אנקרדי ונק׳ ביצי הפיל ([Arab.] *balādhur*, i.e, the fruit of *anacardium* (marking nut tree), and [in Hebr.] *beṣei ha-pil*). Hebr. ביצי הפיל does not feature in the current dictionaries.

בַּיִת • **מבית** · **on the inside**: Arab. من داخل · Ibn al-Jazzār, *Zād al-musāfir wa-qūt al-ḥādir* · trans. Moses ibn Tibbon, *Sefer Ṣedat ha-Derakhim*, bk. 2, ch. 20: או יקח עפצים ואלום ימאני וקלפת הגלנטץ וקלפת רמונים מ״א חלק יודק וינופה ויחבש בו שרשי השנים והככים מבית ומחוץ (Or take one part each of acorns, Yemenite alum, acorn shells, and pomegranate peels, pound and sieve these, and apply [the substance] as a poultice to the roots of the teeth and to the gums on the inside and outside). In the sense of 'on the inside,' Hebr. מבית is only attested for in the current dictionaries as a biblical term (cf. BDB 110; BM 536; EM 160).

• *Plur.* **בתים • בתי הזיעה** · **armpits**: Lat. *ascellae* (Arab. إبطان) · Constantinus Africanus, *Viaticum* · trans. Do'eg ha-Edomi, *Sefer Ya'ir Netiv*, bk. 3, ch. 16: ט״ז מבואשת בתי הזיעה

35 Cf. esp. G. Bos, '*Balādhur* (Marking-nut): A Popular Medieval Drug for Strengthening Memory,' *Bulletin of the School of Oriental and African Studies* 59, no. 2 (1996): 229–236.

(Ch. 16: On stinking armpits). Hebr. בית הזיעה, *Plur.* בתי הזיעה, is not attested for in the current dictionaries. Moses ibn Tibbon translates the parallel Arabic term نتن الإبطين as סרחון השחי.

[בכר] • *Part. Pi'el f.* **מְבַכֶּרֶת** · **woman who has given birth for the first time**: Lat. *primariola* (DMLBS 2810) · Guillaume de Congenis, *Treatise on Surgery* · trans. Isaiah, fol. 57[a]: וזאת נקראת מבכרת שלא היה לה עוד ולד (That [woman] is called *mevakkeret* [i.e., a woman who has given birth for the first time], who did not have a child yet). Hebr. מְבַכֶּרֶת features in BM 542 in an attestation from Rabbinic literature (*Mishnah Ḥulin* 4.2) in the context of an animal that has a young for the first time.

[בלבל] • *Hitpalpel* **הִתְבַּלְבֵּל** · **to be mixed**: Arab. اختلط · Ibn al-Jazzār, *Zād al-musāfir wa-qūt al-ḥādir* · trans. Abraham ben Isaac, *Sefer Ṣedah la-Oreḥim*, bk. 1, ch. 23: תדוך הכל ותכביר ותלוש בדבש שהוסר קצפו ותלוש בטוב יפה יפה ותנענעיהו עד שיתבלבל בטוב (Pulverize all these [ingredients], sieve them, and knead them together with skimmed honey; knead and stir them well until they are thoroughly mixed). In the sense of 'to be mixed,' Hebr. התבלבל is coined after Aramaic איבלבל, which is attested for in Rabbinic literature; cf. JD 171; LW 1:231; SDA 220. Moses ibn Tibbon translates Arab. اختلط as התערב.

בָּלָה · **to putrefy**: Lat. *putresco* (Arab. حدث ورم وصديد) · Constantinus Africanus, *Viaticum* · trans. Do'eg ha-Edomi, *Sefer Ya'ir Netiv*, bk. 3, ch. 7: והרופאים נחלקו בנגעי הריאה כי האחרים אומרים שאין להם עזר והעיר גיאלינוס ואמר: אם איזה רופא יעזור אל ⟨בעל⟩ פריפליומוניא קודם שהנפח יתעכב שם ויבלה יתרפא הנפח (The physicians disagree [in the matter of] pneumonia. Some of them say that it cannot be cured. Galen remarks and says that if a physician treats a pneumonia [patient] before a tumor settles in and putrefies, he [lit., the tumor] can be cured). Hebr. בָּלָה only features in the current dictionaries in the sense of 'to be worn.' Moses ibn Tibbon renders Arab. حدث ورم وصديد as התחדש בו מורסא ומוגלא. Hebr. בָּלָה features in the anonymous translation of Maimonides, *Commentary on Hippocrates' Aphorisms* 6.27 (319) (BMHA 1:589), in the sense of 'to develop pus' for Arab. تقيّح (cf. BCD 35 (NM 3:35)).

• *Part. Pass.* **בָּלוּי** · **putrid**: Lat. *putrescens* (Arab. فاسد) · Constantinus Africanus, *Viaticum* · trans. Do'eg ha-Edomi, *Sefer Ya'ir Netiv*, bk. 2, ch. 22 (fols. 37[a]–37[b]): וכאשר יסבול בשר השינים מוכרח כל הגוף לסבול עמו ויסבול מהליחות הבלויות (When the gums are affected, the whole body is necessarily affected as well, as it suffers from putrid humors). Hebr. בָּלוּי features in Rabbinic literature in the sense of 'outworn;' cf. JD 172. Moses ibn Tibbon renders Arab. فاسد as נפסד.

• **דבר בלוי** → **דָּבָר**.

• *Pi'el* **בִּלָּה** · **to cause putrefaction**: Lat. *putrefacio* · Constantinus Africanus, *Viaticum* · trans. Do'eg ha-Edomi, *Sefer Ya'ir Netiv*, bk. 3, ch. 7: ונעשה בג' ענינים או מן הליחות האדומות יורדות מהראש או מהלבנות והמלוחות עומדות בעצם הריאה ומנגעות אותה בפנים ומבלות אותה (It [i.e., phthisis] can be caused by three things: by choleric humors that descend from the head, by phlegmatic, salty humors that settle in the substance of the lungs and that cause ulceration and putrefaction …). Hebr. בָּלָה features in BM 546 in the sense of 'to consume, to destroy' only.

בָּלֶה ‣ **putrid; putrefying; decaying:** Lat. *putrescens* · Constantinus Africanus, *Viaticum* · trans. Do'eg ha-Edomi, *Sefer Ya'ir Netiv*, bk. 2, ch. 25: ואלו העדשים יכולים להרפא במשיחות לבד אבל אותם אשר יקרו בפתע אל הזכרים או בסבת חולי הם קשים לעזור כי בהולדם מהאדומה השחרחורת והיא אינה בלה אז תתחלפנה איכויות העור (These freckles can be cured by means of salves alone, but those that suddenly appear on men or [appear] because of an illness are hard to cure. When these originate from black[36] bile that is not putrid, the qualities of the skin become different). Hebr. בָּלֶה only occurs in the current dictionaries as a biblical and modern term in the sense of 'worn;' cf. BM 546; EM 170.

בָּלוּי (*Part. Pass.*) → בָּלָה.

בִּלּוּי • בלויי[37] ‣ **I. pus:** Lat. *sanies* (Arab. قيح) · Constantinus Africanus, *Viaticum* · trans. Do'eg ha-Edomi, *Sefer Ya'ir Netiv*, bk. 2, ch. 10: מבלויי האזנים לפעמים סובלות האזנים מדבר בלוי ואם יהיה הכאב רב מאד תחל לעזור עם רפואות מכבות הכאב (On pus in the ears. Sometimes the ears suffer from pus, and if the pain is severe begin to treat it with remedies that alleviate the pain). Hebr. בִּלּוּי only features as a modern term in EM 170 in the sense of השחתה or אבוד. The term also features in the *Sefer Agur*, i.e., Do'eg ha Edomi's translation of a Latin version of Hippocrates' *Aphorisms*, in the sense of 'irritation,' and in the combination בלוי הטיט in the sense of 'pus,' while the anonymous translator of Maimonides' *Commentary on Hippocrates'* Aphorisms 7.20 (372) (BMHA 1:599) uses בִּלּוּי to render Arab. تقيّح ('suppuration') (cf. BCD 36 (NM 3:35–36)).

‣ **II. putrefaction:** Lat. *putretudo* (Arab. عفونة) · Constantinus Africanus, *Viaticum* · trans. Do'eg ha-Edomi, *Sefer Ya'ir Netiv*, bk. 2, ch. 22: בשר השינים יסבול לפעמים מרוב ענינים כמו מבלוי (The gums can suffer from many [diseases], such as putrefaction …). Moses ibn Tibbon translates Arab. عفونة as עפוש.

‣ **III. putrid matter:** Lat. *putredo* · Guillaume de Congenis, *Treatise on Surgery* · trans. Isaiah, fol. 48b: דע כשהחוטם[38] נקוב בסבת פישטולאה והבלוי יוצא דרך הנחירים (Know that when the nose is perforated by a fistula and the putrid matter streams from the nostrils …).

‣ **IV. aphthae:** Lat. *ulcerationes* (Arab. قلاع) · Constantinus Africanus, *Viaticum* · trans. Do'eg ha-Edomi, *Sefer Ya'ir Netiv*, bk. 2, ch. 24: ואם הבלוי יקרה ליונקים האם תקח העדשים ומוח[39] הפת והאמידום מזוג במים חמים עם זעפרן וזרע ורד ותניח עליהם (If babies suffer from aphthae, the mother should take lentils, [a bit] of bread and

36 'black bile' (האדומה השחרחורת): Cf. entry אֲדָמָה: האדומה השחרחורת above.
37 See also entry דָּבָר: דבר בלוי.
38 כשהחוטם: Ms[1] כשהוח? Ms.
39 ומוח: *micam* L.

starch, mix this with hot water, saffron, and seeds of roses, and put it on them). Moses ibn Tibbon transcribes Arab. قلاع as קלאע.

• *Plur.* **בלויים • בלויי עב טיט** · **putrid matters:** Lat. *putretudines* · Constantinus Africanus, *Viaticum* · trans. Do'eg ha-Edomi, *Sefer Ya'ir Netiv*, bk. 2, ch. 20: לפעמים ינועו השנים בסבת הליחות אשר בשרשיהם ואם הליחות חדות הכרח הוא שיתנקבו ותאספו שם בלויי עב טיט (The teeth may become loose because of the moistures in their roots. If those moistures are sharp, the teeth will unavoidably be affected by holes and accumulation of putrid matters). Hebr. *Sing.* בלוי עב טיט features in BCD 36 (NM 3:36–37) in Do'eg ha-Edomi's *Sefer Agur* in the sense of 'suppuration' or 'empyema,' while עב טיט features in the *Sefer Agur* in the sense of 'pus;' cf. BCD 196 (NM 3:172).

בָּלוּל (*Part. Pass.*) → **בָּלַל**.

בָּלַל • בלל ונענע[40] · **to stir:** Arab. ضرب · Ibn al-Jazzār, *Zād al-musāfir wa-qūt al-ḥādir* · trans. Abraham ben Isaac, *Sefer Ṣedah la-Oreḥim*, bk. 1, ch. 17: ושים עמהן שמן זנבק ויניחהו בשמן י׳ ימים ויבללהו וינענעהו בבל יום בבלי זכוכית ואחר כן תצלילהו וקח מן אופיאו כפי הצורך וכותשנו ושימנו באותו שמן ועוד יערבבהו וינענעהו עשרה ימים ואחר כן תחזיר הכל אל השמרים ויוסיף על הכל עוד אופייו וינענעהו בכל יום (Add saffron oil to [the mentioned ingredients], leave it in the oil for ten days, mix it and stir it every day in a glass flacon and purify it. Take opium as much as you need, pound it and add it to the oil. Stir it for [another] ten days, then return everything to the lees [from which it was purified before], and add again opium. Stir this every day ...). Hebr. בלל ונענע does not feature in the current dictionaries. Moses ibn Tibbon translates Arab. ضرب as הכה, Do'eg ha-Edomi translates the parallel Latin term *moveo* as הניע.

• *Part. Pass.* **בָּלוּל** · **turbid:** Lat. *turbidus* · Constantinus Africanus, *Viaticum* · trans. Do'eg ha-Edomi, *Sefer Ya'ir Netiv*, bk. 3, ch. 7: ואם יתראה שיהיה טוב להקיזו פעם שלישית נעשה רק שנתבונן שהדם יהיה בלול וגס (If it is clear that it is good to bleed [the patient] for a third time, one should do so, but only if his blood is turbid and thick). Hebr. בָּלוּל does not feature in this sense in the current dictionaries; cf. BDB 117; JD 173; BM 551, EM 170.

בֵּן • אב טרם הבן → **אָב**.

בַּעַל • *Plur.* בעלים • בעלי הלבנה · **persons full with phlegm:** Lat. *flegmatici* · Constantinus Africanus, *Viaticum* · trans. Do'eg ha-Edomi, *Sefer Ya'ir Netiv*, bk. 1, ch. 19: ואם השכור קר בתולדתו יתנו לו אוקשימל לפני המרחץ וישן אחרי המרחץ ויגרדו רגליו במים חמים ובמלח והאישנץ טוב מאד אל השכורים אם הם בעלי הלבנה (If a drunken person has a cold nature one should give him oxymel before bathing and then he should sleep; his feet should be rubbed with hot water and salt; absinth wormwood is very good for drunken persons when they are full with phlegm). Hebr. *Sing.* בעל הלבנה, *Plur.* בעלי הלבנה, does not feature in the current dictionaries. The term לבנה on its own features

---

40 See also entry עִרְבֵּב: ערבב ונענע.

in the sense of 'phlegm' in BM 2612 in a quotation of Nathan ha-Me'ati's translation of Maimonides' *Medical Aphorisms* 10.23 (BMMN 126; cf. BCD 134 (NM 2:55)).

בָּצָל • בצל העכבר · **(lit., mouse (rat) onion); sea squill [*Drimia maritima* (L.) Stearn]:** Arab. بصل الفأر · *Shinnui ha-Shemot ha-Niqra'im Synonimi*, Ms Florence, Biblioteca Laurenziana, Or. 17, fol. 68ᵃ: אסקיוולה היא בצל אלפאר[41] כלומ׳ בצל העכבר לטין אשקיטלה לעז סיבה[42] מרינה ([Rom.] ʾSQYWWLH ('squill'), [Arab.] *baṣal al-fa'r* (cf. MIG 703), [Hebr.] *beṣal ha-ʿakhbar*, [Lat.] ʾŠQYṬLH (**esquitla*), [O.Occ.] SYBH MRYNH (*seba marina*) (cf. SHS 1:130–131 (Bet 3))). Hebr. בצל העכבר is a non-attested loan translation of Arab. بصل الفأر.

בָּקִיעַ • *Plur.* **בקיעים • בקיעי השפתים** · **lip fissures:** Lat. *rimae labrorum* (Arab. تشقيق الشفتين) · Constantinus Africanus, *Viaticum* · trans. Do'eg ha-Edomi, *Sefer Ya'ir Netiv*, bk. 2, ch. 16: מבקיעי השפתים: השפתים לפעמים סובלים בקיעים או אבעבועות או נגעים וזה יקרה מליחות מחודדות (On lip fissures. The lips can be afflicted by fissures, pustules, or ulcers, which is the result of sharp humors). Hebr. בקיעי השפתים is not attested for in the current dictionaries. The term בָּקִיעַ on its own features in BM 594 in the sense of 'fissure' in attestations from the Bible and Rabbinic and liturgical literature. Masie (MD 351) mentions the term in the sense of 'hernia.' Moses ibn Tibbon renders Arab. تشقيق الشفتين as בקיעת השפתים (cf. BCD 38 (NM 4:28)). The same term features in Isaiah's Hebrew translation of Guillaume de Congenis, *Treatise on Surgery*, fol. 50ᵃ (see entry בְּקִיעָה).

בְּקִיעָה • בקיעת השפתים · **lip fissures:** Lat. *fissure labiorum* · Guillaume de Congenis, *Treatise on Surgery* · trans. Isaiah, fol. 50ᵃ: מבקיעת השפתים קח חלב איל אמידום ליטרגיר מעורבים יחד ויעשה משיחה ([A remedy] for lip fissures: Take fat of a ram, starch, litharge; mix these together, prepare a salve from it [, and apply]). Hebr. בקיעת השפתים features in BCD 38 (NM 4:28) in an attestation from Moses ibn Tibbon's *Sefer Ṣedat ha-Derakhim* as a translation of Arab. تشقيق السفتين.

בַּרְזֶל · **1. surgical instrument; surgery:** Lat. *ferrum* (Arab. حديد) · Constantinus Africanus, *Viaticum* · trans. Do'eg ha-Edomi, *Sefer Ya'ir Netiv*, bk. 2, ch. 19: ואם לא ישקוט הכאב בכל אלה יאות להוציאם בברזל (If the pain [in the teeth] does not abate with any of the [remedies that I mentioned], one should extract the [tooth that causes the pain] with a surgical instrument). Hebr. בַּרְזֶל does not feature in this sense in the current dictionaries. Subsequently, Moses ibn Tibbon uses the same Hebrew term for both Arab. حديد and مبضع, i.e., 'scalpel' (cf. BCD 38 (NM 1:54)). Nathan ha-Me'ati uses בַּרְזֶל for Arab. حديد in his translation of Maimonides' *Medical Aphorisms* 15.18 (BMMN 157; cf. BCD 38 (NM 2:33)).

---

41 אלפאר: emendation editor אלפצר Ms.

42 סיבה: emendation editor סינה Ms.

‣ II. **branding iron**: Lat. *ferrum* · Guillaume de Congenis, *Treatise on Surgery* · trans. Isaiah, fol. 57[a]: ואחר יכוה בברזל חם (Then he should cauterize the spot with a hot branding iron). Hebr. בַּרְזֶל does not feature in this sense in the current dictionaries.

• **חרש ברזל** → חָרָשׁ.

בָּרִיא • בריא מן ‣ **free from**: Arab. سليم من · Ibn al-Jazzār, *Zād al-musāfir wa-qūt al-ḥādir* · trans. Moses ibn Tibbon, *Sefer Ṣedat ha-Derakhim*, bk. 3, ch. 1: ומה שהיה ענינו כן מן האסכרה הנה עליון הגרון בו בריא מן החולי (If the angina is such [as I have described] then the larynx is free from illness). Hebr. בריא מן is not attested for in this sense in the current dictionaries.

בְּרִיאוּת ‣ **recovery**: Arab. برء · Ibn al-Jazzār, *Zād al-musāfir wa-qūt al-ḥādir* · trans. Moses ibn Tibbon, *Sefer Ṣedat ha-Derakhim*, bk. 2, ch. 25: והנה יעשו גם כן רפואות מורכבות ומריחות מועילות. ומזה תאר רפואה חברה בן מאסויה לכלף העב ולטהר הפנים וליפותם והיא תמהר הבריאות (When one applies compound remedies and salves, they are also good [as a cure for freckles]. One of these is a recipe of a remedy composed by Ibn Māsawayh that is good for thick freckles, for cleaning and embellishing the face, and that gives a fast recovery). In the sense of 'recovery' (for Lat. *sanitas*), Hebr. בְּרִיאוּת features in BCD 39 (NM 3:39) in an attestation from Hillel ben Samuel's translation of Hippocrates' *Aphorisms* 2.19.

בִּשּׁוּל • בשול יין ‣ **rob (i.e., fruit juice boiled down to syrup)**: Arab. ربّ · Ibn al-Jazzār, *Zād al-musāfir wa-qūt al-ḥādir* · trans. Moses ibn Tibbon, *Sefer Ṣedat ha-Derakhim*, bk. 3, ch. 1: וכאשר עשינו זה תחלה והתבאר לנו כי החומר כבר שכך מהמשך אל האבר אשר בו החולי נשתדל אז להתיך המותר ההוא מן האבר ולהמס אותו כמו שיגרגר בבשול יין תותים (Once we have done this first and it is clear that the humors have been restrained from streaming to the organ in which the illness is located, we turn to dissolving and liquefying the superfluities that are in that organ. [We do so] by prescribing a gargle prepared from a rob of mulberries …). Hebr. בשול יין does not feature in the current dictionaries. In addition to בשול יין, Moses ibn Tibbon renders Arab. ربّ with the Hebrew loan word רב (see entry רֹב). Do'eg ha-Edomi renders the parallel Latin term *sapa* as שפא (see entry). Moses ibn Tibbon's contemporary Shem Tov ben Isaac renders Arab. ربّ as עסיס in the *Sefer ha-Shimmush*, bk. 27 (cf. BCD 205 (NM 4:149)).

[בשל] • *Pi'el* **בִּשֵּׁל** ‣ **to digest**: Lat. *digestibilis* · Constantinus Africanus, *Viaticum* · trans. Do'eg ha-Edomi, *Sefer Ya'ir Netiv*, bk. 2, ch. 1: ואז נצוה אל החולה שלא יזוז ושישן ומראשותיו גבוהים ושיברח מאור הנר ולא ירים קולו בדברו ומאכליו יהיו קרים ונקלים לבשל (And then we tell the patient [suffering from ophthalmia] not to move, and to sleep with his head on a high cushion, to avoid the light of a lamp, not to raise his voice when speaking, and to eat foods that are cool and easy to digest). In the sense of 'to digest,' Hebr. בִּשֵּׁל features in BM 641, a.o., in an attestation from the *Sefer ha-Qanun*.

• *Part. Pu'al* **מְבֻשָּׁל** ‣ **ripe**: Arab. نضيج · Isḥāq ibn 'Imrān, *Treatise on Melancholy* · trans. Anonymous, fol. 52[h] (53[h]): אבל הענבים המבושלים המתוקים מרכך בטנם בחוזק (But sweet, ripe grapes have a strong laxative effect). In the sense of 'ripe,' Hebr. מְבֻשָּׁל is attested for in Rabbinic literature (cf. BM 641, EM 205).

- **חטה מבושלת** → **חִטָּה**.
- **יין מבושל** → **יַיִן**.

בָּשָׂר • **בשר כתוש** · **pulp**: Lat. *medulla* (Arab. دماغ) · Constantinus Africanus, *Viaticum* · trans. Do'eg ha-Edomi, *Sefer Ya'ir Netiv*, bk. 3, ch. 1: ונתן לו לאכול במדה מועטת מאיזה מרק או מזרע מילונש ואבטיחים או בשרם כתוש וכן אמידום דרגגן עם שמן שקדים מכל אלה יעשה מרק שינתן לו בצום או אמידום עם חלב ועם פניס (We let him eat a little bit of broth from common melon seed, watermelon, or their pulp. Similarly from starch, gum tragacanth with almond oil. The broth prepared from all these ingredients should be given to the patient on an empty stomach. One can also make it from starch with milk and sugar candy). In the sense of 'pulp,' Hebr. בָּשָׂר alone features in BM 645 in later attestations only, a.o., from the *Sefer ha-Qanun*. Moses ibn Tibbon translates Arab. دماغ as מוח.

- **בשר עודף** · **excrescence; keloid:**[43] Lat. *caro superflua* (Arab. نابت; *Plur.* نوابت) · Constantinus Africanus, *Viaticum* · trans. Do'eg ha-Edomi, *Sefer Ya'ir Netiv*, bk. 2, ch. 13: ואם גרב[44] או פורי או בשר עודף יולדו בנחירים העזר הנכון הוא החתוך (If pustules, or polyps, or excrescences appear in the nose, the right therapy is to cut them). Hebr. בשר עודף does not feature in the current dictionaries. Moses ibn Tibbon translates Arab. نوابت as בשר נוסף (cf. BCD 40 (NM 4:29)).
- **בשר השינים** · **gums**: Lat. *gingivae* (Arab. لثة) · Constantinus Africanus, *Viaticum* · trans. Do'eg ha-Edomi, *Sefer Ya'ir Netiv*, bk. 2, ch. 22: כ״ב מבשר השינים (Ch. 22: On the gums). In the sense of 'gums,' Hebr. בשר השנים features in BCD 40 (NM 3:41) in a later attestation from Hillel ben Samuel's translation of Hippocrates' *Aphorisms* 3.25. Moses ibn Tibbon translates Arab. لثة as Aram. כַּכָּא and explains this term as בשר השנים (see entry כַּכָּא).
- **עדיפת הבשר** → **עֲדִיפָה**.
- **הרפואה המעלה הבשר** → **רְפוּאָה**.

---

43 See also entry עֲדִיפָה: עדיפת הבשר.

44 גרב או פורי: *pustule porri* L نواسير a.

גַּבְהוּת · **boiling; seething**: Arab. فوران · Ibn al-Jazzār, *Zād al-musāfir wa-qūt al-ḥādir* · trans. Abraham ben Isaac, *Sefer Ṣedah la-Oreḥim*, bk. 1, ch. 18: ויהיו פניו אדומים מחמת הרתחת דם הלב וגבהותו (His face will be red because of the boiling and seething of the blood of the heart). Hebr. גַּבְהוּת does not feature in this sense in the current dictionaries; cf. BM 674. Moses ibn Tibbon translates Arab. فوران as התגברות.

גְּבוּל • יום הגבול → יוֹם.

[גבן] • *Part. Hitpaʿel* מִתְגַּבֵּן · **coagulating; coagulated**: Arab. متجبّن · Ibn al-Jazzār, *Zād al-musāfir wa-qūt al-ḥādir* · trans. Moses ibn Tibbon, *Sefer Ṣedat ha-Derakhim*, bk. 3, ch. 15: ואם היתה המוגלא לבנה יתערב בה מראה עפרורית נדע שהיא מחלב מתגבן מעופש (If the pus [of a tumor in the breasts] consists of phlegm that has a dusty color, we know that [the tumor] originates from putrid, coagulated milk). In the sense of 'to coagulate,' Hebr. הִתְגַּבֵּן, features in BM 683 in a later attestation from Simeon ben Zemah Duran, *Sefer Magen Avot*. Do'eg ha-Edomi translates the parallel Latin term *coagulatio* as קבוץ.

גָּבַר • **גבר על** · **to soak; to cover (a liquid)**: Arab. غمر · Ibn al-Jazzār, *Zād al-musāfir wa-qūt al-ḥādir* · trans. Moses ibn Tibbon, *Sefer Ṣedat ha-Derakhim*, bk. 3, ch. 11: תאר רפואה מועילה לשעול אשר תגבה ממנו הנשימה מהירת ההצלחה: יקח לבונה לבנה ודרגגן מ״א ב׳ דר׳ אנזרות דר׳ יושם זה במים שעור מה שיגברו עליו ויניחהו לילה עד עלות השחר ואח״כ ישים בו מעט דבש וישתה חצי המשקל הזה בשלש אוקי׳ עד שש מחלב שנחלב מיד (Recipe of a medicine that works quickly and that is good for cough that comes with shallow breathing [lit., breathing that is high (in the chest)]: Take two *dirham*s each of white incense, gum tragacanth, one *dirham* of sarcocol, put this in a quantity of water that is sufficient to cover it, leave it for one night until dawn, put some honey in it, and take a dosis that is half the weight of the ingredients with three to six ounces of fresh milk). Hebr. גבר על does not feature in this sense in the current dictionaries.

גָּדוֹל • צרי הגדול → צֳרִי.

גִּדּוּל · **nutrition; regimen**:[45] Lat. *nutrimentum* (Arab. تدبير) · Constantinus Africanus, *Viaticum* · trans. Do'eg ha-Edomi, *Sefer Ya'ir Netiv*, bk. 1, ch. 22: ואם יחל מיום הולדו הנה הוא מגדול רע או מסבה אחרת רעה וזרה ונעזור לו כפי אשר יסבול כחו ועתו (If [epilepsy] develops from the moment of [a child's] birth, it is caused by a bad regimen or by something else that is bad and external and we treat him according to his strength and age). Hebr. גִּדּוּל features in the current dictionaries in the sense of 'growth, rearing of children' with attestations from Rabbinic literature (JD 235; BM 696–697).

• **גדול הלבנה** · **waxing of the moon**: Lat. *luna crescens* (Arab. زيادة القمر) · Constantinus Africanus, *Viaticum* · trans. Do'eg ha-Edomi, *Sefer Ya'ir Netiv*, bk. 1, ch. 22: איפלמסיא

45 See also entry סֵדֶר.

הבאה בגדול הלבנה יראה טבעה להיות לחה מאד כי כל דבר לח יגדל בגדול הלבנה והבאה בחסור הלבנה היא קרה מאד ואולם היא לחה קצת (As for epileptic fits occurring when the moon waxes, the matter [that causes them] appears extremely moist. For all moist things grow when the moon waxes. As for [epileptic fits] that occur at waning moon, [the matter that causes them] is extremely cold and a little bit moist). Hebr. גדול הלבנה is not attested for in the current dictionaries. Moses ibn Tibbon and Abraham ben Isaac translate Arab. زيادة القمر as תוספת הירח, a term also featuring in Maimonides' *Moreh Nevukhim* (trans. Samuel ibn Tibbon).

[גדל] • *Pi'el* **גִּדֵּל** · **to feed**: Lat. *nutrio* (Arab. غذّا) · Constantinus Africanus, *Viaticum* · trans. Do'eg ha-Edomi, *Sefer Ya'ir Netiv*, bk. 3, ch. 7: ואם בתחלת החולי ימצא בו דם רב יאות לחסר דמו בתחלה כפי כחו לסבול ויאות לגדלו במאכלים מדקדקים וממהרים לבשל כמו הטיבשנא העשויה עם קרנקש הנמצאים בנהרות (If we find that in the beginning of the illness [i.e., phthisis] the patient has much blood, we should first bleed him according to what his strength endures and we should feed him with food that has a thinning effect and that is quickly digested, such as a drink or liquid food made from barley prepared with river crabs). Hebr. גִּדֵּל does not feature in this sense in the current dictionaries. Moses ibn Tibbon translates Arab. غذّا as זן.

• *Part. Hitpa'el* **מִתְגַּדֵּל** • **הדג המתגדל בין הסלעים** → דָּג.

גְּדְמוּת · **leprosy**: Arab. جذام · Shem Tov ben Isaac, *Sefer ha-Shimmush*, bk. 29, list 1 (SHS 1:158 (Gimel 18)): גדמות ב״ה ג׳דאם וב״ל מדיל (*gidmut*; Arab. *judām*, vern. *MDYL* [i.e., O.Occ. *mesel/mezel* or O.Cat. *mesell* for 'leprous']). In the sense of 'leprosy,' Hebr. גְּדְמוּת features in BM 703 in later attestations, a.o., from the *Sefer ha-Qanun*.

גּוֹזֵר (*Part.*) → גָּזַר.

גווייש · **dyspnea (i.e., shortness of breath); orthopnea**: Arab. ربو (UWS 1:180, s.v. ἄσθμα: 'Atemnot, Keuchen;' ibid. 1:791–792, s.v. ὀρθόπνοια: 'Engbrüstigkeit bei der man nur in aufrechter Stellung atmen kann') · Ibn al-Jazzār, *Zād al-musāfir wa-qūt al-ḥāḍir* · trans. Moses ibn Tibbon, *Sefer Ṣedat ha-Derakhim*, bk. 3, ch. 11: ואולם הנשימה הגבוהה היא אשר יצטרך האדם להניע החזה שלו כלו תנועה תכופה והנשימה הזאת היא הנקראת רבו ר״ל גווייש ונשימת הזקיפה (Difficulty of breathing [lit., breathing high (in the chest)] is [a condition] in which the patient has to move his whole chest frequently; this [kind of] breathing is called [in Arabic] *rabwun*; i.e., [O.Occ.] **gois*, and 'orthopnea'). Hebr. גווייש is a non-attested loan word from O.Occ. **gois*, which is formed through aphaeresis from the adj. *engois* (cf. RL 2:88b); the latter term hails from Lat. *angustia*(*re*). In our texts, the term **gois* denotes a noun in the sense of Lat. *angustia*: (1) 'narrowness, cramped space; slightness, weakness; (2) pressure; affliction, anguish' (DMLBS 113).[46] The term גווייש also occurs in Shem Tov ben Isaac, *Sefer ha-Shimmush*,

46 For the interpretation of גווייש in a personal communication between Patrick Sauzet and Guido Mensching I thank both colleagues.

bk. 29, list 1, as a translation of Arab. بُهْر (cf. Lane 265: 'the state of being out of breath;' UW 139, s.v. ἄσθμα: 'Atemnot, Keuchen'); cf. SHS 1:159 (Gimel 22).[47] Do'eg ha-Edomi transcribes the parallel Latin term *orthomia* as אורטומיא.

גּוּף • חוסר הגוף → חָסֵר.

גָּזַר • *Part.* גּוֹזֵר · **decisive**: Arab. قطعي · Maimonides, *Medical Aphorisms* 25.72 · trans. Nathan ha-Me'ati (BMMN 269): ותחקור מה שיחייבהו לאדם בהחזיקו בסברתו. וממה שראוי שתתעורר עליו שאלו נתאמת מה שזכרו היה[48] לו טענה גוזרת לבטל בה סברת אריסטו' בשהתחלת החוש והתנועה מן הלב (Consider to what consequences a person is necessarily lead when he wants to support his opinion. One of the things that should be pointed out is that if what [Galen] says is correct, it would not[49] be a decisive argument for refuting Aristotle's opinion that the principle of sensation and motion comes from the heart). In the sense of 'decisive,' Hebr. גּוֹזֵר is a non-attested calque from Arab. قطعي. Zeraḥyah Ḥen translates Arab. قطعي as נֶחְתָּךְ (see entry [חתך]).

גִּיד · **nerve**: Lat. *neruus* · Constantinus Africanus, *Viaticum* · trans. Do'eg ha-Edomi, *Sefer Ya'ir Netiv*, bk. 1, ch. 24: ואם המצוק ההוא ירד בגיד אחד לבדו נעשה הליחות[50] באותו אבר לאשר אותו הגיד משרת (If the obstruction occurs only to one nerve, the moisture[51] only affects the organ that is served by that nerve). Hebr. גִּיד features in the sense of 'nerve' in BCD 45 (NM 1:18) in a later attestation from the *Sefer ha-Keritut* by Hillel ben Samuel. Abraham ben Isaac translates the parallel Arabic term عصبة as הגיד הדק (see below), and Moses ibn Tibbon as עצב.

• **הגיד הדק** · **nerve**: Arab. عصبة · Ibn al-Jazzār, *Zād al-musāfir wa-qūt al-ḥāḍir* · trans. Abraham ben Isaac, *Sefer Ṣedah la-Oreḥim*, bk. 1, ch. 23: ואם יקרה החולי באבר אחד יקרה[52] על שם האבר ההוא בלבד בעבור כי הסתימה אם יהיה בשורש אחד מהגידים הדקים ויהיה שאר הגידים הקרובים סביביו בלא הזק כלום אז יהיה ההזק והרפיון באותו האבר אשר יעבור אותו הגיד הדק (If the illness [i.e., apoplexy] befalls one [specific] organ, it is named[53] after that [specific] organ. For—if such an obstruction befalls the root of a single nerve and the other surrounding nerves remain sound—harm and looseness occur only in the organ that nerve passes through). Hebr. הגיד הדק does not feature in the current dictionaries. Moses ibn Tibbon translates Arab. عصبة as עצב. Do'eg ha-Edomi translates Lat. *neruus* as גִּיד (see above).

• **הגיד העליון** · **the cephalic vein**: Arab. القيفال · Ibn al-Jazzār, *Zād al-musāfir wa-qūt al-ḥāḍir* · trans. Moses ibn Tibbon, *Sefer Ṣedat ha-Derakhim*, bk. 2, ch. 20: ואם היה הלחות

47 Our interpretation of the term in SHS 1 should be corrected according to this entry.
48 היה לו: لا كان له a (= לא היה לו).
49 'not be': Trans. after a.
50 הליחות: *mollities* L استرخاء a.
51 'moisture': 'softness' L 'looseness' a.
52 יקרה: نسب a = יקרא.
53 'named': Trans. after a.

ההוא חד נצוה להקיז הגיד העליון או לשים כלי המציצה בעורף אחרי הצואר (If that moisture is sharp, we order to bleed the cephalic vein or to put a cupping glass on the nape of the neck). Hebr. הגיד העליון is not attested for in the current dictionaries. For גִּיד in the sense of 'vein,' cf. BCD 44 (NM 1:81). Shem Tov ben Isaac translates Arab. القيفال as גיד הראש (cf. BCD 45 (NM 1:82)). See also Nathan's glossary to the *Sefer ha-Qanun* (NM 2:113, 138 (Ḥet 12)).

• **גיד הערוה** · **penis**: Lat. *virga virilis* · Guillaume de Congenis, *Treatise on Surgery* · trans. Isaiah, fol. 56b: מן מכה בגיד הערוה נקרא מטה: כנגד פיק[54] במטה תחלה תקשרנו בחוט משי או בחוט[55] הבהמה (On an injury of the penis that is called *maṭṭeh*: If there is a tumor on the penis, one should first of all tie it off with a thread from silver or with the hair of a horse[56] ...). Hebr. גיד הערוה is not attested for in the current dictionaries. For the term גִּיד on its own in the sense of 'penis,' cf. BM 752; BCD 44 (NM 1:18). See also entry מַטֶּה.

• **הגיד השומע** · **the auditory (i.e., acoustic) nerve**: Lat. *neruus audibilis* (Arab. العصب الذي يجري فيه السمع) · Constantinus Africanus, *Viaticum* · trans. Do'eg ha-Edomi, *Sefer Ya'ir Netiv*, bk. 2, ch. 7: ואם הנקבים יתראו בריאים ואין שם דבר מכל זה יש להבין כי הגיד השומע סובל החולי (But if the openings [of the ears] look healthy and [we do not notice] anything of what we mentioned, it should be concluded that the auditory nerve is affected by the illness). Hebr. הגיד השומע does not feature in the current dictionaries. Moses ibn Tibbon translates Arab. العصب الذي يجري فيه السمع as העצב אשר בו ילך השמע (cf. BCD 206 (NM 4:150)).

• **הגיד התחתון** · **the basilic vein**: Arab. الباسليق · Ibn al-Jazzār, *Zād al-musāfir wa-qūt al-ḥādir* · trans. Moses ibn Tibbon, *Sefer Ṣedat ha-Derakhim* bk, 3, ch. 6: וכאשר תרצה לרפאת מי שקרה לו שעול הנה ראוי תחלה שנעיין מאיזה סבה קרה השעול וכאב החזה ואם היה מפני חום והורנו על זה מה שימצא החולה עם השעול מנחירות החזה וצמא וחוזק כאב וימצא מנוחה בשאפו אויר קר נצוה החולה אז להקיז הגיד התחתון ולהוציא הדם ממנו כפי שעור הכח (If you want to cure someone suffering from cough you should first of all examine why he suffers from cough and pain in the chest. If it is because of heat and this is indicated if in addition to cough the patient suffers from a rough chest, from thirst and severe pain, and finds relief from inhaling cold air, we tell the patient that he should have venesection from the basilic vein and that blood should be extracted as much as he can endure). Hebr. הגיד התחתון is not attested for in the current dictionaries. Subsequently, in their translations of Maimonides, *Medical Aphorisms* 12.23, 29, 33, 35, Nathan ha-Me'ati transcribes Arab. باسليق as באסליק/באסליקא (BMMN 141–143) and Zeraḥyah Ḥen renders it as באסיליק/בסיליק/הגיד הבסיליק/גיד הנקרא בסיליק (BMMZ 139–141); see also BCD 30 (NM 4:23). Do'eg ha-Edomi translates Lat. *basilica*

---

54 פיק: *ficus* L.
55 הבהמה: *equus* L.
56 'horse': Trans. after L.

vena as המקור הנקרא בשיליקא. Note that in *Shinnui ha-Shemot ha-Niqra'im Synonimi*, Ms Florence, Bibliotheca Laurenziana, Or. 17, fol. 69[a], the term הגיד התחתון stands for Arab. الأكحل; i.e., 'median cubital vein': אלכאחל שם לגיד התחתון מגידי הזרוע ('LK'ḤL [read 'L'KḤL, *al-akḥal*], a name for *ha-gid ha-taḥton*, of the *gidei ha-zero'a* (veins of the arm)).

• *Plur.* גידין • קבוץ הגידין → קִבּוּץ.

גימטריאה[57] • *Plur.* **גימטראות** ‣ **arithmetic**: Arab. حساب · Isḥāq ibn 'Imrān, *Treatise on Melancholy* · trans. Anonymous, fol. 44[a] (45[a]): גימטריאות הנק' בלשון יוני ארמאטיקי (Arithmetic, called 'R⟨Ṭ⟩M'TYQY [i.e., ἀριθμητική] in Greek). Hebr. גימטראות, from Gr. γεωμετρία or γραμματεία (cf. HM 79), is attested for in Rabbinic literature in the sense of 'the use of letters as numerals, numerology' (cf. JD 239) and in medieval scientific literature (e.g., Maimonides) in the sense of 'geometry' (cf. SM 208).

גיעול → גְּעוּל.

גִּיר ‣ **mucilage**: Arab. لعاب · Ibn al-Jazzār, *Zād al-musāfir wa-qūt al-ḥādir* · trans. Abraham ben Isaac, *Sefer Ṣedah la-Oreḥim*, bk. 1, ch. 3 (Ms Jerusalem, National Library of Israel, Fr. 95, fol. 85b): וכאשר יתבאר לך כי תוספת יסוד החמימות כלתה וחדותה נכנעה אז נחזור למשוח בו משיחות למרך בהם כדי לקרר החמימות ולרטב השיער כגון הגיר של זרע איפשיליאו הוא בזר קוטוני שתערב אותו בשמן ויאולטו ותמרך בו עור השיער (When it is clear that the element of heat does not increase any more and that its sharpness has gone, we should turn to rubbing salves on it [i.e., the head] in order to cool the heat and to moisten the hair with [ingredients] such as mucilage of fleawort seed, i.e., Arab. *bizr quṭūnī* [read: *bizrqaṭūnā*], mixed with violet oil and rub the skin [below] the hair with it). Hebr. גִּיר features in the current dictionaries as a Rabbinic term in the sense of 'froth, foam [of wine]' (JD 241; BM 759). Moses ibn Tibbon translates Arab. لعاب as ריר. Abraham ben Isaac (Ms Florence, Biblioteca Medicina Laurenziana, Plut. 88.37) also uses the latter term instead of גִּיר as it features in the Jerusalem Ms.

גִּירְסָא (*Aram.*) ‣ **recollection; memory**: Arab. حفظ · Ibn al-Jazzār, *Zād al-musāfir wa-qūt al-ḥādir* · trans. Abraham ben Isaac, *Sefer Ṣedah la-Oreḥim*, bk. 1, ch. 14: דע כי יושר הגירסא שיגרוס האדם ולא ישכח הוא יזכיר הדברים הטמונים בלב (Know that a good memory, i.e., that one learns and one does not forget, [but] remembers the things hidden in the heart ...). Aram. גִּירְסָא is attested for in Rabbinic literature in the sense of 1. 'learning, study; 2. reciting, recitation; 3. textual tradition' (cf. SDA 283–284). Moses ibn Tibbon translates Arab. حفظ as שמירה. Do'eg ha-Edomi translates the parallel Latin term *memoria* as זכרונות.

גְּלוּלָה • *Plur.* **גלולות** ‣ **pills**: Arab. حبّ · Ibn al-Jazzār, *Zād al-musāfir wa-qūt al-ḥādir* · trans. Abraham ben Isaac, *Sefer Ṣedah la-Oreḥim*, bk. 1, ch. 23: וזה ריקוח הגלולות הסרוחות הנקראות בלשון ישמעאל חב אל מנתן מאת אשר ריקח סבאור המועילות מן חולי הפלג

57 Variant readings: גימטרייה/גימטריה/גימטריא, *Plur.* גימטריאות.

ועיוות הפה וכאב כל פרקי הגוף והפודגרא והרוחות העבות החזקות בכל הגוף ולחולי קוליקום ולליחה העבה ולכאב הגידים ולרפיון ויתיר דם הנדות וכבר ניסינוהו (Recipe of the 'stinking pill,' called in Arab. *ḥabb al-muntin*, composed by Sābūr,[58] which is beneficial for hemiplegia, facial paralysis, joint pain [i.e., arthritis], gout, strong coarse winds throughout the body, colic, thick humors, neuralgia, and looseness; it also stimulates menstruation. We have tested it). Hebr. גְּלוּלָה, Plur. גלולות, features in BM 776 and EM 244 in an attestation from the *Sefer Asaph ha-Rofe*.[59] Moses ibn Tibbon translates Arab. حبّ as גרגרים. Do'eg ha-Edomi transcribes the parallel Latin term *fetidi pilluli* as פילולש פטידש.

גַּלִּי • הדפק הגליי → דֹּפֶק.

גְּמִיאָה • **mouthwash**: Arab. مضمضة • Ibn al-Jazzār, *Zād al-musāfir wa-qūt al-ḥāḍir* • trans. Moses ibn Tibbon, *Sefer Ṣedat ha-Derakhim*, bk. 2, ch. 23: תואר גמיאה לכמו זה (Recipe of a mouthwash similar to this one [i.e., the one prescribed before, which is good for strengthening the gums and lips, for a good breath, and for making the teeth beautiful]). Hebr. גְּמִיאָה is attested for in Rabbinic literature in the sense of 'quaffing, full draught;' cf. JD 252; BM 799 (see also BCD 47, s.v. גָּמָא (NM 4:33)).

גְּמָר/גֶּמֶר • **perfection**: Arab. تمام • Isḥāq ibn 'Imrān, *Treatise on Melancholy* • trans. Anonymous, fol. 49[a] (50[a]): אבל גמר השחוק הוא[60] פירו' הנפש עת השחוק על ענינו (Laughing becomes perfect when[61] the soul grasps its [deeper] meaning when one laughs). Hebr. גְּמָר/גֶּמֶר features in Rabbinic literature in the sense of 'finishing, last touch, consummation' (cf. JD 255, s.v. גְּמָר; BM 805). The standard translation for Arab. تمام in Medieval Hebrew literature is שלמות. Constantine the African translates Arab. تمام as *complementum*.

גַּס • **fat**: Lat. *crassus* (Arab. غليظ) • Constantinus Africanus, *Viaticum* • trans. Do'eg ha-Edomi, *Sefer Ya'ir Netiv*, bk. 2, ch. 23: וירחיק מכל מיני דגים גם מכל בשר גס ומעשבים מולידים הלבנה (He [i.e., someone suffering from bad breath] should avoid taking all kinds of fish, fat meat, vegetables producing phlegm). In the sense of 'fat,' Hebr. גַּס is a non-attested semantic borrowing from Lat. *crassus*. Moses ibn Tibbon translates Arab. غليظ as עב.

גְּעוּל • **1. sordes (i.e., earwax)**: Lat. *res mucidae* (Arab. وسخ / Gr. ῥυπος)[62] • Constantinus Africanus, *Viaticum* • trans. Do'eg ha-Edomi, *Sefer Ya'ir Netiv*, bk. 2, ch. 7: ואם יראה שם

---

58 I.e., Sābūr ibn Sahl; cf. Ibn Sahl, *Dispensatorium Parvum* (*Al-Aqrābādhīn al-ṣaghīr*), ed. Kahl (Leiden 1994), no. 114 (99); and O. Kahl (ed. and trans.), *Sābūr ibn Sahl's Dispensatory in the Recension of the 'Aḍudī Hospital* (Leiden 2009), no. 173 (186).

59 For the composition of the 'stinking pill,' see also Ibn Sahl, ibid.

60 הוא פירו' הנפש עת השחוק על ענינו: فوقوف النفس عند الضحك على معناه a.

61 'when the soul grasps its [deeper] meaning': Trans. after a.

62 Cf. Ḥunayn's translation of Galen's *De simplicium medicamentorum temperamentis ac facultatibus* 10.2.17, ed. Kühn, 12:290 l. 14: ὁ ἐν τοῖς ὠσὶ ῥύπος; Arab. Ms Escurial 793, fol. 165[b] l. 16: *al-wasakhu l-khāriju mina l-udhni*.

נפח או אבעבוע או וירוגא או הם מליאות גיעול או איזה דבר חיצון (And if we [look inside the ear and] see a tumor or pustule or wart, or [see] that it is full with sordes (earwax) or something that comes from the outside ...). In the sense of 'earwax,' Hebr. גְּעוֹל is a non-attested indirect semantic borrowing from Gr. ῥύπος via Arab. وسخ and Lat. *res mucidae*. Moses ibn Tibbon translates Arab. وسخ as לִכְלוּךְ (see entry). The same term features as לכלוך האוזן in Ibn Tibbon's translation of وسخ الأذن in *Sefer Ṣedat ha-Derakhim*, bk. 7, ch. 27.3 (cf. IJZ 169).

‣ II. **blemish; fault; defect**: Lat. *macula* · Constantinus Africanus, *Viaticum* · trans. Do'eg ha-Edomi, *Sefer Ya'ir Netiv*, bk. 2, ch. 17: ואם הלשון בריאה בלא שום גיעול והדבור אפס ונעדר (If the tongue is healthy without any defect, but one cannot speak ...). Hebr. גְּעוֹל does not feature in this sense in the current dictionaries. Moses ibn Tibbon translates the parallel Arabic term علّة ظاهرة as חולי.

גֶּפֶן • ורד הגפן → וֶרֶד.

גַּרְגַּר • *Plur.* **גרגרים** • **גרגרי החשמנה** ‣ **fattening seeds; hemp seeds**: Arab. حبّ السمنة (cf. M 348 (Meyerhof); s.v. *qinnab* (hemp [*Cannabis sativa* L.]): 'C'est *as-šāhranağ*; on dit aussi *šāhdanağ al-barr* ('chanvre sauvage'); c'est *ḥabb as-samna* ('graine pour engraisser,' ou 'graine de graisse')') · *Shinnui ha-Shemot ha-Niqra'im Synonimis*, Ms Munich, Bayerische Staatsbibliothek, Cod. hebr. 8, fol. 198[b]: חב אלסמנה[63] גרגרי החשמנה ([Arab.] *ḥabb al-samna*; [i.e., Hebr.] *gargerei ha-hashmanah*). Hebr. גרגרי החשמנה does not feature in the current dictionaries.

• **גרגרים ירוקים** ‣ **fruits of the turpentine tree** [*Pistacia terebinthus* L.]: Arab. حبّة خضرا (IBF 570; DT 1:35 (117)) · *Shinnui ha-Shemot ha-Niqra'im Synonimis*, Ms Munich, Bayerische Staatsbibliothek, Cod. hebr. 8, fol. 198[b]: חבה כצרה גרגרים ירוקום והוא פרי האיבנוס ([Arab.] *ḥabba khaḍrā*; [i.e., Hebr.] *gargarim yeruqqim*; i.e., the fruit of [Lat.] *ebenus*). Hebr. גרגרים ירוקום does not feature in the current dictionaries. Hebr. איבנוס is possibly a corruption of טירבינטוס ('terebinth').

• **גרגרים מתוקים** ‣ **anise**: Arab. حبّ الحلوة · *Shinnui Shemot ha-Niqra Ṣinonimas*, Ms Leiden, Universiteitsbibliotheek, Or. 4719, fol. 31[a]: אניסון הוא אניס ונקרא עוד בער' חבה חלוה כלומ' גרגרים מתוקי' ונקרא שומר רומי (Anise, that is 'NYS; it is also called in Arab. ḤBH ḤLWH; i.e., sweet grains, and it is called ŠWMR RWMY). In the sense of 'anise,' Hebr. גרגרים מתוקים is a non-attested calque from Arab. حبّ الحلوة.

גרגרישמי ‣ **gargles**: Lat. *gargarismus*, Plur. *gargarismi* (Arab. غرغرة) · Constantinus Africanus, *Viaticum* · trans. Do'eg ha-Edomi, *Sefer Ya'ir Netiv*, bk. 3, ch. 1: אחרי העשות כל אלה והליחות תכבינה נשוב אל הליחות שאינם נתרות ואשר נסגרות באברי החולה ונעשה גרגרישמי שפא מתותי העץ (Once we have done all these things and the [heat of] the humors has been extinguished, we turn to the humors that have not been dissolved and that are enclosed within the organs of the patient and apply gargles prepared

63 אלסמנה: emendation editor אלחנא Ms.

from a rob of mulberries ...). Hebr. גרגרישמי is a non-attested loan word from Lat. *gargarismi*. Moses ibn Tibbon translates Arab. غرغرة as גרגר.

[גרד] • *Pi'el* גֵּרֵד › **to rub**: Lat. *frico* (Arab. دلك) · Constantinus Africanus, *Viaticum* · trans. Do'eg ha-Edomi, *Sefer Ya'ir Netiv*, bk. 1, ch. 19: והרופא יקח עצה לישנו בעבור העשות בשול היין ואחר כך יכינו לו מרחץ מזוג ונגרד רגליו (And the physician will contrive [i.e., exercise his skill] to let him sleep so that the wine can be digested, then a moderately hot bath should be prepared for him and his feet should be rubbed). In the sense of 'to rub' (for Arab. حكّ), Hebr. גֵּרֵד features in BCD 49 (NM 1:134) in a later attestation from Zeraḥyah Ḥen's translation of Maimonides, *Medical Aphorisms* 22.53 (BMMZ 213).[64] Moses ibn Tibbon translates Arab. دلك as חפף and Abraham ben Isaac as הכניס (= Arab. أدخل).

• *Hitpa'el* הִתְגָּרֵד › **to be rubbed**: Lat. *fricor* (Arab. دُلِكَ) · Constantinus Africanus, *Viaticum* · trans. Do'eg ha-Edomi, *Sefer Ya'ir Netiv*, bk. 1, ch. 16: ויאות לעיין תחילה אם החולי הזה הוא מקרירות או מלחות המוח וכמעט שאין לו עזר ואם נתבונן שהוא עשוי מלחות המוח נעזור אליו כן: ישימו רגליו במים חמים ויתגרדו במלח (One should first look whether this illness [i.e., torpor] originates from cold or moisture of the brain, in which case there is hardly any cure for it; and if we see that it originates from the moisture of the brain, we treat it as follows: we put the feet [of the patient] in hot water and rub them with salt ...). Hebr. הִתְגָּרֵד features in the current dictionaries with attestations from the Bible and Rabbinic literature in the sense of 'to scrape, scratch oneself' (cf. BDB 173; BM 834; EM 263). Moses ibn Tibbon renders the parallel Arabic term دُلِكَ as חפף.

גָּרוֹן • עליון הגרון → עֶלְיוֹן.

• הרוח החמוץ היוצא מן הגרון → רוּחַ.

• הרוח הנדחה מהגרון → רוּחַ.

גְּרִידָה › **peel**: Arab. جرادة · i. Ibn al-Jazzār, *Zād al-musāfir wa-qūt al-ḥādir* · trans. Abraham ben Isaac, *Sefer Ṣedah la-Oreḥim*, bk. 1, ch. 10 (Ms Jerusalem, National Library of Israel, Fr. 95, fol. 90a): ואחר שנטהר אם נעטשהו במי פרפחינים או במי גרידת הדלעת עם שמן בנפסג' או שמן נינופר (After the cleansing [of his body], the patient should be caused to sneeze with common purslane juice, or juice of pumpkin peels together with oil of violets or of water lily). In a medical context, Hebr. גְּרִידָה features in BCD 50 in the sense of 'abrasion' (cf. NM 3:48), 'scarification' (cf. NM 1:19), and 'shred' (cf. NM 1:134–135).

ii. Ibn al-Jazzār, *Zād al-musāfir wa-qūt al-ḥādir* · trans. Moses ibn Tibbon, *Sefer Ṣedat ha-Derakhim*, bk. 3, ch. 11: וימשח החזה מחוץ בשמן ויאולד או בשמן זרע קרא או בשמן נינופר או בשמן ורדים אחר שימזגהו במי גרידת קרא (He should rub his chest on

64 In the same sense it features in the anonymous *Sefer ha-Yosher* (Ms Oxford, Bodleian Library, Opp. 180 (cat. Neubauer 2134), fol. 21a). This text quotes many recipes from the *Sefer Ya'ir Netiv*.

the outside with violet oil or pumpkin seed oil or water lily oil or rose oil once it has been mixed with juice from pumpkin peels).

גְּרִישָׁה ‣ **vomiting (spitting)**: Lat. *reiectio* · Constantinus Africanus, *Viaticum* · trans. Do'eg ha-Edomi, *Sefer Ya'ir Netiv*, bk. 3, ch. 8: גרישת הדם נעשת בשני ענינים עם שעול או עם דחוי זה רישקאסיון (Vomiting (spitting) of blood occurs in two ways: with coughing or with clearing[65] one's throat; i.e. [Lat.] *rascatio*). Hebr. גְּרִישָׁה features in BM 842 in the sense of 'expulsion.' As a medical term it features, without any further explication, in an attestation from Me'ir Aldabi, *Shevilei Emunah*: ועוצר (האתרוג) הגרישה והקיא הבא מן האדומה. Moses ibn Tibbon translates the parallel Arabic term نفث الدم as רקיקת הדם.

[גרש] • *Pi'el* **גֵּרֵשׁ** ‣ **to insufflate**: Lat. *insufflo* (Arab. نفخ) · Constantinus Africanus, *Viaticum* · trans. Do'eg ha-Edomi, *Sefer Ya'ir Netiv*, cf. bk. 2, ch. 15: ואם הדם לא יעצור בכל אלה יאות לרפאתו בדברים עוצרים ונגרש שם קליפת ביצים שרופות (But if all these [means] do not stop the bleeding [from the nose], we should treat it with astringent [remedies] and insufflate [i.e., into the nose] burnt egg shells). Hebr. גֵּרֵשׁ does not feature in this sense in the current dictionaries. Moses ibn Tibbon renders Arab. نفخ as נפח.

גרשׁא (*Aram.*) • עשה גרשא → עָשָׂה.

גרשׁה • עשה גרשה → עָשָׂה.

65 'clearing one's throat': Cf. entry דִּחוּי.

ד

דְּאָבוֹן · **wasting; marasmus** · Isḥāq ibn ʿImrān, *Treatise on Melancholy* · trans. Anonymous, fol. 51^b (52^b): ואני אומר שהשרטן הנהריי צלויים או מבושלים במי השעורים או במים ומלח יועילם כי מכח הסרטן להועיל מן הדאבון והחולי היבש (I say that river crabs, roasted or cooked in barley water or in water and salt, are good for them [i.e., for those suffering from melancholy] because [river] crab is, by its [specific] property, beneficial for wasting and for phtisis). Hebr. דְּאָבוֹן features in the Bible in the sense of 'faintness, languishing' (BDB 178), or as a synonym of דאבה 'faintness, failure of mental energy, dismay' (BDB 178; BM 861–862). Ben-Yehuda also mentions it in the sense of 'weakness and collapse of an organ of the body' in an attestation from the *Mordechai*, composed by Mordechai ben Hillel (ca. 1250–1298). Constantine the African translates Arab. الذبول والسلّ as *phthisicos et macilentos*.[66]

[דבק] • *Hifʿil* הִדְבִּיק · **I. to apply**: Arab. ألزق (cf. WKAS 2a:542) · Ibn al-Jazzār, *Zād al-musāfir wa-qūt al-ḥādir* · trans. Abraham ben Isaac, *Sefer Ṣedah la-Oreḥim*, bk. 1, ch. 6 (Ms Jerusalem, National Library of Israel, Fr. 95, fol. 87^a): או קח שריגי תאנים כשהן לחין או מעליו כשהן לחין וכתשם במים היטב ותדביק במקום (Or, take fresh fig branches or fresh leaves, thoroughly pound them with water, and apply this on [the spot]). In the sense of 'to apply,' Hebr. הִדְבִּיק is a non-attested semantic borrowing from Arab. ألزق. For its meaning in the sense of 'to cause to heal up,' cf. BCD 53 (NM 2:36). Moses ibn Tibbon translates Arab. ألزق as הִדְבִּיק as well.

· **II. to make something thick, viscous, adhesive**: Arab. لزّج · Ibn al-Jazzār, *Zād al-musāfir wa-qūt al-ḥādir* · trans. Moses ibn Tibbon, *Sefer Ṣedat ha-Derakhim*, bk. 3, ch. 7: ואם היה הדם בתחלת החולי הזה רב והיה כחו חזק נקיזהו בתחלת החולי ויוציא מן הדם שעור הסיפוק ונזונהו במה שיקרר וידביק ויתבשל מהר כמו מי שעור מתוקן המלאכה (If in the beginning of this illness [i.e., pneumonia] there is a large quantity of blood and [the patient] is strong, we extract a sufficient amount of blood and then give him food that has a cooling and adhesive effect and that is digested quickly, such as barley gruel that has been well prepared). Hebr. הִדְבִּיק features as *Part. Hifʿil* מַדְבִּיק in the sense of 'agglutinant' in BCD 188, s.v. סַם (NM 4:125) in an attestation from an anonymous translation of Ibn Sīnā's *K. al-Adwiya al-qalbiya*. Do'eg ha-Edomi does not translate Constantine's parallel Latin term *solido*.

• *Part. Hifʿil* **מַדְבִּיק** • **מדביק הזהב** · **chrysocolla**: Arab. لصاق الذهب or لزاق الذهب (cf. KM 2:950–952) · Shem Tov ben Isaac, *Sefer ha-Shimmush*, bk. 29, list 1 (SHS 1:332–333 (Mem 63)): מדביק הזהב ב״ה תנכאר וב״ל בורייש (*madbiq ha-zahav*; Arab. *tinkār*;[67]

66 Cf. entry חֳלִי: החלי היבש.

67 For the (incorrect) equation of Arab. تنكار ('borax') with لزاق الذهب featuring in several Arabic sources, cf. KM 1:348.

O.Occ. *borais*). In the sense of 'chrysocolla,' Hebr. מדביק הזהב features in BCD 54 (NM 2:57) in a later attestation from Nathan ha-Me'ati's translation of Maimonides, *Medical Aphorisms* 23.101 (BMMN 232).

• **הרפואה המדביקה** → רְפוּאָה.

דָּבֵק · **viscous:** Arab. لزج · Ibn al-Jazzār, *Zād al-musāfir wa-qūt al-ḥādir* · trans. Moses ibn Tibbon, *Sefer Ṣedat ha-Derakhim*, bk. 2, ch. 13: ואם היו הנגעים ההם או השחין יבש ראוי שירטיבם בשמן ויאולד עם הרירים הדבקים (And when those tumors or ulcers are dry, they should be moistened with violet oil and other [oils] that are viscous). In the sense of 'viscous,' Hebr. דָּבֵק features in BM 873 as an abbrevation for ליחה דבקה ('viscous fluid') in an attestation from Nathan ha-Me'ati's translation of Maimonides, *Medical Aphorisms* 13.54 (BMMN 152). Do'eg ha-Edomi translates the parallel Latin term *viscosus* as יש לו הדבקה (see entry הַדְבָּקָה).

• **החלק הדבק** → חֵלֶק.

דֶּבֶק · **mucilage:** Arab. لعاب · Ibn al-Jazzār, *Zād al-musāfir wa-qūt al-ḥādir* · trans. Moses ibn Tibbon, *Sefer Ṣedat ha-Derakhim*, bk. 3, ch. 2: או יעשה הרפואה הזאת כי היא מהר ובדקות והוא שיקח ריר זרע חבושים ודבק זרע מלוישקלי (He can also apply the following remedy as it works quickly and easily: Take mucilage of quince seed and mucilage of common marshmallow seed ...). Hebr. דֶּבֶק is attested for in the sense of 'glue, paste' in Rabbinic literature (cf. JD 278; EM 279). As a synonym of דֶּבֶק, Moses ibn Tibbon uses the term ריר as it features in the same passage (see also BCD 262 (NM 1:68)).

דְּבֵקוּת · **viscosity; glutinosity:** Arab. تغرية · Ibn al-Jazzār, *Zād al-musāfir wa-qūt al-ḥādir* · trans. Moses ibn Tibbon, *Sefer Ṣedat ha-Derakhim*, bk. 3, ch. 8: תואר עוגות חברתים קבצתי כחות רבים מן הקביצות והנגוב והדבקות והסתום[68] (A recipe for pastilles that I composed and [in which are] concentrated many astringent, drying, glutinizing, and strengthening[69] powers). In the sense of 'viscosity,' Hebr. דְּבֵקוּת features in BM 873 in a later attestation form the *Sefer ha-Qanun*.

דָּבָר • **דבר בלוי** · **putrid or filthy liquid; corrupt discharge:** Lat. *lues* (Arab. رطوبة غليظة لزجة) · Constantinus Africanus, *Viaticum* · trans. Do'eg ha-Edomi, *Sefer Ya'ir Netiv*,[70] cf. bk. 1, ch. 7: ויצא דבר בלוי כדמות דבש (A putrid or filthy liquid exudes [i.e., from the small openings in the skin of the head in the case of honeycomb]). Hebr. דבר בלוי does not feature in this sense in the current dictionaries.

• *Plur.* **דברים** • **דברים מישנים** · **soporifics:** Lat. *res somnum facientes* (Arab. مرقّد) · Constantinus Africanus, *Viaticum* · trans. Do'eg ha-Edomi, *Sefer Ya'ir Netiv*, cf. bk. 1, ch. 17: ובבא התעורה ממאכל ומשקה חם יעזור אליו כפי הנראה אל הרופא הבקי עם דברים מישנים כמו אופי קשטור זעפרן גושקיאמי ליבור שחור מנדראגולא זרע פאפאבר (If hot foodstuffs

---

68 והסתום: التشديد a.

69 'strengthening': Trans. after Arab. التشديد.

70 Cf. entry בָּלוּי and the anonymous *Sefer ha-Yosher* (Ms Oxford, Bodleian Library, Opp. 180 (cat. Neubauer 2134), fol. 18ᵃ): שער לשחין האוזן כשתיגר מן האוזנים מוגלא ודבר בלוי.

or hot drinks are the cause of insomnia, it can be treated in accordance with the opinion of the expert physician with soporifics such as opium, castoreum, saffron, hemlock, black hellebore, mandrake, and poppy seeds). In the sense of 'soporific,' Hebr. מְיַשֵּׁן features in BCD 122 (NM 2:59) in a later attestation from Nathan ha-Me'ati's translation of Maimonides' *Medical Aphorisms* 8.38 (BMMN 97) as a translation of Arab. منوّم. Moses ibn Tibbon and Abraham ben Isaac translate Arab. مرقّد as מרדים.

• **הדברים המפליגים · restraining remedies:** Lat. *repugnativa* (Arab. أدوية ردّاعة) · Constantinus Africanus, *Viaticum* · trans. Do'eg ha-Edomi, *Sefer Ya'ir Netiv*, bk. 2, ch. 24: וזה יתכן לעשות בתחלה ויותר באמצע החולי והדברים המפליגים אל הליחות והמיבשים נחבר כסדר (This can be done in the beginning of the illness, but better in the middle by composing [and administering] in the right order remedies that restrain and dry [the humors]). Hebr. הפליג features in the current dictionaries a.o. in the sense of 'to divert' (cf. BM 4928), but not in a medical context. Moses ibn Tibbon translates Arab. الأدوية التي تعرف بالردّاعة as הרפואות אשר יודעו במשככות (cf. BCD 265 (NM 1:61–62)).

דְּבַשׁ • **דבש מקוצף · skimmed honey**: Arab. عسل منزوع الغروة · Ibn al-Jazzār, *Zād al-musāfir wa-qūt al-ḥāḍir* · trans. Abraham ben Isaac, *Sefer Ṣedah la-Oreḥim*, Adaptation, bk. 1, ch. 14 (Ms Berlin, Staatsbibliothek Preußischer Kulturbesitz, Or. fol. 1058, fol. 94[a]): וישתה מן האבק ב׳ דרמ׳ ואם תלוש בדבש מקוצף אז ישתה ממנו ד׳ דרמ (Take two *dirhams* from this powder, but when it is kneaded with skimmed honey one should take four *dirhams*). In the sense of 'skimmed honey,' Hebr. דבש מקוצף features in BCD 55 (NM 1:20) in an attestation from Hillel ben Samuel's *Sefer Keritut*. The same term features in Abraham ben Isaac, *Sefer Ṣedah la-Oreḥim*, Ms Florence, Biblioteca Medicina Laurenziana, Plut. 88.37, fol. 97[b], in a marginal note quoting the composition of a syrup composed by Don Benveniste, the physician of Don Manuel, the brother of the king of Castile. Moses ibn Tibbon and Abraham ben Isaac translate Arab. عسل منزوع الغروة as דבש שהוסר קצפו. A corresponding term is missing in the *Viaticum* and *Sefer Ya'ir Netiv*.

• **מי דבש** → **מַיִם**.

• **שמן הדבש** → **שֶׁמֶן**.

דָּג • **הדג המתגדל בין הסלעים · rockfish**: Arab. سمك الصخور · Maimonides, *Medical Aphorisms* 17.25 · trans. Zeraḥyah Ḥen (BMMZ 172): הדג המתגדל בין הסלעים מהר הוא מתעכל ועם מהירות התעכלו הוא בתכלית השבח וניאות מאד לשמירת בריאות גוף האדם מפני שהוא מוליד דם ממוצע העצמות אינו דק ורקיק ולא גס (Rockfish is rapidly digested. Together with its high digestibility, it is extremely good and beneficial in preserving the health of a human body since it produces blood of an intermediate consistency, neither thin and fine nor thick). Hebr. הדג המתגדל בין הסלעים does not feature in the current dictionaries. A variant reading featuring in Zeraḥyah's translation is דג הצורים (see below). Nathan ha-Me'ati translates Arab. سمك الصخور as הדג הסלעי׳ (see below).

• **הדג הסלעי** ‣ **rockfish**: Arab. سمك الصخور · Maimonides, *Medical Aphorisms* 17.25 · trans. Nathan ha-Me'ati (BMMN 174): הדג הסלעי הוא מהיר העכול ועם מהירות עכולו הוא בתכלית הטוב והאותות לשמירת הבריאות לגוף האדם מפני שהוא מוליד דם ממוצע העצם איננו דק ורקיק ולא עב וגס (Rockfish is rapidly digested. Together with its high digestibility, it is extremely good and beneficial in preserving the health of a human body since it produces blood of an intermediate consistency, neither thin and fine nor thick). Hebr. הדג הסלעי features in BM 886 in a quotation of this particular aphorism.

• **דג הסלעים** ‣ **rockfish**: Arab. السمك الصخور · Maimonides, *Medical Aphorisms* 8.25 · trans. Nathan ha-Me'ati (BMMN 95): הנה נתחבר בתועלות כשך השעורים שמחזק הכח ומזכך כלי הנשימה מן הליחות הרעות בחתוך והרטבה ולא יתקבצו אלו התועלות כלם בדבר זולתו. וכשיתעב החולה כשך מהשעורים הנה הנכון והטוב שבמזונות אחריו הוא דג הסלעים במים וכרתי ושבת ומלח ושמן בשוה (Barley groats have the combined beneficial effects of invigorating one's strength and cleansing the respiratory organs of bad humors through cutting and moistening. These beneficial effects cannot be found together in any other substance. If a patient dislikes barley groats, the next best food is rockfish with water, garden leek, dill, salt, and a moderate amount of olive oil). Hebr. דג הסלעים does not feature in the current dictionaries. Zeraḥyah Ḥen translates Arab. السمك الصخور as דג הצורים (see entry).

• **דג הצורים** ‣ **rockfish**: Arab. السمك الصخور · Maimonides, *Medical Aphorisms* 8.25 · trans. Zeraḥyah Ḥen (BMMZ 90): נתקבץ בתועלת גרישי השעורים שהוא יחזק הכח וינקה כלי הנשימה מן הליחות הרעות בחיתוך ובלחלוח ולא נתקבצו אילו התועלות בזולתו. וכל זמן שירחיק[71] החולה השעורים האילו המזון הטוב שהוא תחתיו הוא דג הצורים במים וכרתי אניט ומלח ומעט שמן (Barley groats have the combined beneficial effects of invigorating one's strength and cleansing the respiratory organs of bad humors through cutting and moistening. These beneficial effects cannot be found together in any other substance. If a patient dislikes[72] barley groats, the next best food is rockfish with water, garden leek, dill, salt, and a moderate amount of olive oil). Hebr. דג הצורים is not attested for in the current dictionaries. A variant reading featuring in Zeraḥyah's translation is הדג המתגדל בין הסלעים (see entry above). Nathan ha-Me'ati translates Arab. السمك الصخور as דג הסלעים (see entry above).

דּוּדָא/דּוּדַי • *Plur.* **דודאים** ‣ **violets**: Lat. *violae* (Arab. بنفسج) · Ibn al-Jazzār, *Zād al-musāfir wa-qūt al-ḥādir* · trans. Abraham ben Isaac, *Sefer Ṣedah la-Oreḥim*, Adaptation, bk. 1, ch. 10 (Ms Berlin, Staatsbibliothek Preußischer Kulturbesitz, Or. fol. 1058, fol. 92^{b}): ואחר כן תשלשלהו באיפיזימא של תמרינדי וברוניי יינצובי דודאים צמוקים קסיאה פישטולה מנה ודומיהן (After this, we purge him with a decoction made from tamarinds, plums, common jujubes, violets, raisins, pulp of purging cassia, manna, and the like). Bibl. Hebr.

---

71 שירחיק: كره a.
72 'dislikes': Trans. after a.

דודאים (cf. Gen 30:14) only features in the current dictionaries in the sense of 'mandrakes [*Mandragora officinarum* L.]' (cf. BDB 188; BM 900). The adapter possibly interpreted the term דודאים as 'violets' following Rashi on Gen 30:14: דודאים סיגלי ובלשון ישמעאל יסמין (*duda'im*, i.e., SYGLY; in Arab. YSMYN).[73] Aram. סיגלא, *Plur.* סיגלי, can mean both 'violet' and 'nutgrass, root of *Cyperus rotundus* L.' (cf. SHS 1:374–375 (Samekh 44)). Do'eg ha-Edomi transcribes Lat. *violas* as ויאולש; the same term is used by Moses ibn Tibbon for Arab. بنفسج. Abraham ben Isaac transcribes Arab. بنفسج as בנפסג'.

דוחק → דחק.

דופק → דפק.

דוֹקֵר (*Part.*) → דָּקַר.

[דחה] • *Nif'al* נִדְחָה • הרוח הנדחה → רוּחַ.

• הרוח הנדחה מהגרון → רוּחַ.

דִּחוּי · **clearing one's throat (i.e., hawking)**: a) Lat. *rascatio* (cf. DMLBS 3010: 'expulsion of phlegm') (Arab. تنخنخ) · Constantinus Africanus, *Viaticum* · trans. Do'eg ha-Edomi, *Sefer Ya'ir Netiv*, bk. 3, ch. 8: גרישת הדם נעשת בשני ענינים עם שעול או עם דחוי זה רישקאסיון (Vomiting (spitting) of blood occurs in two ways: with coughing or with clearing one's throat; i.e., RYŠQ'SYWN). Hebr. דִּחוּי features in BM 915–916 only as a synonym of דחיה in the sense of 'adjournment.' Moses ibn Tibbon renders Arab. تنخنخ as נחנח. Arab. تنخنخ features once again in bk. 3, ch. 9; Do'eg once again renders Lat. *rascatio* as דִּחוּי and Moses ibn Tibbon translates Arab. تنخنخ as נחנח, with the exception of Ms London, British Library, Ar. Or. 26, fol. 98[b], which has the same term as Do'eg: דִּחוּי.

b) Lat. *screatus* (cf. DMLBS 3331: '(act of) clearing the throat, expectoration, discharge of phlegm by hawking and spitting') · Constantinus Africanus, *Viaticum* · trans. Do'eg ha-Edomi, *Sefer Ya'ir Netiv*, bk. 3, ch. 11: ואם הוא חומד מאד האויר למשכו והחזה ימלא בעובי גדול מהנשימה אז נבין כי קוצר כלי הרוח הם. ואם הוא מהנפח יהיה זה כאשר ישעול בדחוי (If he has a strong need to frequently inhale air and fill the chest we know that this is because of the narrowness in [one of] the respiratory channels. If [the narrowness] is caused by a tumor his coughing will be accompanied by hawking). Moses ibn Tibbon translates the parallel Arabic term يقذف به مادّة as ישליך עמו לחה.

דָּחוּק (*Pass. Part.*) → דָּחַק.

דְּחִיקָה · **narrowness**: (no parallel Arabic term) · Ibn al-Jazzār, *Zād al-musāfir wa-qūt al-ḥāḍir* · trans. Abraham ben Isaac, *Sefer Ṣedah la-Oreḥim*, bk. 1, ch. 2 (Ms Florence, Biblioteca Medicina Laurenziana, Plut. 88.37, fol. 87[a]): ואם יקרה מחמת עובי העור ודחיקת סימפוניו אז יעשה הרפואות הפותחין הסימפונות (If it [i.e., the loss of hair] hap-

73 See also the refutation of Rashi's interpretation of the term דודאים in Nachmanides' commentary on Gen 30:14.

pens because of the thickness of the skin and the narrowness of its pores we apply remedies that open the pores). Hebr. דְּחִיקָה features in the current dictionaries in the sense of 'pushing, pressure' (cf. BM 917). The adaptation of this text featuring in Ms Berlin, Staatsbibliothek Preußischer Kulturbesitz, Or. fol. 1058, has צרות.

דָּחַק • *Pass. Part.* **דָּחוּק** · **narrow:** (no parallel Arabic term) · Ibn al-Jazzār, *Zād al-musāfir wa-qūt al-ḥādir* · trans. Abraham ben Isaac, *Sefer Ṣedah la-Oreḥim*, bk. 1, ch. 2 (Ms Florence, Biblioteca Medicina Laurenziana, Plut. 88.37, fol. 87[b]): ואחר כן תשים הכל בכלי שפיו דחוק (Then put all [these ingredients] in a pot with a narrow opening). Hebr. דָּחוּק does not feature in this sense in the current dictionaries. The adaptation of this text featuring in Ms Berlin, Staatsbibliothek Preußischer Kulturbesitz, Or. fol. 1058, has צר.

דֹּחַק • **דוחק** · **pressure; compression:** Arab. تضاغط (Gr. θλῖψις; cf. UWS 1:468) · Maimonides, *Medical Aphorisms* 10.22 · trans. Zeraḥyah Ḥen (BMMZ 122): ולא ימצא דוחק הדפק או דוחק החמימות בזולתי העפושית ואין זה מיוחד בה לבדה (One does not find compression of the pulse or of the heat in non-putrid [fevers]. Nevertheless, [their occurrence] is not specific for [putrid fevers] alone). Hebr. דֹּחַק features in BM 919–920 in the sense of 'need, distress' only. Nathan ha-Me'ati translates Arab. تضاغط as לחיצה.

דַּיְסָה · **porridge [made from wheat or barley]:** Arab. حسو · Ibn al-Jazzār, *Zād al-musāfir wa-qūt al-ḥādir* · trans. Moses ibn Tibbon, *Sefer Ṣedat ha-Derakhim*, bk. 3, ch. 6: וישתה בשול אישוף או משקה ג'וג'ובש ושבשתן או משקה שליום וישתה אחר שתית מה שספרנו בשלש שעות דיסת שעור בשמן שקדים ומעט פניס או סוכר (Let him take a decoction of hyssop or a potion of common jujube and sebesten, or of fleawort, and then three hours later he should take porridge made from barley with almond oil, a small amount of sugar candy or sugar). Hebr. דַּיְסָה features in BM 930–931 (s.v. דיס) in a later attestation from Me'ir Aldabi, *Shevilei Emunah*. The Aramaic counterpart דַּיְסָא also features in Moses ibn Tibbon's translation (cf. entry לֵב), and in Shem Tov ben Isaac's *Sefer ha-Shimmush*, bk. 27, where it features as a translation of Arab. هريسة (cf. BCD 56 (NM 4:38)). Do'eg ha-Edomi renders the Latin counterpart *ptisana* as טיבשנא (see entry).

דָּם • **דם העינים** · **hyposphagma (i.e., bloodshot eyes):** Lat. *sanguis in oculis* (Arab. طرفة; cf. MMT 195) · Constantinus Africanus, *Viaticum* · trans. Do'eg ha-Edomi, *Sefer Ya'ir Netiv*, bk. 2, ch. 3: מדם העינים (On hyposphagma (bloodshot eyes)). Hebr. דם העינים is not attested for in the current dictionaries. In addition to דם העינים, Do'eg ha-Edomi renders the parallel Latin term *crustula* as קְלִפָּה (see entry). Moses ibn Tibbon translates Arab. طرفة as אודם אשר באחת קצוות העין (see entry אֹדֶם).

• **דם שני האחים** · **dragon's blood (i.e., the resin of the Socotra dragontree [*Dracaena cinnabari* Balf. f.]):** Arab. دم الأخوين (cf. MIG 73) · Ibn al-Jazzār, *Zād al-musāfir wa-qūt al-ḥādir* · trans. Moses ibn Tibbon, *Sefer Ṣedat ha-Derakhim* (Ms Munich, Bayerische Staatsbibliothek, Cod. hebr. 19, fol. 66[a], and Ms London, British Library, Ar. Or. 26, fol. 93[b]), bk. 3, ch. 7: ואם התבאר לנו מה שזכרנו כי הנגעים אשר בריאה כבר נתכו לכלוכם

ונתנגבו לחויותיהם ונפסק חמרם נצוה החולה אז לעשות רפואות מיבשות הנגעים כדי שידביקם כמו ורדים ובלושטיאש ואכסיאה ודרגגן ומשתיק וקהרבי הוא כהרבא בערבי ובול ארמיני וגומא ארביקא ודם שני האחים הוא שנק דדרגון (When it has become clear to us from what we mentioned, that the putrid matter of the tumors in the lung has dissolved and is gone, and that their humors have dried up, we tell the patient to take ingredients that dry the tumors [even more] so that they heal, such as roses, rose or blossom of the wild pomegranate, acacia gum, gum tragacanth, mastic, amber, i.e., KHRBʾ in Arabic, Armenian bole, gum Arabic, and dragon's blood, i.e., [Rom.] SNQ DDRGWN). In the sense of 'dragon's blood,' Hebr. דם שני האחים is a non-attested loan translation of Arab. دم الأخوين. Doʾeg ha-Edomi translates the parallel Latin term *sanguis draconis* as דם תנין (cf. SHS 1:168 (Dalet 2)).

- **הזלת הדם** → הֲזָלָה.
- **חיסר דם** → [חסר].
- **חסור הדם** → חִסּוּר.
- **נזלת דם הנחירים** → נַזֶּלֶת.

[דמה] • *Hitpaʿel* **הִתְדַּמָּה** · **to be in doubt; to be doubtful**: (Arab. اشتبه) · Ibn al-Jazzār, *Zād al-musāfir wa-qūt al-ḥāḍir* · trans. Moses ibn Tibbon, *Sefer Ṣedat ha-Derakhim*, ck. 3, ch. 9: והרבה שיתדמה הענין לרופאים אבל כי הם כשיתבאר להם כי סבת רקיקת הדם עלוקה שנבלעה יצוו החולה לעמוד כנגד השמש ופיו פתוח ואם ראו העלוקה נתלית בחיך ימשכו אותה בחכה דקה משיכה דקה[74] (Physicians are often doubtful in this matter [i.e., that of bloodspitting resulting from the ingestion of a leech through drinking water]. However, when it is clear to them that the cause of the bloodspitting is a leech that has been swallowed, they tell the patient to stand opposite the sun and to open his mouth. If they see the leech hanging from the palate they pull it out softly with a fine hook). In the sense of 'to be in doubt,' Hebr. הִתְדַּמָּה is a non-attested semantic borrowing from Arab. اشتبه.

דְּמוּת · **color**: Arab. لون · Ibn al-Jazzār, *Zād al-musāfir wa-qūt al-ḥāḍir* · trans. Abraham ben Isaac, *Sefer Ṣedah la-Oreḥim*, bk. 1, ch. 1 (Ms Jerusalem, National Library of Israel, Fr. 95, fol. 82b): ואם יהיה דמות המקום ההוא אדום דע כי החולי ההוא בא לו מחמת דם רע (If the color of that spot [on the head] is red, understand that the illness [i.e., alopecia] is caused by bad blood). Hebr. דְּמוּת does not feature in this sense in the current dictionaries; cf. BM 957–958; KTP 1:139. Doʾeg ha-Edomi translates the parallel Latin term *color* as צבע; Moses ibn Tibbon translates Arab. لون as מראה.

• **לדמות** · **like; resembling; similar to**: a) Lat. *in modum* (Arab. أمثال) · Constantinus Africanus, *Viaticum* · trans. Doʾeg ha-Edomi, *Sefer Yaʾir Netiv*,[75] bk. 2, ch. 6: ותעשה

---

74 דקה (= Ms London, British Library, Ar. Or. 26): רבה Ms Oxford, Bodleian Library, Poc. 353, Uri Heb. 314.

75 For a synonym used by Doʾeg ha-Edomi, cf. entry מִדָּה: למדת.

גרגרים לדמות עדשים (And make pills resembling lentils). Hebr. לדמות does not feature in the current dictionaries. Moses ibn Tibbon translates Arab. أمثال as כמו. See also entry דִּמְיוֹן below.

b) Lat. *similis* · Constantinus Africanus, *Viaticum* · trans. Do'eg ha-Edomi, *Sefer Ya'ir Netiv*, bk. 1, ch. 25: ומכל אלה הענינים יש רפואה אחת זהו שנתן לו דברים מחממים להתיר ולחסר שפעת הליחות כמו גירא לוגודיאון טאודוריטון ודומיהם ושמנים ומשיחות לדמות הנזכרים למעלה (For all these [afflictions] there is one remedy, namely, to administer [the patient] heating ingredients, which dissolve and diminish the surplus of superfluities. [Such ingredients are]: the Logadion hiera, the Theodoretus, and the like. [One can also apply different kinds of] oils and salves similar to those mentioned before).

דִּמְיוֹן · **species; kind**: Lat. *species* (Arab. نوع) · Constantinus Africanus, *Viaticum* · trans. Do'eg ha-Edomi, *Sefer Ya'ir Netiv*, bk. 2, ch. 1: והחיצונה יש לה שני דמיונים זהו גדולה וקטנה והקטנה נפרדת מהגדולה כי היא אין לה איזה דמיון מהנפח (The external [cause of ophthalmia] consists of two kinds; i.e., major and minor; the minor [cause] differs from the major insofar as it is not a kind of inflammation). Hebr. דִּמְיוֹן features in medieval philosophical literature in the sense of 'imagination, fantasy, likeness, example, analogy, appearance, metaphor' (KTP 1:140; EF 25).

• **כדמיון** · **like; resembling**: Arab. أمثال · Ibn al-Jazzār, *Zād al-musāfir wa-qūt al-ḥādir* · trans. Moses ibn Tibbon, *Sefer Ṣedat ha-Derakhim*, bk. 3, ch. 4: ויעשה ממנו גרגרים כדמיון הפולים (And make pills of them resembling beans). Do'eg ha-Edomi does not translate the parallel Latin term *in modum* in this passage, but in bk. 2, ch. 6, he renders the Latin term as לדמות (see entry דְּמוּת above), whereas Moses ibn Tibbon renders Arab. أمثال as כמו.

דְּמָמָה · **apoplexy**: Arab. سكات · Isḥāq ibn 'Imrān, *Treatise on Melancholy* · trans. Anonymous, fol. 43[a] (44[a]): ובאורך הזמן יבואון לידי חולי זה וזולתו מן החליים הקשים כגון רעש האברים והפאליג' והדממה (Eventually they [i.e., those who frequently drink old wine in the morning and evening] will suffer from this illness [i.e., melancholy], in addition to other severe illnesses, such as tremors, hemiplegia, and apoplexy). Hebr. דְּמָמָה does not feature in this sense in the current dictionaries. Constantine the African renders Arab. سكات as *apoplexia*. Zeraḥyah Ḥen translates the same Arabic term as תרדמה in his translation of Maimonides' *Commentary on Hippocrates'* Aphorisms 3.16 (122) (BMHA 1:450; cf. BCD 298 (NM 3:247)).

דָּמַע • *Part.* דּוֹמֵעַ · **full of tears; tearful**: Lat. *lacrimosus* (Arab. تكثر الدموع) · Constantinus Africanus, *Viaticum* · trans. Do'eg ha-Edomi, *Sefer Ya'ir Netiv*, bk. 2, ch. 1: והפנימית מעלה נפח והכאב והיא קשה ודומעת ומקורותיה מלאים (The internal [cause of ophthalmia] produces swelling and pain. It is severe, [it comes with] many tears and full vessels). Hebr. דּוֹמֵעַ is not attested for Hebrew medical literature in the current dictionaries; cf. BM 965. Moses ibn Tibbon translates Arab. تكثر الدموع as רבוי דמע.

דַּעַת • שלא מדעתו · **involuntary**: Lat. *preter voluntatem* (Arab. بغير إرادة) · Constantinus Africanus, *Viaticum* · trans. Do'eg ha-Edomi, *Sefer Ya'ir Netiv*, bk. 1, ch. 22: ולפעמים ישתתפו עם זה החולי האיסטניסות[76] והתוצאות והשתן יוצא שלא מדעתו (Sometimes this illness [i.e., epilepsy] comes with [pollution,[77] i.e., involuntary emission of sperm] and involuntary excretion [of feces] and [emission of] urine). Hebr. שלא מדעתו does not feature in this sense in the current dictionaries. Moses ibn Tibbon translates Arab. بغير إرادة as מבלי רצון.

דַּף • *Plur.* דפים · **membranes**: Lat. *pelliculae* (cf. DMLBS 2525) (Arab. سفاقات) · Constantinus Africanus, *Viaticum* · trans. Do'eg ha-Edomi, *Sefer Ya'ir Netiv*, bk. 1, ch. 18: פרינישין הוא צמח נולד בתוך דפי המוח הוא הקרום ומן הצמח ההוא יחולו בכל עת תעורה וזרות המחשבה (Phrenitis; i.e., an inflammation originating in the membranes of the brain, i.e., QRWM [membrane], and from that inflammation always hails sleeplessness and aberration of the mind [i.e., delirium]). Hebr. דַּף, *Plur.* דפים, does not feature as a medical term in the current dictionaries. Hebr. QRWM (קרום) is the standard term for 'membrane,' which also features in Moses ibn Tibbon's *Sefer Ṣedat ha-Derakhim* as *Plur.* קרומות, for the parallel Arabic term سفاقات.

• **הדפים הסובבים הלב** · **pericardium**: Lat. *circumdantes et cor pelliculae* (Arab. الطبقة المحيطة بالقلب) · Constantinus Africanus, *Viaticum* · trans. Do'eg ha-Edomi, *Sefer Ya'ir Netiv*, bk, 3, ch. 13: פלצות הלב הוא מהליחות המקובץ בדפים הסובבים הלב (Palpitation is caused by moisture that collects in the pericardium). Hebr. הדפים הסובבים הלב does not feature in the current dictionaries. Moses ibn Tibbon translates Arab. الطبقة المحيطة بالقلب as המכסה המקיף הלב.

דְּפִיקָה · **tension**: Lat. *tentio* (= *tensio*) (Arab. تمدّد) · Constantinus Africanus, *Viaticum* · trans. Do'eg ha-Edomi, *Sefer Ya'ir Netiv*, bk, 2, ch. 1: ואם הוא מליחות גסות וקרות או מרוח ירגישו הדפיקה בעינים זהו טיטאנוס (And if it [i.e. ophthalmia] is caused by crude, cold humors or wind, [the patient] will feel tension, i.e., ṬYṬ'NWS, in his eyes). Hebr. דְּפִיקָה features in medieval medical literature in the sense of 'pulsation' (cf. BM 977). Moses ibn Tibbon translates Arab. تمدّد as משיכה. The latter term is used by him for Arab. تمدّد in the sense of 'tetanus' in his translation of Maimonides' *Commentary on Hippocrates'* Aphorisms 4.57 (194) (BMHA 1:370; cf. BCD 165 (MN 3:146)), where Do'eg ha-Edomi's *Sefer Agur* has דפק הגידים for Lat. *tetanus* (cf. BCD 59 (NM 3:53–54)).

דֹּפֶק • הדפק הגליי · **the undulatory pulse**: Arab. النبض الموجي · Maimonides, *Medical Aphorisms* 4.33 · trans. Nathan ha-Me'ati (BMMN 60): כמו[78] שמשאיר אחריו הדפק הגליי כשיקטן וימעט הדפק התולעי כן משאיר[79] אחריו התולעי כשיבטלו תנועותיו הרבות ונשארה בו תנועה אחת והוא הדפק הנמלי והיא תנועה מעטה מאד דומה לשריצת הנמלים ויש בו באמת

---

76 האיסטניסות: *pollutio* L.

77 '[pollution]': Cf. Lat. *pollutio.*

78 כמו שמשאיר אחריו: كما يعقب a.

79 משאיר אחריו: يعقب a.

התחלפות אך בשביל קטנו לא ישיג החוש התחלפותיו (As the undulatory pulse, when it becomes small and little, is followed by the vermicular one, so the vermicular pulse, when most of its motions stop and only one motion is left, is followed by the ant-like pulse, which is a very small motion similar to the crawling of an ant. It is actually unequal, but because it is so small, the senses cannot distinguish its inequality). Hebr. הדפק הגלי(י) features in BM 779, s.v. גלי, in an attestation from the *Sefer ha-Qanun*. See also MD 610, s.v. 'pulse, undulating.' Zeraḥyah Ḥen translates Arab. النبض الموجي as הדפק הגלי.

• **הדפק הנק׳ זנב העכבר** · **the pulse called 'mousetail'**: Arab. النبض المسمّى ذنب الفأرة · Maimonides, *Medical Aphorisms* 4.11 · trans. Nathan ha-Me'ati (BMMN 57): תחלת מדרגות חולשת הכח והפחותה שבהם ישים הדפק יותר נוסף קוטן ונוסף חולש. והמדרגה הנלות לזאת מחולשה היא אותה שתשימהו שיכבידהו עם זה הנחת האצבעות אשר יונחו על העורקים ותשים הדפק הנק׳ זנב העכבר החוזר פעם שניה ואם יתש הכח ויתך יותר מזה ישים הדפק זנב העכבר הקיים. (The first and lowest degree of weakness of the faculty makes the pulse smaller and fainter. The next degree of weakness is that in which one's fingers put on the artery are a burden for the faculty. It turns one's pulse into the recurrent one called 'mousetail.' When the faculty is wasted and dissolved [even] more than this, it turns one's pulse into the permanent 'mousetail'). Hebrew הדפק הנק׳ זנב העכבר features in MD 610, s.v. 'pulsus myurus'. Zeraḥyah Ḥen translates Arab. النبض ذنب الفأرة المسمّى as הדפק הנק׳ זנב העכבר as well.

• **הדפק המגרי** · **the serrated pulse**: Arab. النبض المنشاري · Maimonides, *Medical Aphorisms* 6.54 · trans. Zeraḥyah Ḥen (BMMZ 67): המקרים הדבקים לבעלי חולי הצד ולא יבדילוהו הם חמשה הקדחת החדה והכאב הנושך בצד והניפוש הקטן המתואתר[80] והדפק המגרי והשעול והוא ברוב עם רקיקה צבועה (The symptoms that always accompany pleurisy are five [in number]: acute fever, goading pain in the side, shallow and frequent respiration, serrated pulse, and cough, mostly accompanied by colored sputum). Hebr. הדפק המגרי features in BM 2791, s.v. מגרי, in an attestation from Tuviah ha-Kohen, *Ma'aseh Tuvyah*; see also MD 610, s.v. 'pulsus, formicans.' Nathan ha-Me'ati translates Arab. النبض المنشاري as דפק משורי (cf. BCD 59 (NM 2:63)).

• **הדפק המתרעד** · **the vibratory pulse**: Arab. النبض المرتعد · Maimonides, *Medical Aphorisms* 4.12 · trans. Zeraḥyah Ḥen (BMMZ 51): הדפק החזק יחבוט לעולם חבטה גדולה וכן מין הדפק הקשה יחבוט חבטה גדולה כמו הדפק המתרעד והדפק המתואתר (A strong pulse always strikes a forceful beat. Similarly, a hard type of pulse strikes a forceful beat just like the vibratory and spasmodic pulses). Hebr. הדפק המתרעד is not attested for in the current dictionaries. Masie (MD 609–610) mentions the term דפק בלתי קבוע as a synonym for 'vibrating pulse,' which is equal to the 'jerky pulse.' Nathan ha-Me'ati translates Arab. النبض المرتعد as הדפק הנרעד (see entry below).

80 המתואתר: المتواتر a.

• **הדפק הנמלי** · **the ant-like pulse**: Arab. النبض النملي · Maimonides, *Medical Aphorisms* 4.33 · trans. Zeraḥyah Ḥen (BMMZ 54): כמו שהדפק הגלי כשיתקטן ויתמעט יבוא אחריו הדפק התולעי כן התולעי כשיתבטלו תנועותיו המרובות ונשארה בו תנועה אחת יבוא אחריו הדפק הנמלי והיא תנועה מועטה מאד דומה להליכת הנמלה ובו באמת שינוי אבל לקטנותו לא ישיג החוש שינויו (As the undulatory pulse, when it becomes small and light and little, is followed by the vermicular one, so the vermicular pulse, when most of its motions stop and only one motion is left, is followed by the ant-like pulse, which is a very small motion similar to the crawling of an ant. It is actually unequal, but because it is so small, the senses cannot distinguish its inequality). Hebr. הדפק הנמלי features in BM 3679, s.v. נמלי, in an attestation from Tuviah ha-Kohen, *Ma'aseh Tuvyah*; see also MD 610, s.v. 'pulsus, serratus.' Nathan ha-Me'ati translates Arab. النبض النملي as הדפק הנמלי as well.

• **הדפק הנרעד** · **the vibratory pulse**: Arab. النبض المرتعد · Maimonides, *Medical Aphorisms* 4.12 · trans. Nathan ha-Me'ati (BMMN 57): הדפק החזק יהלום לעולם הלימה כבדה וכן מין הדפק הקשה יהלום הלימה כבדה כמ דפק הנרעד והדפק הנמתח[81] (A strong pulse always strikes a forceful beat. Similarly, a hard type of pulse strikes a forceful beat just like the vibratory and spasmodic[82] pulses). Hebr. הדפק הנרעד is not attested for in the current dictionaries. Masie (MD 609–610) mentions the term דפק בלתי קבוע as a synonym for 'vibrating pulse,' which is equal to the 'jerky pulse.' Zeraḥyah Ḥen translates Arab. النبض المرتعد as הדפק המתרעד (see entry above).

• **הדפק התולעי** · **the vermicular pulse**: Arab. النبض الدودي · Maimonides, Medical Aphorisms 4.33 · trans. Nathan ha-Me'ati (BMMN 60): כמו[83] שמשאיר אחריו הדפק הגליי כשיקטן וימעט הדפק התולעי כן משאיר[84] אחריו התולעי כשיבטלו תנועותיו הרבות ונשארה בו תנועה אחת והוא הדפק הנמלי והיא תנועה מעטה מאד דומה לשריצת הנמלים ויש בו באמת התחלפות אך בשביל קטנו לא ישיג החוש התחלפותיו (As the undulatory pulse, when it becomes small and little, is followed by the vermicular one, so the vermicular pulse, when most of its motions stop and only one motion is left, is followed by the ant-like pulse, which is a very small motion similar to the crawling of an ant. It is actually unequal, but because it is so small the senses cannot distinguish its inequality). Hebr. הדפק התולעי features in BM 7690 in a quotation of this particular aphorism. Ben-Yehuda's reference to Maimonides, *Medical Aphorisms* 4.11, should be corrected to 4.33. See also MD 610, s.v. 'pulse, vermicular.' Zeraḥyah Ḥen translates Arab. النبض الدودي as הדפק התולעי as well.

דַּק • **הגיד הדק** → **גִּיד**.

• *Plur.* **דקים** · **intestines**: Lat. *interiora* · Guillaume de Congenis, *Treatise on Surgery* · trans. Isaiah, fol. 55b: ממכה שיצאו הדקים: אם מכה תעשה באינטישטינא[85] צריך לחזור הדקים

81 הנמתח: المتواتر a.
82 'spasmodic': Trans. after a.
83 כמו שמשאיר אחריו: كما يعقب a.
84 משאיר אחריו: يعقب a.
85 באינטישטינא: emendation editor בטישטינא Ms.

במקום ויושם בגד טבול במים באשר יבושל בו מירא ורושש ואישניץ (On an injury causing the intestines to protrude: If an injury affects the intestines [and they protrude] one should restore them to their position by putting a cloth on it that has been soaked in water in which myrrh, roses, and absinth wormwood have been cooked ...). In the sense of 'intestines,' Hebr. דקים features in BM 981 with attestations from Rabbinic literature only. The term features in JD 318 in the sense of 'small bowels;' cf. Low XLVI, s.v. דקין: 'Small intestines (intestinuum tenuum) or mesenter, mesenteron membranes.'

דֹּק • דוק ‧ pannus; ailment of the eyes; cataract?: Lat. *pannus* (DMLBS 2455) · Guillaume de Congenis, *Treatise on Surgery* · trans. Isaiah, fol. 48ª: דע כי זה האבק תועיל לדוק שבעין ולבהרת (Know that this powder is useful for pannus of the eyes and for a[86] spot or opaque place on the eye [i.e., leucoma, cataract]). In the sense of 'cataract,' Hebr. דֹּק is attested for in Rabbinic literature; cf. JD 318; Low XLVI. Ben-Yehuda (BM 982) mentions the term with the following meanings: 1) fine cloth; 2) fine membrane; 3) thinness. Possibly also in the sense of 'cataract,' the term דֹּק features as דַּק in Lev 21:20 (cf. KB 229). In addition to דֹּק, Isaiah translates Lat. *pannus* as בֶּגֶד (see entry).

דקוקציאון ‧ decoction: Lat. *decoctio* · Guillaume de Congenis, *Treatise on Surgery* · trans. Isaiah, fol. 45ᵇ: אחר תשים זה על המכה ויפתחנה: מיץ הפיטרווייל ומיץ האפי וכמון ויבושל בדקוקציאון ותשים בנעורת ופושר ויושם שם (Another remedy that should be put on the injury and that will open it: [Take] clover juice, celery juice, and cumin, cook it and make a decoction; put it on chaff, and apply it when it is lukewarm). Hebr. דקוקציאון is a non-attested loan word from Rom. *decoction.*

דָּקַר • *Part.* דּוֹקֵר • כאב דוקר בלב → כְּאֵב.

דַּרְדִּיחַ • *Plur.* דרדיחים ‧ **small flies** · Ibn al-Jazzār, *Zād al-musāfir wa-qūt al-ḥādir* · trans. Abraham ben Isaac, *Sefer Ṣedah la-Oreḥim*, bk. 1, ch. 1: המשיחה הנעשת מן הדרדיחים הם קנטרילי (A salve prepared with small flies called QNṬRYLY [i.e., O.Occ. *cantarilhe*, 'Spanish fly' (from Lat. *cantharis, -idis*)]). Hebr. דַּרְדִּיחַ features in BM 992 in an attestation from *Sefer Asaph ha-Rofe*. The term actually features in Ms Munich, Bayerische Staatsbibliothek, Cod. hebr. 231, fol. 169ᵇ as דרדיחים and in Ms Oxford, Bodleian Library, Opp. 687 (cat. Neubauer 2138), fol. 97ᵇ as דרדיחים הוא קנטריטס. It concerns a pharmacopoeia, which is a parallel version of the list of simples found in the *Sefer Asaph ha-Rofe* and is described as 'medicines for the poor,' arranged by order of maladies from head to toe. This is a list of compound medicines, also arranged by that order, and very similar to the simples list.[87]

---

86 'a spot or opaque place on the eye [i.e., leucoma, cataract]' (Lat. *macula*): See entry בַּהֶרֶת above.

87 I thank Emunah Levi for the references to the Munich and Oxford Mss.

דֶּרֶךְ • דרך אפכא · by opposite means (i.e., ingredients with opposite qualities):[88] Lat. *per contrarios* · Ibn al-Jazzār, *Zād al-musāfir wa-qūt al-ḥādir* · trans. Abraham ben Isaac, *Sefer Ṣedah la-Oreḥim*, Adaptation, bk. 1, ch. 5 (Ms Berlin, Staatsbibliothek Preußischer Kulturbesitz, Or. fol. 1058, fol. 91[a]):[89] וכך נרפאהו דרך אפכא כלומר פירקונטרריאוש בלעז (Thus we treat it [i.e., dandruff] with opposite [remedies]; i.e., *per contrarios* in Latin). Hebr. דרך אפכא, a combination of Hebr. דרך and Aramaic אפכא 'opposite, reverse' (cf. SDA 124, s.v. איפכא) is not attested for in the current dictionaries. Do'eg ha-Edomi renders Lat. *ex contrariis*, as it features in the *Viaticum*, as בדברים שהם הפך להם. A parallel term for דרך אפכא and *per contrarios* is missing in the original Arabic text.

דֶּשֶׁן · ashes: Lat. *ciner* (Arab. رماد) · Constantinus Africanus, *Viaticum* · trans. Do'eg ha-Edomi, *Sefer Ya'ir Netiv*, bk. 1, ch. 20: וכן אלום שרוף ודשן תמריץ ומלח ותשחוק לאבק בשקל שוה ותניח על השינים (Likewise burnt alum, ashes of French tamarisk wood, and salt: Pulverize an equal amount and put this on the teeth). Hebr. דֶּשֶׁן features in the current dictionaries in the sense of 'fatness, fat ashes' (BDB 206; cf. JD 326; BM 1009). Moses ibn Tibbon translates Arab. رماد as אפר.

• **דשן הכסף · silver dross:** Lat. *cathymia* (*cadmia*) (Arab. إقليميا الفضة) · Constantinus Africanus, *Viaticum* · trans. Do'eg ha-Edomi, *Sefer Ya'ir Netiv*, bk. 1, ch. 8: אחר כן תקח ליטרג'יר שירנו דשן הכסף ותמזוג הכל עם שמן ורד ותמשח הראש בו (Then take litharge, ŠYRNW;[90] silver dross, mix everything with rose oil and smear it on the head). Hebr. דֶּשֶׁן features in BM 1009 in the sense of 'fattiness, ashes.' See also BCD 60 (NM 2:11); BMZ 36 (Ḥet 4) for its use in the sense of 'ophthalmia' in Shem Tov ben Isaac's *Sefer Almansur*, i.e., his translation of al-Rāzī's *K. al-Manṣūrī*. Moses Ibn Tibbon translates the parallel Arabic term إقليميا الفضة as סיג כסף and Abraham ben Isaac as כבת (= خبث) אפר כסף אלצפה (= الفضة).

• **דשן הצמר · grease of wool (i.e., lanolin):** Arab. دسم الصوف (cf. MIG 315) · Shem Tov ben Isaac, *Sefer ha-Shimmush*, bk. 29, list 1 (SHS 1:174 (Dalet 10)): דשן הצמר ב"ה זופא אלצוף ובל"ל אישנוסרונטום (Hebr. *deshen ha-ṣemer*; Arab. *zūfā al-ṣūf*; Lat. 'YŠNWSRWNṬWM (**ysopum cerotum*)). Hebr. דשן הצמר is possibly a non-attested calque of Arab. دسم الصوف.

• **מי הדשן → מַיִם.**

88 Cf. the statement *contraria contrariis curantur* (Opposites are cured by opposites). A medical belief of allopathic medicine—the traditional form of medical practice—that seeks to fight a disease by using remedies that produce effects opposite to the effects produced by the disease under treatment.

89 Ms Moscow, Russian State Library, Guenzburg 165, fol. 95[b], has a Hebrew variant: דרך ההפך.

90 ŠYRNW: I.e., Romance for 'ashes;' cf. BMZ 96 (Resh 5). The term is used as a Romance parallel to דֶּשֶׁן.

ה

הַבְדָּלָה • הבדלת האוכל והמשתה · abstention from food and drink: Lat. *abstinentia* (Arab. نقصان الغذاء) · Ibn al-Jazzār, *Zād al-musāfir wa-qūt al-ḥādir* · trans. Abraham ben Isaac, *Sefer Ṣedah la-Oreḥim*, Adaptation, bk. 1, ch. 2 (Ms Berlin, Staatsbibliothek Preußischer Kulturbesitz, Or. fol. 1058, fol. 90[a]): ועל כן העשונים אינם מגיעים למקומם כלומר למקום בשיער ולהשלים צמיחתם מחמת הבדלת האוכל והמשתה אבשטינניציאה בלעז (Because of the abstention from food and drink the vapors cannot reach their place, i.e., their place in the hair for the completion of its growth). Hebr. הבדלת האוכל והמשתה does not feature in the current dictionaries. As a synonym for הבדלת האוכל והמשתה, the anonymous adapter also uses חסרון הפרנוס (see entry חֶסְרוֹן). Do'eg ha-Edomi renders Lat. *abstinentia* as צום. Moses ibn Tibbon renders Arab. نقصان الغذاء as חסרון המזון.

הֲבָרָה · ringing in the ears (i.e., tinnitus): Lat. *sonitus aurium* · Ms Cambridge, T-S K14.14, fol. 4[a]: שער די שוֹנִיטוֹ אבריאום ראוי שתדע שסבת ההברה לפעמי׳ תהיה חיצונית ופעמי׳ תהיה פנימית (Chapter on tinnitus: Know that sometimes the cause of tinnitus is external and sometimes internal). Hebrew הֲבָרָה features in Rabbinic literature in the sense of 1) 'confused sound, noise', and 2) 'report, rumor' (JD 330), in medieval linguistic literature in the sense of 'pronunciaton' or 'syllable' (BM 1029–1030), and in medieval medical literature in the sense of '[intestinal] rumblings (borborygmus)' (BCD 61 (NM 1:86; 4:40)).

• **הברה באזנים · ringing in the ears (i.e., tinnitus)**: Arab. طنين في الأذنين (Gr. συριγμός) (cf. UW 658–659) · Ibn al-Jazzār, *Zād al-musāfir wa-qūt al-ḥādir* · trans. Moses ibn Tibbon, *Sefer Ṣedat ha-Derakhim*, bk. 1, ch. 13: ואם היה החולי מיוחד במוח ימצא החולה קודם זה כובד בראש והברה באזנים (If this disease [i.e., dizziness or vertigo] occurs in the brain only, the patient feels beforehand heaviness in the head and ringing in the ears). Hebr. הברה באזנים does not feature in the current dictionaries. Do'eg ha-Edomi translates the parallel Latin term *sonitus in auditu* as הברת השמע (see entry below). In bk. 2, ch. 8, Moses ibn Tibbon translates the Arabic synonym دويّ (Gr. ἦχος) as צלילה (cf. BCD 229 (NM 4:172)).

• **הברת השמע · ringing in the ears (i.e., tinnitus)**: Lat. *sonitus in auditu* (Arab. طنين في الأذنين) · Constantinus Africanus, *Viaticum* · trans. Do'eg ha-Edomi, *Sefer Ya'ir Netiv*, bk. 1, ch. 13: ואם החולי הזה עשוי במוח לבדו אז ירגיש כובד בחלק הראש מן הראשון והברת השמע (If this disease [i.e., dizziness or vertigo] occurs in the brain only, the patient feels beforehand heaviness in the head and ringing in the ears). Hebr. הברת השמע does not feature in the current dictionaries. Moses ibn Tibbon translates Arab. طنين في الأذنين as הברה באזנים (see entry above) and Abraham ben Isaac as כבדות באזנים.

הַגְמָעָה · giving to sip · Ms Cambridge, T-S K14.14, fol. 4[b]: והגמעת השמן והמים יועילו כי הם מרכבים ומרפים המעברים וזה מורגל אצלינו (Giving [the affected person] to sip olive oil with water is beneficial [in case an object is stuck in the throat] because it makes the passages soft and loose. This is something that is normal with us). Hebrew הַגְמָעָה does not feature in the current dictionaries.

הַדְבָּקָה • יש לו הדבקה · **viscous:** Lat. *viscosus* (Arab. لزج) · Constantinus Africanus, *Viaticum* · trans. Do'eg ha-Edomi, *Sefer Ya'ir Netiv*, bk. 2, ch. 13: ואם הם יבשות יאות לעזור עם שמן ויאולד ועם אחרים אשר יהיה להם הדבקה (And when they [i.e., the tumors in the nose] are dry, they should be treated with violet oil and other [oils] that are viscous). Hebr. הַדְבָּקָה is attested as a medical term in the sense of 'agglutination' in Hillel ben Samuel's *Sefer Keritut*, cf. BCD 62–63 (NM 1:21). For its occurrence as a philosophical term in the additions (supplements) to the *Tagmulei ha-Nefesh* by Hillel ben Samuel (ed. Lyck 1874), fol. 46b, cf. KTP 1:158; BM 1042. Moses ibn Tibbon translates Arab. لزج as דָּבֵק (see entry).

הָדִי • לוזים הודיים → לוּז.

הָדַף • *Part.* **הוֹדֵף • הכח ההודף** → כֹּחַ.

הודי → הָדִי.

הוֹדֵף (*Part.*) → הָדַף.

הוֹרָאָה · **discernment:** Arab. رؤية · Ibn al-Jazzār, *Zād al-musāfir wa-qūt al-ḥāḍir* · trans. Abraham ben Isaac, *Sefer Ṣedah la-Oreḥim*, bk. 1, ch. 19: ואז יירפו האיברים וכל הגידים וייחלשו ההרגשות ותתגבר השינה ויפסיד ההירהור וההוראה (And then all the organs, nerves, and senses become weak, one is overtaken by sleep and the ability to think as well as the discernment is getting corrupted). Hebr. הוֹרָאָה does not feature in this sense in the current dictionaries. Moses ibn Tibbon translates Arab. رؤية as דעת.

הוֹרֵג (*Part.*) → הָרַג.

הַזָּלָה • הזלת הדם · **bleeding:** Lat. *fluxus sanguinis* (Arab. سيلان الدم) · Constantinus Africanus, *Viaticum* · trans. Do'eg ha-Edomi, *Sefer Ya'ir Netiv*, bk. 2, ch. 22: ובסבת הרכות יחול הזלת הדם (Softness [i.e., weakness of the gums] causes bleedings). Hebr. הַזָּלָה features in BM 1065 in the sense of 'flowing (of menstrual blood)' in an attestation from Me'ir Aldabi, *Shevilei Emunah*. In Do'eg ha-Edomi's *Sefer Agur*, the term הזלת הדם features in the sense of 'dysentery' (cf. BCD 64–65 (NM 3:62)). Moses ibn Tibbon renders Arab. سيلان الدم as הגרת הדם. The latter term features in the sense of 'dysentery' in Zeraḥyah Ḥen's translation of Maimonides, *Medical Aphorisms* 6.90 (BMMZ 72) and in the sense of 'hemoptysis' in 9.61 (ibid. 107; cf. BCD 62 (NM 1:138)). • **הזלת הפרחים** · **menstruation:** Lat. *menstrua* · Constantinus Africanus, *Viaticum* · trans. Do'eg ha-Edomi, *Sefer Ya'ir Netiv*, bk. 2, ch. 15: נזלת דם הנחירים אשר לפעמים מועיל ולפעמים לא ⟨המועיל⟩ יקרה בקבשון ובפרינישין ובהזלת הפרחים ובארובות חמות בתנועת התולדת והדם (A nosebleed is sometimes beneficial and sometimes not; the beneficial one occurs during hectic fever, phrenesis, menstruation, and hot catarrhs moved by nature and blood). Hebr. הזלת הפרחים does not feature in the current dictionaries. The term פרחים on its own in the sense of 'menstruation' features in the *Sefer Agur*, i.e., Do'eg ha-Edomi's translation of a Latin version of Hippocrates' *Aphorisms* 5.39 (cf. BCD 223 (NM 3:190)).

הַכְנָעָה · **abatement**: Arab. انكسار · Ibn al-Jazzār, *Zād al-musāfir wa-qūt al-ḥādir* · trans. Abraham ben Isaac, *Sefer Ṣedah la-Oreḥim*, bk. 1, ch. 18: ויש אשר יתבלבל דעתם מחמת כאב המוח בלבד כי הבלבול לאילו יוסיף וירבה מעט מעט ויתמיד בהם לאחרי שקט הכאב והכנעת הקדחת (Some people who suffer from mental confusion [i.e., delirium] because of the pain of the brain in particular, their mental confusion [i.e., delirium] increases and gets gradually worse. It continues even if the pain has already stopped and the fever has abated). Hebr. הַכְנָעָה does not feature in a medical context in the current dictionaries. Moses ibn Tibbon translates Arab. انكسار as השבר. Do'eg ha-Edomi translates Lat. *febris extingitur* as הקדחת תכבה.

הַלְבָּנָה • הלבנת השיער · **grey hair**: Arab. شيب · Ibn al-Jazzār, *Zād al-musāfir wa-qūt al-ḥādir* · trans. Abraham ben Isaac, *Sefer Ṣedah la-Oreḥim*, bk. 1, ch. 4 (Ms Jerusalem, National Library of Israel, Fr. 95, fol. 85[b]): השער הרביעי יזכיר הלבנת השיער והעלילה אשר תשניהו (Chapter four: On grey hair and [ingredients to correct] it). Hebr. הלבנת השיער does not feature in the current dictionaries. In addition to this term, Abraham ben Isaac uses the standard term שיבה (cf. entry קֶרֶב), which is also used by Moses ibn Tibbon. Do'eg ha-Edomi translates the parallel Latin term *cani* as השיער הלבן.

הֶמְשֵׁכִי · **tensive**: Arab. امتدادي (Gr. τονώδης) · Maimonides, *Medical Aphorisms* 6.60 · trans. Zeraḥyah Ḥen (BMMZ 68): ואם יהיה הכאב בקרום אשר תחת העור אשר יהיה נפשט עמו ויתחדש בעבורו כאב המשכי בטוליי (When the pain is in the membrane that lies under the skin and can be stripped off with it, it causes a tensive numb pain). Hebr. הֶמְשֵׁכִי features in medieval philosophical literature in the sense of 'continual' (מטבע ההמשך); cf. KT 1:180; BM 1120. Nathan ha-Me'ati translates Arab. امتدادي as מתפשט (ונמתח).

הֲנָחָה · **mildness; gentleness**: Lat. *mansuetudo* (Arab. رضى) · Constantinus Africanus, *Viaticum* · trans. Do'eg ha-Edomi, *Sefer Ya'ir Netiv*, bk. 1, ch. 20: ואמרו כי אורפיוש אמר: המלכים מקדשים אותי לשולחנם בעבור שיתענגו בי ואני בהיותי מתענג בם אוכל להכריע לבם למה שארצה כמו מכעס להנחה (They said that Orpheus said: Kings invite me to their banquets so that they get delighted by me. I equally get delighted by them. I am able to bend their heart to what I want, like from anger to mildness). Hebr. הֲנָחָה does not feature in this sense in the current dictionaries. Moses ibn Tibbon and Abraham ben Isaac translate Arab. رضى as רצון.

הַנָּחָה • *Plur.* **הנחות • ההנחות העשויות למטה** · **suppositories**: Lat. *supposituræ* · Constantinus Africanus, *Viaticum* · trans. Do'eg ha-Edomi, *Sefer Ya'ir Netiv*, bk. 1, ch. 17: ואמר דיאשקורידש לעשות לו אחת מן ההנחות העשויות למטה עם שמן ותעורר שינה (Dioscurides stated that if one makes a suppository for him [and applies it] with olive oil, it will induce sleep). Hebr. *Sing.* ההנחה העשויה למטה, *Plur.* ההנחות העשויות למטה, does not feature in the current dictionaries. Moses ibn Tibbon and Abraham ben Isaac render the parallel Arabic term فتيلة as פתילה.

הַעֲדָרָה · **absence; lack; want**: Lat. *carentia* (Arab. عدم) · Constantinus Africanus, *Viaticum* · trans. Do'eg ha-Edomi, *Sefer Ya'ir Netiv*, bk. 3, ch. 11: יאות להבין כי הלב לא יוכל

לסבול בשום פנים העדרת משיכת האויר כי אם ינוח כרגע ממשוך האויר יגוע מפני החום (One should understand that [someone's] heart cannot bear in any way to be without inhaled air; if it rests even one moment and does not attract the air, he dies because of the [innate] heat). In the sense of 'absence, lack, want,' Hebr. העדרה is a non-attested synonym of העדר. Moses ibn Tibbon translates Arab. عدم as העדר.

הַעֲטָשָׁה · **the application of a sternutatory**: Lat. *sternutamenta* (Arab. سعوط) · Ibn al-Jazzār, *Zād al-musāfir wa-qūt al-ḥādir* · trans. Abraham ben Isaac, *Sefer Ṣedah la-Oreḥim*, Adaptation, bk. 1, ch. 10 (Ms Berlin, Staatsbibliothek Preußischer Kulturbesitz, Or. fol. 1058, fol. 92[b]): ואם יבוא לו שריפה באפיו אחר העטשתו שים בנחיריו חלב אשה מיניקת זכר (If burning happens after the application of a sternutatory, milk of a mother of a baby boy should be sniffed). Hebr. הַעֲטָשָׁה features as a novel term in EM 390. Do'eg ha-Edomi renders Lat. *sternutamenta* as עטוש, Abraham ben Isaac translates Arab. سعوط as שום בנחיריו, and Moses ibn Tibbon as סמי העיטוש.

הָפוּךְ (*Part. Pass.*) → **הָפַךְ**.

הָפוּךְ • הפוך הבטן · **upset stomach; gripes**: Lat. *tortura ventris* (Arab. غثي) · Ibn al-Jazzār, *Zād al-musāfir wa-qūt al-ḥādir* · trans. Abraham ben Isaac, *Sefer Ṣedah la-Oreḥim*, Adaptation, bk. 1, ch. 10: ואם הסבה מחמת רפש חם חד הנקבץ באצטומכה אלו סימניו: ירגיש היפוך הבטן כלומר טורטרה ווינטריש וכאב דוקר בלב (If it [i.e., the headache] is caused by a hot, sharp superfluity collected in the stomach, these are its symptoms: [the patient] will suffer from an upset stomach, i.e., [Lat.] *tortura ventris*, and cardialgia). Hebr. הפוך הבטן does not feature in the current dictionaries. Moses ibn Tibbon translates Arab. غثي as קבסא (cf. BCD 236 (NM 1:66; 2:78–79; 3:198)); Abraham ben Isaac transcribes it as אל גשי. Do'eg ha-Edomi translates Lat. *tortura ventris* as איסטניסות (cf. BCD 24 (NM 2:30; 3:26; 4:19)).

[הפך] • *Part. Pass.* **הָפוּךְ** • **עפעפים הפוכות** → **עַפְעַף**.

• *Part. Nif'al* **נֶהְפָּךְ** · **upset (re: stomach)**: Arab. منقلب (Gr. ἀνατετραμμένος (cf. LSG 124: 'upset' (stomach))) · Maimonides, *Medical Aphorisms* 9.51 · trans. Zeraḥyah Ḥen (BMMZ 105): וכמו שכל המינים המוסרחים יהפכו הנפש ויעשו קרבונקלי כן כל המינים הטובים בריחם יחזקו האסטומכא וכל שכן אם הם דברים נאכלים שהוא יותר ראוי שיועילו לאסטומכא הנהפכת מפני המגל (Just as all malodorous [spices and seeds] upset the soul and cause nausea, all fragrant ones strengthen the stomach, especially when they belong to the comestibles, for these are most suited to benefit a stomach upset because of that fluid). In the sense of 'upset,' Hebr. נֶהְפָּךְ is a non-attested semantic borrowing from Arab. منقلب. Nathan ha-Me'ati translates Arab. منقلب as מִתְהַפֵּךְ (see entry below).

• *Part. Hitpa'el* **מִתְהַפֵּךְ** · **upset (re: stomach)**: Arab. منقلب (Gr. ἀνατετραμμένος (cf. LSG 124: 'upset' (stomach))) · Maimonides, *Medical Aphorisms* 9.51 · trans. Nathan ha-Me'ati (BMMN 110): וכמו שכל המינים הנבאשים מהפכים הנפש ומעוררים אסטנסות כן כל המינים המבושמים טובי הריח מחזקים האסטומכה וביחוד כשיהיה מן הדברים הנאכלים כי הם

מפני החלודה[91] יותר נכונים להועיל לאסטו' המתהפכת באסטנסות (Just as all malodorous [spices and seeds] upset the soul and cause nausea, all fragrant ones strengthen the stomach, especially when they belong to the comestibles, for these are most suited to benefit a stomach upset[92] because of that fluid). In the sense of 'upset,' Hebr. מִתְהַפֵּךְ is a non-attested semantic borrowing from Arab. منقلب. Zeraḥyah Ḥen translates Arab. منقلب as נֶהְפָּךְ (see entry above).

הַפְסָדָה · **corruption** · Ibn al-Jazzār, *Zād al-musāfir wa-qūt al-ḥādir* · trans. Abraham ben Isaac, *Sefer Ṣedah la-Oreḥim*, Abbreviation, bk. 1, ch. 1 (Ms St. Petersburg, Institute of Oriental Studies of the Russian Academy, B 133): אבל יש ראיה על הפסדת היסוד ראוי שיראה דמות עור הראש (For an indication of the corruption of the humor[93] one should look at the color[94] of the skin of the head). Hebrew הַפְסָדָה is not attested for in Hebrew medical literature. Ben-Yehuda mentions the term in an attestation from Jacob Anatoli, *Malmad ha-Talmidim*, and from Jedaiah Bedersi's commentary on *Psalms* (BM 1157). Even Shoshan (EM 396) mentions it in an attestation from Bahya ibn Paquda, *Ḥovot ha-Levavot*.

הַפְשָׁטָה · **abrasion**: Lat. *excoratio* (= *excoriatio*) (DMLBS 1067) · Guillaume de Congenis, *Treatise on Surgery* · trans. Isaiah, fol. 56b: פינפינילא עם חלב תיש יועיל להפשטת הביצים (Pimpernel [mixed] with goat's fat is good for abrasion of the testicular skin [lit., testicles]). Hebr. הַפְשָׁטָה features in Rabbinic literature in the sense of 'flaying, stripping' (of the skin); cf. JD 363; BM 1163–1164.

הַקְדָּמָה • הקדמת הידיעה · **prognostic**: Arab. تقدمة المعرفة · Ibn al-Jazzār, *Zād al-musāfir wa-qūt al-ḥādir* · trans. Moses ibn Tibbon, *Sefer Ṣedat ha-Derakhim*, bk. 3, ch. 1: וכבר זכר גאלי' בפרושו לספר אבקרט בהקדמת הידיעה כי היותר רע שבמיני האסכרה אשר יגיע מחזקתו שיצטרך החולה להזדקף (Galen said in his commentary on Hippocrates' *Prognostic* that the worst kind of angina is the one that is so severe that the patient needs to stand upright). Hebr. הקדמת הידיעה features in BCD 71 (NM 2:41) in a later attestation from Nathan ha-Me'ati's translation of Maimonides' *Medical Aphorisms* 2.4 (BMMN 35). Do'eg ha-Edomi translates the parallel Latin term *pronostica* as השגחות (see entry הַשְׁגָּחָה).

הַר • אבן ההר → **אֶבֶן**.

הָרַג • *Part.* הוֹרֵג הכלב • הוֹרֵג · **(lit., dog killer); (Ger. *Aufrechter Hundswürger*) [*Cionura erecta* (L.) Griseb]**: Arab. قاتل الكلب (Gr. ἀπόκυνον (DT 4:71 (586–587))) · [*Synonima*], Ms Vatican, Biblioteca Apostolica, ebr. 550, fol. 127b (128b): קאתל[95] אל כלב הוא הורג

91 באסטנסות: om. a.
92 'upset because of that fluid': Trans. according to a.
93 For יסוד in the sense of 'humor,' see entry יְסוֹד: *Plur.* יסודות below.
94 For דמות in the sense of 'color,' see entry דְּמוּת above.
95 קאתל: emendation editor קתאל Ms.

הכלב ([Arab.] *qātil al-kalb*; i.e., [Hebr.] *horeg ha-kelev*). In the sense of *Cionura erecta*, Hebr. הורג הכלב is a non-attested calque from Arab. *qātil al-kalb*.

הַרְגָּשָׁה • נאפסת הרגשתו → [אפס].

• *Plur.* **הרגשות • עיכוב ההרגשות** → עִכּוּב.

הַרְחָבָה · looseness or relaxation (of the stomach or bowels): Lat. *solutio* (Arab. إسهال) · Constantinus Africanus, *Viaticum* · trans. Do'eg ha-Edomi, *Sefer Ya'ir Netiv*, bk. 3, ch. 7: ואם תתארך ההרחבה נתן לו האבק הזה (If the looseness (of the stomach or bowels) lasts for a long time we administer [the patient] the following powder ...). Hebr. הַרְחָבָה does not feature in this sense in the current dictionaries. Moses ibn Tibbon translates Arab. إسهال as שלשול.

• **הרחבת התולדת · softening of the stools; purgation of the bowels**: Lat. *mollicies naturae* (Arab. إحدار الطبيعة) · Constantinus Africanus, *Viaticum* · trans. Do'eg ha-Edomi, *Sefer Ya'ir Netiv*, bk. 3, ch. 12: ויאות להשמר מאד בחולי הזה מהרחבת התולדת (One should be very careful not to soften the stools [i.e., purge the bowels] in this kind of illness [i.e., pleurisy] unless when it is necessary). Hebr. הרחבת התולדת is not attested for in the current dictionaries. Moses ibn Tibbon translates Arab. إحدار الطبيعة as הרחיב הטבע (see entry [רחב]).

הרמוס • אצבעות הרמוס → אֶצְבַּע.

הֶרָפוּת · flabbiness: Arab. استرخاء · Ibn al-Jazzār, *Zād al-musāfir wa-qūt al-ḥādir* · trans. Moses ibn Tibbon, *Sefer Ṣedat ha-Derakhim*, bk. 3, ch. 1: ואם נתילדה המורסא בגרון מפני ליחה לבנה והורה על זה המופת אשר זכרנו מרכות הכאב ורפיונו ונפח הלשון והרפותה (If the swelling in the throat is caused by phlegm according to the indications [i.e., symptoms] I mentioned, namely when the pain is mild and weak, and the tongue is swollen and flabby ...). Hebr. הֶרָפוּת is not attested for in the current dictionaries.

הַרְתָּחָה · boiling: Arab. غليان · Ibn al-Jazzār, *Zād al-musāfir wa-qūt al-ḥādir* · trans. Abraham ben Isaac, *Sefer Ṣedah la-Oreḥim*, bk. 1, ch. 18: והב׳ מחמת הרתחת הדם שבתוך הלב כי דם זה שבלב כאשר ירתח ויתלהב מחמת מרירה האדומה אז יעלה מן הדם בהרתחתו עשן אל הראש ואז יולד במוח הראש צמח חד מרירי (The second [cause of phrenitis] is the boiling of the blood within the heart. When this blood seethes and becomes inflamed because of the yellow bile, vapors arise to the head and cause a sharp bilious swelling). Hebr. הַרְתָּחָה does not feature in the current dictionaries in a medical context (cf. BM 1201; EM 411). Moses ibn Tibbon translates Arab. غليان as רתיחה. Do'eg ha-Edomi uses the same term to render Lat. *ebullitio*.

הַשְׁגָּחָה • *Plur.* **השגחות • ספר ההשגחות · the Book [called] *Prognostic***: Lat. *pronostica* (Arab. تقدمة المعرفة) · Constantinus Africanus, *Viaticum* · trans. Do'eg ha-Edomi, *Sefer Ya'ir Netiv*, bk. 3, ch. 1: מאשר אמר גלינוס על ספר ההשגחות מאבוקראט (... as Galen said in [his commentary] on Hippocrates' *Prognostic*). Hebr. השגחות is not attested for in this sense in the current dictionaries. Moses ibn Tibbon translates the parallel Arabic term تقدمة المعرفة as הקדמת הידיעה (see entry הַקְדָּמָה).

הַשְׁחָתָה · **[bodily] defect**: Lat. *vitium* (Arab. حالات مرضة) · Constantinus Africanus, *Viaticum* · trans. Do'eg ha-Edomi, *Sefer Ya'ir Netiv*, bk. 1, ch. 21: העיטוש נולד מליחות משתנות כי לפעמים התולדת פועל בחזקתו לדחות הליחות המקובצות או עשן המוח אותם שהם סבת חולי או סבת ההשחתה העתידה לבא (Sneezing may originate from various fluids, for sometimes nature becomes active to repel with all its force the humors or vapors that are aggregated in the brain and are the cause of the [current] illness or of the bodily defects that will occur later on). Hebr. הַשְׁחָתָה features in the current dictionaries in the general sense of 'destruction' only (cf. JD 369; BM 1206; EM 1414). Moses ibn Tibbon translates Arab. حالات مرضة as ענינים מחליאים and Abraham ben Isaac as חלאים אחרים.

הַשְׁמָנָה • **גרגרי החשמנה** → **גַּרְגֵּר**.

הִשְׁתַּטְּחוּת · **stretching**: Lat. *extensio* (*distensio*) (Arab. تمدّد) · Constantinus Africanus · trans. Do'eg ha-Edomi, *Sefer Ya'ir Netiv*, bk. 3, ch. 8: חתוך המקורות הוא פנימי או חיצון. החיצון הוא מנגעים או מהשתטחותם והנגעים הם ממכה או מנפילה ההשתטחות הוא מדלוג או מצעקה גדולה (Veins burst by an external cause or an internal cause. The external [cause] is a wound or stretching; a wound results from a blow, or from a fall. Stretching results from a jump or a loud cry). Hebr. הִשְׁתַּטְּחוּת features in EM 418 as השתטחות על הקרקע or השתטחות על קברי אבות (To stretch oneself on the earth, on the graves of the forefathers). Moses ibn Tibbon translates Arab. تمدّد as משיכה (cf. BCD 165 (NM 3:146)).

הִתְאַבְּנוּת · **calcification**: Arab. تحجّر · Maimonides, *Medical Aphorisms* 23.89 · trans. Nathan ha-Me'ati (BMMN 230): הרופאים מנהגם לאמר מוטחלים מאותם שימצאם קושי בטחולם והתאבנות מבלי מורסא (When speaking of 'spleen patients,' physicians usually mean those patients whose spleen is affected by induration and calcification without an inflammation). Hebr. הִתְאַבְּנוּת features in BM 1216 in attestations from the *Sefer ha-Qanun*. Zeraḥyah Ḥen translates Arab. تحجّر as אַבְנִינוּת (see entry).

הִתְדּוֹמְמוּת · **end (i.e., abatement of a fever)**: Arab. إقلاع · Maimonides, *Medical Aphorisms* 10.20 · trans. Zeraḥyah Ḥen (BMMZ 122): ובהיותה בלתי מתדוממת ולא נבדלת אבל תעשה עונותיה בכל יום על עניין אחד דומה וזו היא התמידית אשר עונותיה בכל יום ולא תתבאר בה התדוממות (And [the type of fever] that does not end nor depart but occurs every day in the same way is the [so-called] continuous quotidian fever. This fever does not have a clear end). Hebr. הִתְדּוֹמְמוּת does not feature in the current dictionaries. Nathan ha-Me'ati translates Arab. إقلاع as הסתלקות.

הִתְפַּשְּׁטוּת · **dilatation (of the palpebral membrane)**: Arab. انتشار (D 2:671) · Maimonides, *Medical Aphorisms* 23.69 · trans. Nathan ha-Me'ati (BMMN 227): המים המתקבצים בעין והם הקוראים הרופאים התפשטות יתקבץ בין הלחות הגלדיית והקרום הקרניי. בעשירי בתועלות (The cataract that occurs in the eye and which the physicians call 'extension [i.e., dilatation]' lies between the crystalline humor and the horn-like tunic). Hebr. הִתְפַּשְּׁטוּת does not feature in this sense in the current dictionaries. In addition to הִתְפַּשְּׁטוּת, Nathan ha-Me'ati renders the same Arabic term as הִתְרַחֲבוּת

in Maimonides, *Medical Aphorisms* 22.40 (BMMN 214; see next entry). Zeraḥyah Ḥen translates Arab. انتشار as פישוט.

הִתְרַחֲבוּת · dilatation of the palpebral membrane: Arab. انتشار (D 2:671) · Maimonides, *Medical Aphorisms* 22.40 · trans. Nathan ha-Me'ati (BMMN 214): הכחילה במשקה וורדים סוכרי מחזק הראות ויבריא התמדת זה מההתרחבות. נתאמת זה בניסיון ואיני סר מעשותו לחזק הראות (The anointment of the eyelids with rose syrup made with sugar strengthens vision. Its permanent use cures dilatation of the palpebral membrane. This has been verified by experience; I have not ceased to use it for strengthening vision). Hebr. הִתְרַחֲבוּת features in BM 1249 in an attestation from the *Sefer ha-Qanun* without further explication. In addition to הִתְרַחֲבוּת, Nathan ha-Me'ati translates the same Arabic term as הִתְפַּשְּׁטוּת in Maimonides, *Medical Aphorisms* 23.69 (BMMN 227; see previous entry). Zeraḥyah Ḥen (a.l.) translates Arab. انتشار as פשוט הראות (see entry פִּשּׁוּט).

וולון • הוולון המבדיל · **diaphragm**: Arab. الحجاب الفاصل · Ibn al-Jazzār, *Zād al-musāfir wa-qūt al-ḥādir* · trans. Abraham ben Isaac, *Sefer Ṣedah la-Oreḥim*, bk. 1, ch. 18: או חולי הבראסם הנקר׳ מחמת הוולון המבדיל ונק׳ בלש׳ ישמעאל אלחג׳אב אלפצאל (… or the illness of phrenitis that occurs because of [an inflammation of] the diaphragm, which is called in Arabic *al-ḥijāb al-faṣṣāl*). In the sense of 'diaphragm,' the term הוולון המבדיל is a non-attested combination of Lat. *velum* and Hebr. מבדיל. Moses ibn Tibbon translates Arab. الحجاب الفاصل as המסך המבדיל. Do'eg ha-Edomi renders the parallel Latin term *diafragma* as קרב (cf. BCD 249 (NM 3:207)).

וינטושא • עשה וינטושא → עָשָׂה.

וֶסֶת · **habit**: Arab. عادة · Ibn al-Jazzār, *Zād al-musāfir wa-qūt al-ḥādir* · trans. Abraham ben Isaac, *Sefer Ṣedah la-Oreḥim*, bk. 1, ch. 10 (Ms Jerusalem, National Library of Israel, Fr. 95, fol. 89[b]): וצריך הרופא שיבין גם עיתי השנה להנחיל החולאים כתיקון וכפי כח האויר אם חום ואם קור גם שני עיתי החולה אם הוא בחור אם נער אם זקן או סריס או אשה גם ישים לבו על ווסתו שלחולה (The physician should also consider the seasons of the year in order to treat the patient correctly, according to the severity of the weather, whether it is warm or cold, and according to the age of the patient [and] whether the patient is a young man, a boy, an elderly, or eunuch, or woman. He should also pay attention to the habits of the patient). Hebr. וֶסֶת does not feature in the current dictionaries in the sense of 'habit' in medieval medical literature; cf. BM 1268–1269. Moses ibn Tibbon translates Arab. عادة as מנהג. Do'eg ha-Edomi translates the parallel Latin term *consuetudo* as הנהגה.

וֶרֶד • ורד הגפן · **bean clover** [*Anagyris foetida* L.] Arab. ينبوت (cf. MIG 427) · *Shinnui ha-Shemot ha-Niqra'im Synonimis*, Ms Munich, Bayerische Staatsbibliothek, Cod. hebr. 8, fol. 199[a]: ינבות הוא וורד הגפן ([Arab.] *yanbūt*; i.e., [Hebr.] *wered ha-gefen*). Hebr. ורד הגפן does not feature in the current dictionaries.

• *Plur.* **ורדים • ורדי החמורים** · **(lit., roses of donkeys); peony** [*Paeonia officinalis* L.]: Arab. ورد الحمير · Shem Tov ben Isaac, *Sefer ha-Shimmush*, bk. 29, list 1 (SHS 1:195 (Waw 2)): ורדי החמורים ב״ה ורד אלחמיר וב״ל ג׳נשקולא (*wardei ha-ḥamorim*; Arab. *ward al-ḥamīr*; vern. ǦNŠQWL' [perhaps M.Lat. **genestula* or O.Cat. **ginestola* [*Genista tinctoria* L.]]). Hebr. *Sing.* ורד החמור is a non-attested calque of Arab. ورد الحمير.

ז

זְאֵב · **lupus (i.e., erosive lesions that were reminiscent of a wolf's bite)**: Lat. *lupus* (DMLBS 2019: 'skin disease, ulcer, 'lupus'') · Guillaume de Congenis, *Treatise on Surgery* · trans. Isaiah, fol. 49[b]: כנגד זאב:[96] דבש ומלח ושעור יחד שרוף בקדרה חדשה ואבק מובחרת תעשה ותשים עליו (Against lupus: [Take] honey, salt, and barley, [put them] together and burn them in a new pot, prepare a fine powder and put it on the spot [of the lupus]). As an illness, Hebr. זְאֵב features in BM 1276 only in the sense of 'a ravenous hunger,' in an attestation from Judah al-Ḥarizi, *Mahberot Itiel*. The term לובאט featuring in the marginal gloss is possibly O.Fr. *louvet* (since 13th cent.); M.Fr. *louvat* (since 1340; Ger. *Wolfsjunges* (FEW 5:458a)); or O.Occ. *lobat* (RL 4:107a) or *lobet* (RL 4:416a) with the same meaning.[97]

זֶבֶל · **feces**: a) Arab. خراء · Ibn al-Jazzār, *Zād al-musāfir wa-qūt al-ḥādir* · trans. Moses ibn Tibbon, *Sefer Ṣedat ha-Derakhim*, bk. 3, ch. 1: או יגרגר חלב עזים החלוב עם מעט זבל כלב לבן (He [i.e., someone suffering from angina] may also gargle with fresh goat's milk with some feces of a white dog). In the sense of 'feces,' Hebr. זֶבֶל is only attested for in Rabbinic literature (cf. BM 1285). Do'eg ha-Edomi translates the parallel Latin term *stercus* as צואה.

b) Arab. زبل · Isḥāq ibn ʿImrān, *Treatise on Melancholy* · trans. Anonymous, fol. 52[b] (53[b]): אבל[98] שהפירות יועילום לאכול מהם התאנים היבשים ולהמעיט מהם מפני שהוא מוציא הזבל בסוף הלילה במיהור (But to eat fruit, e.g., dried figs, is good for them [i.e. those who suffer from melancholy], but [one should only eat] a small amount because they quickly expel the feces at the end of the night). Nathan ha-Me'ati and Zeraḥyah Ḥen both use the same Hebrew term for Arab. زبل in their translations of Maimonides, *Medical Aphorisms* 22.21 (BMMN 212; BMMZ 209).

• **זבל היונים** · **(lit., pigeons' droppings); alkali plant**: Arab. أشنان (cf. MIG 7): *Shinnui Shemot ha-Niqra Synonimas*, Ms Leiden, Universiteitsbibliotheek, Or. 4719, fol. 68[a]: אושנאן הוא זבל היונים בלשונם אשטירקו קולובינו[99] (*ushnān*; i.e., pigeons' droppings, in their language [Rom./Lat.] ʾYŠṬYRQW QWLWBYNW). In the sense of 'alkali plant,' Hebr. זבל היונים is a calque of Lat./Rom. ʾYŠṬYRQW QWLWBYNW. Note that the regular synonym for 'alkali plant' in Arabic sources, e.g., Ibn Sīnā, *K. al-Qānūn fī al-ṭibb* 1:254, is *khuruʾ al-ʿaṣāfīr* ('sparrows' droppings'), which is translated by Zeraḥyah Ḥen, *Sefer ha-Qanun*, as זבל הצפורים ('birds' droppings') (see entry below).

• **זבל העפורים** · **(lit., birds' droppings); alkali plant**: Arab. أشنان (cf. MIG 7): Ibn Sīnā, *K. al-Qānūn fī al-ṭibb* · trans. Zeraḥyah Ḥen, *Sefer ha-Qanun* (Ms Oxford, Bodleian

---

96 זאב: לופוש נקרא בהמון לובאט Ms[1].

97 I thank my colleague and friend Guido Mensching for this explanatory note.

98 אבל שהפירות: emendation editor אבל שימי הפירות Ms.

99 קולובינו: emendation editor קולומינו Ms.

Library, Opp. Add. Fol. 12, fol. 174^{a}), fol. 173b: אשְנַאן המהות הם מינים היותר דק הוא הלבן ונקרא זבל הצפורים ואחד מהם הוא הירוק (*oshnan* [i.e., *ushnān*], nature [...] [it has different] species; the white [species] is the finest; it is called 'birds' droppings;' [another] of these [species] is the green one). Hebr. זבל הצפורים does not feature in this sense in the current dictionaries. A synonymous term is זבל היונים (see entry above).

זָהָב • מדביק הזהב → [דבק].

זוֹב • זוב טפת הזרע ‣ **flow of sperm (i.e., ejaculation)**: Arab. سيلان المني · Isḥāq ibn 'Imrān, *Treatise on Melancholy* · trans. Anonymous, fol. 49^{b} (50^{b}): ויארע להם החנוק וזוב טפת הזרע ויציאת הצואה והשתן מבלי חפץ (And they [i.e., those who suffer from epilepsy] will also suffer from suffocation, and unvoluntary flow of sperm [i.e., ejaculation], defecation, and urination). Hebr. זוב טפת הזרע is not attested for in the current dictionaries. The synonym הגרת הזרע features in Moses ibn Tibbon's *Sefer Ṣedat ha-Derakhim* (cf. BCD 41 (NM 4:41)).

זולאבי ‣ **I. julep**: Arab. جلّاب · Ibn al-Jazzār, *Zād al-musāfir wa-qūt al-ḥādir* · trans. Abraham ben Isaac, *Sefer Ṣedah la-Oreḥim*, bk. 1, ch. 18: וישקהו בערב מי רימונים עם זולאבי או עם מי צוקרו (Or, administer in the evening juice of pomegranates together with julep or crystalline sugar). The term זולאבי is a non-attested loan word from the Italian, i.e., *giulebbe* ('rosewater') (FEW 19:59b), derived from Arab. *julāb*. Moses ibn Tibbon translates Arab. جلّاب as משקה סוכרי (cf. BCD 166 (NM 4:109–110)); Do'eg ha-Edomi renders the parallel Latin term *scirupus* as אישרוף (see entry).

‣ **II. beverage; wine; potion; juice; syrup**: Arab. شراب · Ibn al-Jazzār, *Zād al-musāfir wa-qūt al-ḥādir* · trans. Abraham ben Isaac, *Sefer Ṣedah la-Oreḥim*, bk. 1, ch. 10: ותשקהו מי שעורים עם מי רימונים מתוקים וערב במים שישתה זולאבי שליינצובי או זולאבי שלבנפסג ([The patient] should be administered barley water together with juice of sweet pomegranates. The [barley] water may also be mixed with syrup of common jujubes, or syrup of violets). Moses ibn Tibbon translates Arab. شراب as משקה.

זַיִת • זיתי המים ‣ **(lit., water olives); green, unripe olives**: Arab. زيتون الماء (MIG 336: زيتون الماء هو الغضّ الأخضر الذي لا يعقد زيتًا ولا دهنًا عن الإسرائيلي ('Water olive' is a fresh and green [olive] from which neither oil nor ointment can be extracted according to al-Isrā'īlī)) · *Shinnui ha-Shemot ha-Niqra'im Synonimis*, Ms Munich, Bayerische Staatsbibliothek, Cod. hebr. 8, fol. 197^{b}: זיתי המים הם פגי זתים אשר לא יגיעו לבישול שיעשה מהם שמן ושבם? שמנוני ולפי קצת המחברים הם כבושים ('Water olives' are green, olives that are not ripe so that no oil and no ointment can be made from them; according to some authors they are olives that have been preserved). In the sense of 'green, unripe olives,' Hebr. זיתי המים is a non-attested calque from Arab. زيتون الماء.

זְמַן • יש לו/לה הרבה זמן ‣ **to become chronic**: Arab. تقادم · Ibn al-Jazzār, *Zād al-musāfir wa-qūt al-ḥādir* · trans. Abraham ben Isaac, *Sefer Ṣedah la-Oreḥim*, bk. 1, ch. 14: ואם יש לחולי זה הרבה זמן אז נצוהו שישתה בכל יום שקל קשטורנו במים חמין (If the illness becomes chronic, we tell the [the patient] to take every day one *sheqel* of castoreum with hot water). Hebr. יש לו/לה הרבה זמן does not feature as a medical term in the current dictionaries. Do'eg ha-Edomi translates the parallel Latin term *inveterasco* as הִזְקִין (see entry [זקן]).

זָנָב • זנב העכבר • הדפק הנק׳ זנב העכבר → דֹּפֶק.

זֵעָה • בתי הזיעה → בַּיִת.

• כלי מיודע להעלות זיעתו → כְּלִי.

זְקִיפָה • נשימת הזקיפה → נְשִׁימָה.

[זקן] • *Hif'il* הִזְקִין · **to become chronic**: Lat. *inveterasco* (Arab. تقادم) · Constantinus Africanus, *Viaticum* · trans. Do'eg ha-Edomi, *Sefer Ya'ir Netiv*, bk. 1, ch. 14: ואם יזקין החולי ינתן לו בכל יום דרמכ׳ קשטור בחמים (If the illness becomes chronic, we give [the patient] every day one *dirham* of castoreum with hot water). In the sense of 'to become chronic,' Hebr. הִזְקִין features in BCD 85 (NM 3:77) in a later attestation from Hillel ben Samuel's translation of Hippocrates' *Aphorisms* 3.28. Moses ibn Tibbon translates Arab. تقادم as נתישן and Abraham ben Isaac as יש לו/לה הרבה זמן (see entry זְמַן).

זָרוּת · **sadness; sorrow**: Arab. وحشة (VL 4:444) · Ibn al-Jazzār, *Zād al-musāfir wa-qūt al-ḥādir* · trans. Moses ibn Tibbon, *Sefer Ṣedat ha-Derakhim*, bk. 3, ch. 13: ואם היה מדם או מרה כרכומית יהיה עם הדפיקה ההיא חום וצמא ונשימה גבוהה ואם היה מדם עב שחורי יהיה עם הדפיקה ההיא זרות ופחד ורעדה ודאגה מבלתי סבה ומעוט צמא ועצלה (If they [i.e., palpitations] occur because of blood or yellow bile, they are accompanied by fever, thirst, difficult breathing [lit., breathing high (in the chest)]; if they occur because of thick, melancholic blood, they come with sadness, fear, trembling, worry for no reason, slight thirst, indolence). Hebr. זָרוּת does not feature in this sense in the current dictionaries.

• זרות המחשבה · **mental aberration**: Lat. *alienationes* (Arab. هذيان واختلاط عقل) · Constantinus Africanus, *Viaticum* · trans. Do'eg ha-Edomi, *Sefer Ya'ir Netiv*,[100] bk. 1, ch. 18: פרינישין הוא צמח נולד בתוך דפי המוח הוא הקרום ומן הצמח ההוא יחולו בכל עת תעורה וזרות המחשבה (Phrenitis; i.e., an inflammation originating in the membranes of the brain, i.e., QRWM [membrane], and from that inflammation always hail sleeplessness and aberration of the mind [i.e., delirium]). Hebr. זרות המחשבה does not feature in the current dictionaries. Moses ibn Tibbon translates Arab. هذيان واختلاط عقل as שגעון וערבוב השכל and Abraham ben Isaac as בילבול וטרוף דעת.

• זרות הרוח · **mental aberration**: Lat. *alienationes* (Arab. هذيان واختلاط عقل) · Constantinus Africanus, *Viaticum* · trans. Do'eg ha-Edomi, *Sefer Ya'ir Netiv*,[101] bk. 1, ch. 18: ונולד בשני ענינים או משלהבת האדומה עולה אל המוח או מרתיחת הדם בלב. והעשן ההוא בעלותו אל המוח נעשה צמח ויחולו מזה התעורה וזרות הרוח וכאב (It [i.e., phrenitis] may occur for

100 Do'eg ha-Edomi renders the same Latin term as זרות הרוח; cf. next entry.

101 Do'eg ha-Edomi renders the same Latin term as זרות המחשבה; cf. previous entry.

two reasons: either from the burning of the yellow bile, which arises to the brain, or from the boiling of the blood in the heart. When the resulting smoke arises to the brain it causes a swelling, which results in sleeplessness and mental aberration and pain). Moses ibn Tibbon translates Arab. هذيان واختلاط عقل as שגעון וערבוב שכל and Abraham ben Isaac as בילבול וטרוף דעת.

זַרְנִיךְ · **orpiment**: Lat. *auripigmentum* · Guillaume de Congenis, *Treatise on Surgery* · trans. Isaiah, fol. 56^b: ולסרטן[102] ולפישטולא: קח זרניך ירוק הנחשת איירמן שליימא קרן איל שרוף עצם ארנבת שרוף צואת אדם שרופה שוק השומים שרוף (Against cancer and fistulas: Take orpiment, verdigris, vitriol, rock salt, burnt horn of a ram, burnt bone of a hare, burnt human feces, burnt fibrous top of garlic …). For the identification of Hebr. זַרְנִיךְ, commonly meaning 'arsenic,' as 'orpiment', cf. SHS 1:353 (Samekh 2).

זֶרַע • **זוב שפת הזרע** → **זוֹב**.

זֵרְעוֹן • *Plur.* **זרעונים** · **chickpeas** [***Cicer arietinum*** **L.**]: Lat. *ciceres* · Constantinus Africanus, *Viaticum* · trans. Do'eg ha-Edomi, *Sefer Ya'ir Netiv*, bk. 3, ch. 6: ויאות גם כן לתת לו מרק חטה עם שמן שקד גם להאכילו בטנים תאנים שקדים וישתה מליקרט עם ארומטיקש ויאכל מרק זרעונים עם צמוקים (One should also let him eat broth prepared from wheat with almond oil, and pine cones, figs, and almonds. He should drink hydromel with spices and eat a broth prepared from chickpeas and raisins). In the sense of 'chickpeas,' Hebr. זרעונים features in BCD 86 (NM 1:71) in a later attestation from Moses ibn Tibbon, *Sefer Ṣedat ha-Derakhim*, bk. 7, ch. 16.3 (IJZ 153).

---

102 ולסרטן: Ms[1].

ח

חִבּוּר · **temperament:** Lat. *complexio* (Arab. مزاج) · Constantinus Africanus, *Viaticum* · trans. Do'eg ha-Edomi, *Sefer Ya'ir Netiv*, bk. 2, ch. 17 (Ms Oxford, Bodleian Library, Can. Or. 26, fol. 267[a]): ואם החבור הרע והחם יהיה בלשון יאות להקיז שני המקורות אשר תחת הלשון (If the bad, hot temperament is in the tongue, one should bleed the two veins that are beneath the tongue). Hebr. חִבּוּר does not feature in this sense in the current dictionaries. Moses ibn Tibbon translates Arab. مزاج with the standard term מזג.

חֶבֶל • **חבל העניים** · **(lit., poor men's rope); binding material from twiners for poor people:** Arab. حبل المساكين (DT 4:35 (548, n. 6): 'Bindfadenersatz für arme Leute'; M 104 (Meyerhof): 'un nom designant plusieurs plantes volubiles') · *Shinnui ha-Shemot ha-Niqra'im Synonimis*, Ms Munich, Bayerische Staatsbibliothek, Cod. hebr. 8, fol. 198[b]: חבל[103] אלמסאכין הוא חבל העניים[104] ([Arab.] *ḥabl al-masakīn*; i.e., [Hebr.] *ḥevel ha-ʿaniyyim*). Hebr. חבל העניים does not feature in the current dictionaries.

חָבַר • *Part.* **חוֹבֵר** • **הכתונת החוברת** → **כְּתֹנֶת**.

• *Part. f.* **חוֹבֶרֶת** · **conjunctiva:** Lat. *coniunctiva* (Arab. الملتحم) · Constantinus Africanus, *Viaticum* · trans. Do'eg ha-Edomi, *Sefer Ya'ir Netiv*,[105] bk. 2, ch. 3: הקליפה[106] היא דם היורד אל הכתונת החוברת זהו קונגוקטיבא ואל[107] הארטיריאש שלה בהבקעם ונעשה משני ענינים מהכאת העין ומבקיעת החוברת או בעבור הנפח הנולד בחוברת (Hyposphagma[108] is blood that streams to the conjunctiva, i.e., [Lat.] QWNGWQṬYB', [from][109] blood vessels torn in it. It is caused either by a blow to the eye or by a tear in the conjuctiva or by a tumor originating in the conjunctiva). Hebr. חוֹבֶרֶת features in Masie (MD 179), s.v. 'conjunctiva,' referring to Me'ir Aldabi, *Shevilei Emunah* (cf. KDS 93). Moses ibn Tibbon translates Arab. ملتحم as לובן. For *Part. Puʿal* מְחֻבָּר in the sense of 'compounded,' see BCD 89 (NM 1:161).

• *Piʿel* **חִבֵּר** · **1. to compose [a medicine]:** Arab. ألّف · Ibn al-Jazzār, *Zād al-musāfir wa-qūt al-ḥāḍir* · trans. Abraham ben Isaac, *Sefer Ṣedah la-Oreḥim*, bk. 1; ch. 10 (Ms Jerusalem, National Library of Israel, Fr. 95, fol. 92[a]): וזה מעשה ריקוח אצטומטיכון בעל עשרה סמים אשר חיבר יצחק בן עמרן (This is the recipe of the stomachic consisting of ten ingredients composed by Isḥāq ibn ʿImrān). Hebr. חִבֵּר is not attested for in a medical sense in the current dictionaries; cf. BM 1431–1432. Moses ibn Tibbon renders

---

103 חבל: emendation editor חב Ms.

104 העניים: העיניים Ms.

105 As synonyms of חוֹבֶרֶת (Lat. *coniunctiva*), we find החלק הדבק and החלק המחוברת (see entry חֵלֶק), and הכתונת החוברת (see entry כְּתֹנֶת).

106 הקליפה: *crustula* L طرفة a.

107 ואל הארטיריאש: *a suis arteriis* L.

108 'Hyposphagma': See entry קְלִפָּה.

109 '[from]': Trans. according to Lat. *a*.

Arab. أَلَّه إسحاق بن عمران as לאסחק בן עמראן. Subsequently, Hebr. חִבֵּר features in the same sense in the translations by Nathan ha-Me'ati and Zeraḥyah Ḥen of Maimonides, *Medical Aphorisms* 13.13; 22.35; 24.44; 25.25, 59, 61 (BMMN 147, 213, 240, 249, 261–262; BMMZ 145, 211, 239, 249, 261–262).

‣ II. **to mix**: Lat. *iungo* (Arab. خلط) · Constantinus Africanus, *Viaticum* · trans. Do'eg ha-Edomi, *Sefer Ya'ir Netiv*, bk. 1, ch. 23: ואם תרצה לחמם וליבש יותר תחבר שם אבפורבי קשטור (If you want that [the mentioned ingredients] will be more hot and dry, you have to mix them with [the weight of one *dirham* each of] resin spurge and castoreum). Moses ibn Tibbon translates Arab. خلط as עירב, and Abraham ben Isaac as הוסיף בריקוחם.

‣ III. **to add**: Lat. *addo* · Constantinus Africanus, *Viaticum* · trans. Do'eg ha-Edomi, *Sefer Ya'ir Netiv*, bk. 3, ch. 6: מרקחת אחר זה מועיל אל השעול הקר ולרוח ולנשימת החזה: ריקליציא זרע פשתן חרוך שקד מתוק דרכמ׳ פניס י׳ אניש מראטרי אישופו קפיליוינירידי פרשי ו׳ דרכמ׳ זעפרן זנגביל קלימנט ד׳ ותכתוש לאבק ותחבר שם דבש די ספקו ותתן ב׳ דרכמ׳ (Another remedy, beneficial for cold cough, winds, and [difficulty of] breathing: [Take] one *dirham* each of licorice, roasted common flax seed, and sweet almonds; ten *dirhams* of sugar candy; six *dirhams* each of anise, fennel, hyssop, maidenhair fern, white horehound; four *dirhams* each of saffron, ginger, mint; pound these ingredients, add a sufficient amount of honey, and administer two *dirhams* to [the patient]).

• *Part. Pu'al* מְחֻבָּר • **החלק המחוברת** → חֵלֶק.

חָבֵר • **המקור העומד בין האצבע הקטון לחבירו** → מָקוֹר.

• **העורק אשר בין האצבע הקטן וחברו** → עוֹרֶק.

חָבֶשׁ ‣ **plaster; poultice**: Arab. ضماد · i. Ibn al-Jazzār, *Zād al-musāfir wa-qūt al-ḥāḍir* · trans. Abraham ben Isaac, *Sefer Ṣedah la-Oreḥim*, bk. 1, ch. 10 (Ms Jerusalem, National Library of Israel, Fr. 95, fol. 89ᵇ): או ישים על המצח והצדעים חובש מן סנדלי לבנים ושושנים וקאפורא וקמח שעורים (Or apply to the forehead and the temples a poultice made from white sandalwood, roses, camphor, and barley flour). In the sense of 'poultice,' Hebr. חָבֶשׁ is only attested for in Hebrew medieval (liturgical) poetry (cf. BM 1439; EM 501). According to Muntner (MM 137) the term also features in the *Sefer Asaph ha-Rofe*. Another term for 'plaster, poultice,' derived from the same root חבש, is חִבּוּשׁ; cf. BCD 87 (NM 1:44–45). Moses ibn Tibbon translates Arab. ضماد as תחבושת. Do'eg ha-Edomi translates the parallel Latin term *unguo* as משח.

ii. Ibn al-Jazzār, *Zād al-musāfir wa-qūt al-ḥāḍir* · trans. Abraham ben Isaac, *Sefer Ṣedah la-Oreḥim*, Adaptation, bk. 1, ch. 10 (Ms Berlin, Staatsbibliothek Preußischer Kulturbesitz, Or. fol. 1058, fols 93[a]–93[b]): או נעשה לו חובש זה אחר הטהרו בהקזה ובשלשול קח סנדלי אדומים סולטרו עלי ערבה דודאים קמח שעור ודומיה (Once [the body] has been cleansed through bleeding and purging, we should apply the following poultice: take red sandalwood, black nightshade, willow leaves, violets, barley flour, and the like ...). Abraham ben Isaac translates Arab. ضمّد 'to apply a plaster' as עשה תחבושת. Do'eg ha-Edomi translates the parallel Latin term *cataplasma impono* as חוּבַּשׁ.

[חדד] • *Part. Pu'al* מְחֻדָּד • **מחודד מאד** · **very acute**: Lat. *peracutus* · Constantinus Africanus, Viaticum · trans. Do'eg ha-Edomi, *Sefer Ya'ir Netiv*, bk. 3, ch. 1: ובעבור שהוא מחודד מאד וממית פתאום (Since it [i.e., angina] is a very acute [illness] and kills all of a sudden). In a medical sense, Hebr. מְחֻדָּד features in MD 11, s.v. 'acuminate.'

חִדּוּשׁ · **accident**: Arab. حادث (Lat. *passio*) · Ibn al-Jazzār, *Zād al-musāfir wa-qūt al-ḥādir* · trans. Moses ibn Tibbon, *Sefer Ṣedat ha-Derakhim*, bk. 3, ch. 11: וכשיהיו כלי הנשימה בריאים והצורך אליהם ממוצע והכח שלם אז תהיה הנשימה הטבעית אשר זכרנו ואם התחדש שום חדוש בענין מאלו הכלים הנה בלא ספק שיקרה הנזק בנשימה (But when the respiratory organs are healthy and there is a moderate need for them [i.e., breathing is moderate] and the strength is sound, then breathing will be natural, as I mentioned, but if an accident occurs in one of the respiratory organs, then breathing will—without any doubt—be harmed). In the sense of 'accident,' Hebrew חִדּוּשׁ features in medieval philosophical literature in an attestation from Moses ibn Tibbon's translation of Themistius' *Paraphrase of Metaphysica Lambda* (cf. PESHAT, s.v. חִדּוּשׁ, entry 6).[110] Do'eg ha-Edomi translates the parallel Latin term *passio* as חולי.

• **חדוש הנפש** · **that which affects the soul (h.l., anxiety; unrest)**: Arab. حديث النفس (cf. D 1:259: كلّ ما يحدّث به الانسان نفسه من خير وشرّ 'il se prend donc dans le sens d'espoir et dans celui de crainte, inquietude …') · Ibn al-Jazzār, *Zād al-musāfir wa-qūt al-ḥādir* · trans. Moses ibn Tibbon, *Sefer Ṣedat ha-Derakhim*, bk. 3, ch. 13: תאר אבק חברו אסחק בן עמרם יועיל לתחלת המלנקוניה ויחזק הלב ויסיר חדוש הנפש והדפיקה והשטות הכוזב (Recipe of a powder that was composed by Isḥāq ibn 'Imrān and that is good for the beginning of melancholy and that strengthens the heart and takes away anxiety, palpitations, and delusions). Hebrew חדוש הנפש does not feature in the current dictionaries.

חֶדֶר • *Plur.* **חדרים** · **ventricles (of the brain)**: Arab. بطون · Ibn al-Jazzār, *Zād al-musāfir wa-qūt al-ḥādir* · trans. Abraham ben Isaac, *Sefer Ṣedah la-Oreḥim*, cf. bk. 1, ch. 22: דע כי החולי הזה הנקרא בלשון יון איפילינישיאה והוא אל צרע רטיבות מונעת[111] תסגור חדרי המוח שלראש סגירות חזקה (Know that this disease that is called in Greek ʾYPYLYNYŠYʾH [i.e., ἐπιληψία], i.e., [Arab.] ʾL ṢRʿ [i.e., الصرع], [originates] from a viscous[112] fluid, which completely closes the ventricles of the brain). In the sense of 'ventricles (of the brain),' Hebr. חדרים features in BCD 90 (NM 4:61) in a later attestation from Nathan ha-Me'ati's *Sefer ha-Qanun*. Do'eg ha-Edomi translates Lat. *ventriculi* as בטנים (see entry בֶּטֶן); the same term is used by Moses ibn Tibbon for Arab. بطون.

---

110 PESHAT, https://peshat.gwiss.uni-hamburg.de (accessed October 2021).

111 מונעת (= مانعة): ميّاعة a.

112 'viscous': Trans. after a.

חוֹבֵר (*Part.*) → חָבַר.
חוֹבֶרֶת (*Part. f.*) → חָבַר.
חובש → חֹבֶשׁ.
חוטם → חֹטֶם.
חולשה → חֲלְשָׁה.
חוסר → חֹסֶר.
חור → חֹר.
חורפה → חֲרְפָּה.
חוֹתָם • חותם שלמה · (the plant called) 'Solomon's Seal' (Sigillum Salomonis); or angular Solomon's Seal [*Polygonatum odoratum* (Mill.) Druce] (cf. DN 449): Arab. شقاقل (i.e., the species of parsnip called secacul, *Pastinaca sekakul* DC. (cf. MIG 985))[113] · *Shinnui ha-Shemot ha-Niqra'im Synonimi*, Ms Florence, Bibliotheca Laurenziana, Or. 17, fol. 68ª: אשקקל הם רינצי פ"א אשקאקל החותם שלמה ('ŠQQL; [Rom.] RYNṢY;[114] read 'ŠQ'QL [i.e., Arab. *ishqāqul*, or ŠQ'QL, i.e., Arab. *shaqāqul*]; [Hebr.] 'Solomon's Seal').
חָזֶה • חלל החזה → חָלָל.
חֲזָז • *Plur.* חזזים · scabby, scaly eruptions on the skin: Arab. قواب · Isḥāq ibn 'Imrān, *Treatise on Melancholy* · trans. Anonymous, fol. 49ª (50ª): ובעבור כי לפעמים יראה בגופות המלאנכו' דברים אחרים ר"ל הג' מיני' הבוהק השחור או חזזים קטנים או חבורות קטנות ויש להם תועלת בהם (When the bodies of those who suffer from melancholy show other [symptoms], [those] consist of three kinds: black *bahaq*,[115] small scabby, scaly eruptions on the skin, and small tumors; it is beneficial for them). Hebr. חזזים features in BM 1482 in an attestation from the *Sefer ha-Qanun*, and is defined by Ben-Yehuda as עפרורית כעין סובין בראש ('Kopfschinnen, pellicules'). It is a loan word of Arab. حزاز, a skin disease that is identified as 'a lichen-like eruption on the skin' (Gr. λειχήν), cf. UW 385; or 'bran-like eruptions on the skin, scurf, dandruff' (Gr. πίτυρον), cf. UW 530–531; IJZ, 53, 113. For the parallel Arabic term قوباء, Plur. قواب, cf. UW 385–386: 'a lichen-like eruption on the skin' (Gr. λειχήν); see also IJZ 47, 105, n. 182. Constantine the African translates Arab. قواب as *impetigo*.
חֲזִירִי • לחם חזירי → לֶחֶם.
[חזק] • *Hitpa'el* הִתְחַזֵּק · I. to become inveterate, chronic: Arab. استحكم · Ibn al-Jazzār, *Zād al-musāfir wa-qūt al-ḥādir* · trans. Abraham ben Isaac, *Sefer Ṣedah la-Oreḥim*,

113 As a parallel term for Arab. *shaqāqul*, Hebr. *ha-ḥotam Shlomoh* features as שין שילמה (LA שאיל) in LF 3:450.

114 RYNṢY: I.e., purple starthistle [*Centaurea calcitrapa* L.], but often identified with secacul; cf. G. Ineichen (ed.), *El Libro Agregà de Serapiom*, vol. 2: *Volgarizzamento di frater Jacobus Philippus de Padua* (Florence 1966), 189, s.v. 'rinçi.' (I thank Sebastian Lauschus for this reference).

115 '*bahaq*': For this skin disease, three kinds of which are distinguished by Ibn al-Jazzār (dust-colored, white, and black), cf. IJZ 49–53, 108–113.

bk. 1, ch. 18: דע כי ראוי תחילה להקיז בעל החולי הזה הנקרא ברסאם ובלשון יון פראניטיס כדי שלא יתחזק החולי (You should know that first of all one should bleed a patient suffering from this disease that [in Arab.] is called *birsām* [i.e., برسام, phrenitis] and in Gr. *phrenitis* [i.e., φρενῖτις] so that it does not become chronic). Hebr. הִתְחַזֵּק does not feature in this sense in the current dictionaries. Moses ibn Tibbon translates Arab. استحكم as נגמר (cf. BCD 47 (NM 4:33)).

‣ II. **to be forced:** Lat. *cogi* · Constantinus Africanus, *Viaticum* · trans. Do'eg ha-Edomi, *Sefer Ya'ir Netiv*, bk. 3, ch. 11: ונוכל להבין להקרא האורטומיא כי הסובלים אותה מתחזקים לעמוד זקופים (We can understand why [this illness] is called 'orthopnea' because those who suffer from it are forced to stand upright). Hebr. הִתְחַזֵּק does not feature in this sense in the current dictionaries.

חֲזֶרֶת • חזרת החמור ‣ (lit., donkey's lettuce); dandelion [*Taraxacum officinale* Webb] · *Shinnui ha-Shemot ha-Niqra'im Synonimis*, Ms Munich, Bayerische Staatsbibliothek, Cod. hebr. 8, fol. 197[a]: הופילוס הוא אחד משמות חזרת החמור (HWPYLWS (cf. StH 1991; IB 2255: هرفلوس); i.e., one of the names of dandelion). Hebr. חזרת החמור, a calque from Arab. خسّ الحمار (cf. MIG 1062) features in BM 1499 in a reference from the *Sefer ha-Qanun*; however, Ben-Yehuda does not give its meaning.

חִטָּה • חטה מבושלת ‣ porridge cooked with [meat and] grains: Arab. هريسة (*harīsa*)[116] · Ibn al-Jazzār, *Zād al-musāfir wa-qūt al-ḥāḍir* · trans. Moses ibn Tibbon, *Sefer Ṣedat ha-Derakhim*, bk. 3, ch. 8: ואם היהה הרקיקה מסדיקת העורק או חתוך נצוה שיעשה רפואות שהם דבקות וקובצות מעט בלא עקיצה ולא חדוד ... ויזון בחטה מבושלת ומנודטץ (If the spitting of blood is caused by the rupture or cut of a vein, we tell [the patient] to use remedies that are slightly viscous and astringent but are not acrid or sharp [...] and to feed himself with porridge cooked with [meat and] grains and noodles). Hebr. חטה מבושלת does not feature in this sense in the current dictionaries. Shem Tov ben Isaac renders Arab. هريسة as דיסא in the *Sefer ha-Shimmush*, bk. 27 (cf. BCD 56 (NM 4:38)).

חֹטֶם • קנה החוטם → קָנֶה.

חַי ‣ raw: Arab. نيء · Isḥāq ibn ʿImrān, *Treatise on Melancholy* · trans. Anonymous, fol. 43[a] (44[a]): ואין מי שינצל ממנה מפני שטבע הבלגם החי להאריך החולי לפי שאינו מתבשל אלא לאחר זמן ארוך ואינו מתמסס אלא מעט מעט (No one can escape from it [i.e., from the semi-tertian fever] because it is in the nature of the raw phlegm to prolong the disease since it is only concocted after a long time and only dissolved little by little). In the

116 On *harīsa*, cf. FL 4:384: 'Spissi pulmenti species, quod ex cocto tritico, coctosque carnibus, simul contusis multum, conficitur' (A kind of thick dish, prepared from cooked wheat and cooked meats that are thoroughly pounded together); NA 606–607: 'smooth porridge cooked with meat and grains such as rice or wheat'. See also Maimonides, *On Coitus* 6 (BMC 40): 'It is prepared from sheep's meat or rooster testicles, and spiced with the spices that we have mentioned; one may [also] sprinkle cinnamon (cassia) over it;' for a variety of recipes cf. ISW 128–140 (ch. 50) (Arab.); NA 256–258 (Engl.).

sense of 'raw,' Hebr. חַי features in BM 1515–1516 in attestations from the Bible and Rabbinic literature.

• **סיד חי** → סִיד.

חיסור → חִסּוּר.

חָכָם • נפשות חכמות ממללות → נֶפֶשׁ.

חָכְמָה • חכמת התכנית · **geometry**: Arab. علم الهندسة · Isḥāq ibn ʿImrān, *Treatise on Melancholy* · trans. Anonymous, fol. 44[a] (45[a]): והמעיינים בחכמת[117] התכנית והוא שאומ׳ לה בערבי הנדשה (… and those who study the science of geometry, which is called *handasah* in Arabic). Hebr. חכמת התכנית is not attested for in this sense in the current dictionaries; the term תכנית features in the Bible in the sense of 'measurement, proportion' (cf. BDB 1067).

• **חכמת הקווים** · **geometry**: Arab. علم الخطوط · Isḥāq ibn ʿImrān, *Treatise on Melancholy* · trans. Anonymous, fol. 44[a] (45[a]): וחכמת המדות והוא הנק׳ חכמת הקוים ובלשון רומיים ג׳ומטריא[118] (… and the science of measurements called 'geometry' and in Latin *geometria*). Hebr. חכמת הקוים is not attested for in the current dictionaries. The synonymous חכמת המדות features in KTP 1:295.

חָלָב • חלב חמורה · **ass's milk**: Lat. *lac asininum* (Arab. لبن الأتن) · Constantinus Africanus, *Viaticum* · trans. Do'eg ha-Edomi, *Sefer Ya'ir Netiv*, bk. 3, ch. 1: או עם חלב תישית או חמורה (… or with [a gargle] from goat's milk or ass's milk). Hebr. חֲמוֹרָה features in the current dictionaries with attestations from Rabbinic literature; cf. JD 476, BM 1618, EM 552. Moses ibn Tibbon translates Arab. الأتن as אתון.

• **אבן החלב** → אֶבֶן.

חָלַב • *Pass. Part.* **חָלוּב • חלוב מיד** · **fresh (re: milk)**: Arab. حليب · Ibn al-Jazzār, *Zād al-musāfir wa-qūt al-ḥādir* · trans. Moses ibn Tibbon, *Sefer Ṣedat ha-Derakhim*, bk. 3, ch. 2: הנה ראוי לנו כשראינו מופתי הבשול במורסא המתהוה תוך הגרון וידענו כי כבר קבצה המוגלא שנערים אז ונדקדק לפתחה ולא נעשה לה רפואות חזקות אבל נכון בו בקלות כמו שיגרגר בחלב עז חלוב מיד (Once we see signs that the tumor in the throat has cocted and know that the pus has accumulated, we should use our skill and expertise to open it. However, we should not apply strong medications but light ones, as, for example, a gargle of fresh goat's milk). Hebr. חלוב מיד does not feature in the current dictionaries. In addition to חלוב מיד, Moses ibn Tibbon renders Arab. حليب as נחלב מיד (see entry below). Constantine the African does not translate the term حليب; consequently it is missing in Do'eg ha-Edomi's translation as well.

• *Part. Nif'al* **נֶחֱלָב • נחלב מיד** · **fresh (re: milk)**: Arab. حليب · Ibn al-Jazzār, *Zād al-musāfir wa-qūt al-ḥādir* · trans. Moses ibn Tibbon, *Sefer Ṣedat ha-Derakhim*, bk. 3, ch. 1: או יקח אמידום ויותך בחלב שנחלב מיד וישים נו פניס ושמן שקדים ומעט לב זרע קשואים

---

117 בחכמת: emendation editor בחכמות Ms.

118 ג׳ומטריא: emendation editor ג׳ומטריקא Ms.

שחוק ויאכלנו בעל האסכרה (One can also take starch, dissolve it in fresh milk, add sugar candy, almond oil, and some pounded cucumber seeds without their skin and let the partient suffering from angina eat this). Hebr. נחלב מיד is not attested for in the current dictionaries. In addition to נחלב מיד, Moses ibn Tibbon renders Arab. حليب as חלוב מיד (see entry above). The corresponding term in Shem Tov ben Isaac's *Sefer ha-Shimmush*, bk. 27, is תכף שנחלב (cf. BCD 282, s.v. שְׁפוֹת (NM 4:211)). Constantine the African does not translate the term حليب; consequently it is missing in Do'eg ha-Edomi's translation as well.

• *Hifʿil* הֶחֱלִיב ‣ **to pour out milk**: Arab. حلب · Ibn al-Jazzār, *Zād al-musāfir wa-qūt al-ḥāḍir* · trans. Abraham ben Isaac, *Sefer Ṣedah la-Oreḥim*, bk. 1, ch. 24: ואם יולד אלתשנג' מחמת הריקנות אז ראוי שנחליב על ראש החולה חלב שלאתון או חלב שלעז או חלב של אשה בחורה (If spasms occur because of [the nerves] being empty, one should pour on the patient's head ass's milk, ewe's milk, or milk of a mother of a [baby] girl). Hebr. הֶחֱלִיב is not attested for in the current dictionaries. Moses ibn Tibbon translates Arab. حلب as חלב. Do'eg translates the parallel Latin term *mulgeo* as טבל.

חֶלְבָּא (*Aram.*) • **חלבא דארעא** ‣ **earthworms**: Arab. شحمة الأرض, syn. خراطين (cf. MIG 1045) · Shem Tov ben Isaac, *Sefer ha-Shimmush*, bk. 29, list 1 (SHS 1:221–222 (Ḥet 21)): חלבא דארעא ב"ה שחמה אלארץ' (*ḥelba de arʿa*; Arab. *shaḥma al-arḍ*). In the sense of 'earthworms,' Aram. חלבא דארעא is a non-attested calque of Arab. شحمة الأرض. The reason that the term has been coined in Aramaic instead of Hebrew was possibly in order to distinguish it from Bibl. Hebr. חלב הארץ as featuring in Gen 45:18: ואכלו את חלב הארץ (And you shall live off the fat of the land), which is translated by Onkelos as: טובא דארעא and by Pseudo-Jonathan as: שמנומיתא דארעא.

חָלוּב (*Pass. Part.*) → חָלַב.

חֳלִי • **החלי היבש** ‣ **I. phthisis**: Arab. السلّ · Isḥāq ibn ʿImrān, *Treatise on Melancholy* · trans. Anonymous, fol. 51b (52b): ואני אומר שהשרטן הנהריי צלויים או מבושלים במי השעורים או במים ומלח יועילם כי מכח הסרטן להועיל מן הדאבון והחולי היבש (I say that river crabs roasted or cooked in barley water or in water and salt, are good for them [i.e., for those suffering from melancholy] because [river] crab is, by its [specific] property, beneficial for wasting and for phtisis). Hebr. החלי היבש features in BCD 96 (NM 3:83) in an attestation from the *Sefer Agur*, i.e., Do'eg ha-Edomi's translation of a Latin version of Hippocrates' *Aphorisms* 3.29. Constantine the African translates Arab. الذبول والسلّ as *phthisicos et macilentos*.[119]

‣ II. **wasting diseases**: Arab. الأمراض السلية والذبولية · al-Rāzī, *K. fī al-faṣd* · trans. Anonymous, *Maʾamar ba-haqazah*, Ms Parma, Bibliotheca Palatina, Cod. Parm. 2283,4, fol. 91a: אמ' אבובכר בעבור היות הדם יותר ישר משאר הליחות אשר באדם ובו החמימות הטבעי אשר הוא קיום החיות והוא כמו העצים אל האש והוא ישמין ויבריאהו

119 Cf. entry דְּאָבוֹן.

וישמחהו ויסיר האנחות וימנע ממנו החלי היבש הנק׳ אלסליה או אלדבוליא (Says Abu Bakr: Blood is more balanced than the other humors in the [human body]; it contains the natural heat, which is the foundation of life; it is like wood [that is used] for a fire; it makes a human being bountiful, healthy, and cheerful by taking away sadness; it prevents him from being affected by wasting diseases that are called [in Arab.] *al-silliya* or *al-dhubūliyya*).

• **חלי העינים** · **ophthalmia**: Arab. رمد · Isḥāq ibn ʿImrān, *Treatise on Melancholy* · trans. Anonymous, fol. 42ª (43ª): כגון הברסאם והקדחת השלישית וכאב הצד וחולי העינים והדומה להם (… just as phrenitis, tertian fever, pleurisy, ophthalmia, and the like). Hebr. חולי העינים does not feature in the sense of 'ophthalmia' in the current dictionaries. Nathan ha-Me'ati transcribes Arab. رمد in his translation of Maimonides, *Medical Aphorisms* 9.31 (BMMN 107) as רמד and Zeraḥyah Ḥen renders it as חולי העין הנק׳ רמד. Shem Tov ben Isaac renders Arab. رمد as אפר (*Sefer Almansur*; BMZ 16 (Alef 17)) and אפר העינים (*Sefer ha-Shimmush*, bk. 30) (cf. BCD 26 (NM 1:78)).

• **חלי השחורה** · **melancholy**: Lat. *melancolia* (Arab. مالنخوليا) · Constantinus Africanus, *Viaticum* · trans. Do'eg ha-Edomi, *Sefer Ya'ir Netiv*, bk. 1, ch. 20: ועל כן אם לא יהיה נעזר בענין שיוסרו הרהורי נפשו ומחשבותיו להקל מעל הנפש הנה הוא מוכרח לנפול בחולי מלנקוניא כי כמו שיפלו בסבת רב יגיעת הגוף במדוה גדול וחזק כן ביגיעת הנפש יפלו בחולי השחורה (For this reason, if he [i.e., someone suffering from lovesickness] gets no treatment to lighten his brooding and gloomy thoughts, he will unavoidably fall into a melancholic disease. Just as people will fall into a serious, grave disease from excessive physical exertion, they will fall into melancholy from psychical exertion). Hebr. חלי השחורה features in BCD 98 (NM 3:87) in a later attestation from Joseph Delmedigo's translation of Hippocrates' *Aphorisms* 3.14. Moses ibn Tibbon and Abraham ben Isaac translate Arab. مالنخوليا as מרה שחורה.

• *Plur.* **חלאים** • **חלאי הנפש** · **affections of the soul (i.e., emotions)**:[120] Arab. الآلام النفسانية · Isḥāq ibn ʿImrān, *Treatise on Melancholy* · trans. Anonymous, fol. 50ᵇ (51ᵇ): המאמר ביישור השש סבות על בעלי המלאמקו׳ והיאך תהיה רפואתם והם האויר המקיף והנום והתעורה והמלוי וההרקה והתנועה וההשקט וחלאי הנפש והמזון (Chapter on the equalisation of the six elementary factors [i.e., *sex res non naturales*] for those who suffer from melancholy and how they can be cured. These [six] things are: the surrounding air, sleep and waking, repletion and evacuation, movement and rest, affections of the soul, food [and drink]). Hebr. חלאי הנפש is not attested for in the current dictionaries. Constantine the African translates Arab. الآلام النفسانية as *accidentia animae*.

120 In addition to חלאי הנפש, we find שיחת הנפש for the Arabic synonym الأحداث النفسانية. See entry שיחת הנפש: שִׂיחָה.

חָלָל • חלל החזה › **chest cavity:** Arab. فضاء الصدر (FAL 1225) · Ibn al-Jazzār, *Zād al-musāfir wa-qūt al-ḥādir* · trans. Moses ibn Tibbon, *Sefer Ṣedat ha-Derakhim*, bk. 3, ch. 11: ואולם הנשימה הגבוהה היא אשר יצטרך האדם להניע החזה שלו כלו תנועה תכופה והנשימה הזאת היא הנקראת רבו ר״ל גוייש ונשימת הזקיפה וזה יהיה מאחת מג׳ סבות: אם מחוזק הצורך אל הנשימה כמו שיקרה לבריאים כשיתנועעו תנועה חזקה ואם לצרות חלל החזה כמו שיקרה למי שבו מורסא או יציאה בחזהו ואם לצרות ראש מעבר הנשימה (However, [the condition of] difficult breathing [lit., breathing high (in the chest)] during which someone has to move the whole chest frequently is called 'asthma,' i.e., [Rom.] GWYYŠ or 'orthopnea.' It is caused by one of three things: Either because of a strong need for breath(ing) as happens to healthy people when they move strenuously, or because of the narrowness of the chest cavity as it happens to someone who has a tumor or abscess in his chest, or because of the narrowness of the beginning of the trachea ...). Hebr. חלל החזה features in MD 142, s.v. 'cavity, thoracic.' Do'eg ha-Edomi translates the parallel Latin term *spacio thoracis* as חזה.

• *Plur.* **חללים** › **vessels; channels:** Arab. أوعية · Ibn al-Jazzār, *Zād al-musāfir wa-qūt al-ḥādir* · trans. Moses ibn Tibbon, *Sefer Ṣedat ha-Derakhim*, bk. 3, ch. 12: והסבה בשעול המתמיד כי החומר באברים המושכים רוח הנשימה וכשיהיה אשר ילך בם רוח הנשימה שום דבר שיזיקהו ישתדל הטבע בכל ענין לדחות אותו ולהוציאו ממנו בשעול ורקיקה (The reason that [someone suffering from pleurisy] coughs all the time is that when the matter that is in the organs by which one inhales the air is damaged, nature tries to expel it in any way through coughing and expectoration). Hebr. *Sing.* חָלָל features in the current dictionaries in the sense of 'concavity, empty space, hollow' (JD 470; BM 1580). For different meanings in medieval medical literature, see BCD 99–100.

[חלק] • *Part. Hif'il* **מַחְלִיק • הרפואה המחליקה** → **רְפוּאָה**.

חָלָק • יותר חלק › **milder:** Lat. *lenior* (Arabic أيسر) · Constantinus Africanus, *Viaticum* · trans. Do'eg ha-Edomi, *Sefer Ya'ir Netiv*, bk. 1, ch. 18: ואם החולי יהיה עם דאגה נכלכל הכח תחילה עם דברים יותר חלקים (If the disease is annoying [but not dangerous], we first of all enhance the strength [of the patient] with a treatment that is milder). Hebr. חָלָק features in the current dictionaries in the sense of 'bald, smooth, slippery,' but cf. BCD 101 (NM 1:149): 'soft.' Moses ibn Tibbon translates Arab. أيسر as יותר קל and Abraham ben Isaac as קל.

חֵלֶק • החלק הדבק › **conjunctiva:** Lat. *coniunctiva* (Arab. الحجاب الملتحم)[121] · Constantinus Africanus, *Viaticum* · trans. Do'eg ha-Edomi, *Sefer Ya'ir Netiv*, bk. 2, ch. 1: והסבה כאשר יקרה פנימית וחיצונה החיצונה היא גדולה או קטנה כי סבתה היא העשן וחום השמש או האבק והסבה הפנימית היא מהליחות אשר נזולו אל החלק הדבק[122] (The cause of it [i.e., ophthalmia], when it occurs, is internal or external; the external [cause] is major or minor,

121 As synonyms of החלק הדבק (Lat. *coniunctiva*), we find החלק המחוברת (see entry below), הכתונת החוברת (see entry כֻּתֹּנֶת), and חוֹבֶרֶת (see entry חָבֵר).

122 הדבק: המחוברת Ms Parma, Bibliotheca Palatina, Cod. Parm. 2474, fol. 26b.

i.e., smoke, heat of the sun, or dust; the internal cause is one of the humors that streams to the conjunctiva). Hebr. החלק הדבק does not feature in the current dictionaries. Moses ibn Tibbon translates Arab. الحجاب الملتحم as הירִיעה הלבנה (cf. BCD 121 (NM 4:77)).

• **החלק המחוברת** · **conjunctiva**: Lat. *coniunctiva* (Arab. الحجاب الملتحم) · Constantinus Africanus, *Viaticum* · trans. Do'eg ha-Edomi, *Sefer Ya'ir Netiv*,[123] bk. 2, ch. 1 (Ms Parma, Bibliotheca Palatina, Cod. Parm. 2474, fol. 26[b]): והסבה כאשר יקרה פנימית וחיצונה החיצונה היא גדולה או קטנה כי סבתה היא העשן וחום השמש או האבק והסבה הפנימית היא מהליחות אשר נזולו אל החלק המחוברת[124] ([The cause of it [i.e., ophthalmia], when it occurs, is internal or external; the external [cause] is major or minor, i.e., smoke, heat of the sun, or dust; the internal cause is one of the humors that streams to the conjunctiva). Hebr. החלק המחוברת does not feature in the current dictionaries. Moses ibn Tibbon translates Arab. الحجاب الملتحم as הירִיעה הלבנה (cf. BCD 121 (NM 4:77)).

חֲלָקוּת · **clarity**: Lat. *planitas* (Arab. إبانة) · Constantinus Africanus, *Viaticum* · trans. Do'eg ha-Edomi, *Sefer Ya'ir Netiv*, bk. 3, ch. 4: שפלות הקול הוא מלחות מפריד[125] כלי הקול וזה הלחות מהלבנה או מהדם והוא ברדתו מן הראש יפריד כלי הקול וישחית חלקות הדבור (Hoarseness originates from moisture that pours[126] upon the instruments of the voice. It is moisture consisting of phlegm or blood, when it streams from the head it pours[127] upon the instruments of the voice and destroys clarity of speaking). In the sense of 'clarity,' Hebr. חֲלָקוּת is a non-attested semantic borrowing from Lat. *planitas*. Moses ibn Tibbon translates Arab. إبانة as באור.

חֲלָשׁ · **lacking courage; anxious**: Arab. جبان · Isḥāq ibn 'Imrān, *Treatise on Melancholy* · trans. Anonymous, fol. 45[a] (46[a]): וכמו כן אלו היה מאחר לענות דומם חלש ואחר כך ראינוהו ממהר לענות ומרבה לדבר והראה קלות וגבורה הורנו מעשיו אלו שהגיע זה החולי אליו (Likewise, if someone is slow to answer [a question], silent, lacking courage [i.e., anxious], and then we see that he is quick to answer [a question], talkative, and that he shows courage and bravery, we learn from this that he is affected by this disease [i.e. melancholy]). Hebr. חֲלָשׁ does not feature in this sense in the current dictionaries. Constantine the African translates Arab. جبان as *timidus*.

חֲלְשָׁה • **חולשת הראש** · **indolence**: Lat. *pigritia* (Arab. كسل) · Constantinus Africanus, *Viaticum* · trans. Do'eg ha-Edomi, *Sefer Ya'ir Netiv*, bk. 1, ch. 22 (fol. 22[a]): והנה החרדה והכובד הולכים לפני האפילמסיא מהליחות אשר בראש המוח וחולשת הראש ומחשך העינים (The epilepsy that is caused by superfluities in the front part of the brain is preceded by

---

123 As synonyms of החלק המחוברת (Lat. *coniunctiva*), we find החלק הדבק (see entry above), הכתונת החוברת (see entry כְּתֹנֶת), and חוֹבֶרֶת (see entry חָבֵר).

124 המחוברת: הדבק Ms Oxford, Bodleian Library, Can. Or. 26, fol. 252[b].

125 מפריד: *infundens* L.

126 'pours upon': Trans. after L.

127 'pours upon': Trans. after L.

anxiety, heaviness [in the head], indolence, and loss [lit., darkness] of vision). Hebr. חולשת הראש does not feature in the current dictionaries. Moses ibn Tibbon possibly reads the parallel Arabic term كسل as كسر and translated it as שברון. Abraham ben Isaac renders Arab. كسل as עיכוב ההרגשות (see entry עִכּוּב).

חָמוּץ • הרוח החמוץ היוצא מן הגרון → רוּחַ.

חִמּוּץ • חמוץ המאכלים ‣ **sour foods**: Lat. *acrumines ciborum* (Arab. الأشياء الحامضة) · Constantinus Africanus, *Viaticum* · trans. Do'eg ha-Edomi, *Sefer Ya'ir Netiv*, bk. 2, ch. 20: וכן השנים סובלות לפעמים מחמוץ המאכלים (Sometimes the teeth are affected by [the consumption of] sour foods). Hebr. חִמּוּץ features in Rabbinic literature in the sense of 'becoming sour, fermentation, leavening' (JD 457); for medieval literature it is attested for in an attestation from Me'ir Aldabi, *Shevilei Emunah*, as חימוץ האתרוגים 'the acidic inner part of the lemon' (cf. BCD 103 (NM 1:150)). Moses ibn Tibbon translates Arab. الأشياء الحامضة as דברים חמוצים.

חָמוֹר • חזרת החמור → חֲזֶרֶת.

• *Plur.* חמורים • ורדי החמורים → וֶרֶד.

חֲמוֹרָה • חלב חמורה → חָלָב

חֹמֶץ • חומץ אתרוג ‣ **citron pulp**: Lat. *acetum mali citrini* (Arab. حمّاض الأترجّ) · Constantinus Africanus, *Viaticum* · trans. Do'eg ha-Edomi, *Sefer Ya'ir Netiv*, bk. 1, ch. 19: ויאות לחזקו בתרנוגלים קטנים ופרדיץ ובורטולייגא עם חומץ וירגיל חומץ אתרוג ורמונים גם נשפילש וחבושים ודומיהם (One should strengthen him with young chickens, partridge, and common purslane with vinegar; he should take citron pulp and pomegranate; also common medlars, quinces, and the like). Hebr. חומץ אתרוג does not feature in the current dictionaries. Moses ibn Tibbon translates Arab. حمّاض الأترجّ as חמיצות האתרוג (cf. BCD 103 (NM 4:71)) and Abraham ben Isaac as חומץ אתרוגים. The same Arabic term is translated by Zeraḥyah Ḥen as חימוץ האתרוגים in his translation of Maimonides, *Medical Aphorisms* 22.52 (BMMZ 213; cf. BCD 103 (NM 1:150)).

חִנּוּק ‣ **strangulation**: Arab. اختناق · Isḥāq ibn ʿImrān, *Treatise on Melancholy* · trans. Anonymous, fol. 49[b] (50[b]): ויארע להם החנוק וזוב טפת הזרע ויציאת הצואה והשתן מבלי חפץ (And they [i.e., those who suffer from epilepsy] will also suffer from suffocation, and unvoluntary flow of sperm [i.e., ejaculation], defecation, and urination). Hebr. חִנּוּק only features as a modern term in EM 559 in an attestation from Agnon, *Hakhnasat Kallah*.

[חנך] • *Hitpaʿel* הִתְחַנֵּךְ ‣ **to be rubbed**: Arab. حنّك (cf. D 1:332: 'frotter le palais de l'enfant nouveau-né avec de l'huile d'amande, de l'eau de grenade …') · Ms Cambridge, T-S K14.48, P8 (verso): דבש התחנך בו החיך יועיל מחולי השקדים והאסכרה ויועיל לשעול וישלשל השתן (Honey rubbed on the palate is good for the illness [i.e., swelling] of the tonsils, diphteriah, cough, and dysuria). In the sense of 'to be rubbed,' Hebr. הִתְחַנֵּךְ is a non-attested calque from Arab. حَنَّكَ.

חֶנֶק ‣ **angina**: Arab. ذبحة · Ibn al-Jazzār, *Zād al-musāfir wa-qūt al-ḥāḍir* · trans. Moses ibn Tibbon, *Sefer Ṣedat ha-Derakhim*, bk. 3, ch. 1: וכבר זכר גליינוס כי כל מה שיקרה בגרון

שיעצור הנשימה יקרא אסכרה והוא חנק[128] (Galen has said that everything that occurs to the throat and stops breathing is called 'angina,' i.e., [Hebr.] *ḥeneq*). Hebr. חֶנֶק only features as a medical term in BM 1661 in the sense of 'hysterical suffocation.' In the sense of 'angina,' Hebr. חֶנֶק features in BCD 104–105 (NM 1:151) in later attestations from Zeraḥyah Ḥen's translation of Maimonides, *Medical Aphorisms* 25.11 (BMMZ 245) and his translation of Hippocrates' *Aphorisms* 1.12. Do'eg ha-Edomi transcribes Lat. *sinancia* ('quinsy') as שיגנסיאה. For the variant reading מַחֲנָק, featuring in Ms London, British Library, Add. 27542, cf. entry.

חִסּוּר • חסור הדם · bloodletting: Lat. *diminutio* [*sanguinis*] · Constantinus Africanus, *Viaticum* · trans. Do'eg ha-Edomi, *Sefer Ya'ir Netiv*, bk. 1, ch. 18: בטרם יעלה החולי יתכן להקיזו ולחסר דמו כפי כחו לסבול רק נשמור שלא יעכבו דברים אחרים ואחר חסור הדם נעזור אליו עם קאטרטיקש (Before the illness [i.e., phrenitis] gets worse, it is possible to bleed [the patient] according to his strength, but we should be careful lest other things make this impossible. After the bloodletting we should treat him with cathartic remedies). Hebr. חסור הדם is a non-attested loan translation from Lat. *diminutio* [*sanguinis*]. The term חִסּוּר is attested for in Rabbinic literature in the sense of 'lack, want' (cf. JD 458; BM 1665), and as an arithmetical term in the sense of 'substraction,' a.o., in Abraham ibn Ezra's *Sefer ha-Mispar* (cf. BM 1665; KTP 1:316).

• חיסור הירח · waning of the moon: Arab. نقصان القمر · Ibn al-Jazzār, *Zād al-musāfir wa-qūt al-ḥādir* · trans. Abraham ben Isaac, *Sefer Ṣedah la-Oreḥim*, bk. 1, ch. 22 (Ms Florence, Biblioteca Medicina Laurenziana, Plut. 88.37, fol. 96^{b}): ואת אשר יקרה לו מזה החולי בחיסור הירח יוכיח כי היסוד ההוא שלריאומה הקראסיס שלזה קור הוא גם היא רטיבות קלה ([Epileptic fits] that occur at the waning of the moon prove that the humor [that causes them] has a cold temperament and little moisture). Hebr. חיסור הירח is not attested for in the current dictionaries. Moses ibn Tibbon translates Arab. نقصان القمر as חסרון הירח (see entry חֶסְרוֹן). Do'eg ha-Edomi translates Lat. *luna deficiens* as חסור הלבנה (see next entry).

• חסור הלבנה · waning of the moon: Lat. *luna deficiens* (Arab. نقصان القمر) · Constantinus Africanus, *Viaticum* · trans. Do'eg ha-Edomi, *Sefer Ya'ir Netiv*, bk. 1, ch. 22: איפלמסיא הבאה בגדול הלבנה יראה טבעה להיות לחה מאד כי כל דבר לח יגדל בגדול הלבנה והבאה בחסור הלבנה היא קרה מאד ואולם היא לחה קצת (As for epileptic fits occurring when the moon waxes, the matter [that causes them] is extremely moist. For all moist things grow when the moon waxes. As for [epileptic fits] that occur at the waning of the moon, [the matter that causes them] is extremely cold and a little bit moist). Hebr. חיסור הלבנה is not attested for in the current dictionaries. Moses ibn Tibbon translates Arab. نقصان القمر as חסרון הירח (see entry חֶסְרוֹן), and Abraham ben Isaac as חיסור הירח (see previous entry).

---

128 והוא חנק: ומחנק Ms London, British Library, Add. 27542.

[חסר] • *Pi'el* **חִסֵּר** • **חיסר דם** ‧ **to bleed:** Lat. *minuo* [*sanguinem*] (Arab. فصد) · Constantinus Africanus, *Viaticum* · trans. Do'eg ha-Edomi, *Sefer Ya'ir Netiv*, bk. 2, ch. 25: ואם יתראו בפנים לבד נחסר דם הספליקא ואם יתפשטו בכל הגוף נקיזהו מן המקור האמצעי. (If [the freckles] only appear on the face, we bleed from the cephalic vein, but if they spread over the whole body, we bleed from the median vein). In the sense of 'to bleed,' Hebr. חיסר דם is a non-attested loan translation from Lat. *minuo* [*sanguinem*]. Moses ibn Tibbon translates Arab. فصد as הקיז.

חֹסֶר • **חוסר הגוף** ‧ **meagerness:** Arab. هزال · Isḥāq ibn ʿImrān, *Treatise on Melancholy* · trans. Anonymous, fol. 41ᵇ (42ᵇ): וישיג לגוף מפני שהולכות אחר הנפש נזק גדול מהתמדת התעורה וחוסר הגוף ושיחת[129] הנפש (And since [the afflictions] of the body follow [those of] the soul, severe harm through constant sleeplessness, meagerness, and sorrow[130] affects the body). Hebr. חוסר הגוף is not attested for in the current dictionaries. Constantine the African translates Arab. هزال as *macilentia*.

חֶסְרוֹן • **חסרון הירח** ‧ **waning of the moon:** Arab. نقصان القمر · Ibn al-Jazzār, *Zād al-musāfir wa-qūt al-ḥādir* · trans. Moses ibn Tibbon, *Sefer Ṣedat ha-Derakhim*, bk. 1, ch. 22: ומה שיקרה ממנו בחסרון הירח החומר המחדש הכפיה קר המזג מעט הלחות ([Epileptic fits] that occur at the waning of the moon [prove] that the matter that causes epilepsy has a cold temperament and little moisture). Hebr. חסרון הירח features in KTP 1:318 in an attestation from the *Moreh Nevukhim*, i.e., Samuel ibn Tibbon's translation of Maimonides' *Guide of the Perplexed* 2.10: תוספת הימים והנהרות בתוספת הירח וחסרונם בחסרנו. Abraham ben Isaac translates Arab. نقصان القمر as חיסור הירח (see entry חִסּוּר). Do'eg ha-Edomi translates Lat. *luna deficiens* as חסור הלבנה (see also entry חִסּוּר).

• **חסרון הפרנוס** ‧ **abstinence [from food]; lack of food:** Lat. *abstinentia* (Arab. نقصان الغذاء) · Ibn al-Jazzār, *Zād al-musāfir wa-qūt al-ḥādir* · trans. Abraham ben Isaac, *Sefer Ṣedah la-Oreḥim*, Adaptation, bk. 1, ch. 2 (Ms Berlin, Staatsbibliothek Preußischer Kulturbesitz, Or. fol. 1058, fol. 90ᵃ): אם נראה שנפילת השיער מחמת חסרון הפרנוס כאמור למעלה (When we see that the loss of hair has been caused by lack of food as mentioned above …). Hebr. חסרון הפרנוס does not feature in the current dictionaries. A synonym used by the anonymous adapter is הבדלת האוכל והמשתה (see entry הַבְדָּלָה). Do'eg ha-Edomi renders Lat. *abstinentia* as צום. Moses ibn Tibbon renders Arab. نقصان الغذاء as חסרון המזון and Abraham ben Isaac as חסרון הפרנסה.

• **חסרון הקול** ‧ **hoarseness:** Arab. بحح · Maimonides, *Medical Aphorisms* 22.45 · trans. Zeraḥyah Ḥen (BMMZ 212): אכילת הצנון והכרוביות יסיר חסרון הקול ואכילת הספרגלים הצלויים אחר המזון ישמח.[131] ואכילת קלפת האתרוגים יחזק הלב וזרעו יועיל מהסמום[132] וקלפת

---

129 ושיחת הנפש: والحزن a.
130 'sorrow': Trans. after a.
131 ישמח: ينشط ويفرح a.
132 מהסמום: السموم a.

הלומיא יועיל מהסמום[133] וכן עלי אילנו (The consumption of radish and cabbage eliminates hoarseness and the consumption of roasted quince after meals gives energy and joy. The consumption of citron peel strengthens the heart and its pits are beneficial against poisons. Lemon peel is [also] beneficial against poisons, as are the leaves of its tree). Hebr. חסרון הקול does not feature in the current dictionaries. Nathan ha-Me'ati translates Arab. بحح as צרידות הקול (cf. BCD 234 (NM 3:197)).

• **חסרון השמע** · **loss of hearing**: Lat. *diminutio auditus* (Arab. ثقل السمع) · Constantinus Africanus, *Viaticum* · trans. Do'eg ha-Edomi, *Sefer Ya'ir Netiv*, bk. 2, ch. 7: מחסרון השמע (On hearing loss). Hebr. חסרון השמע is not attested for in the current dictionaries. A Latin synonym to *diminutio auditus*, i.e., *gravitas auditus* is translated by Do'eg ha-Edomi as כובד השמע (see entry כֹּבֶד). Moses ibn Tibbon translates Arab. ثقل السمع as כבדות השמע (see entry כְּבֵדוּת).

חֵפֶץ • **תנועת החפץ** → תְּנוּעָה.

• **תנועות שלא מחפץ** → תְּנוּעָה.

חקנית* • *Plur.* **חקניות**[134] · **clysters**: Arab. حقن · Ibn al-Jazzār, *Zād al-musāfir wa-qūt al-ḥāḍir* · trans. Abraham ben Isaac, *Sefer Ṣedah la-Oreḥim*, bk. 1, ch. 22: אם יצטרכו לו חקניות הם קלישטירי אז יעשה לו חקניות חדות שיש בהן כמומילון ואניתון וקינטוריון ומילולוטה הוא אכליל אלמלך ושחם חנטל והדומה להם (If the patients [suffering from epilepsy] need clysters, i.e., [Rom.] QLYŠṬYRY, they should be given sharp clysters made from camomile, dill, centaury, melilot, i.e., [Arab.] *iklīl al-malik*, colocynth pulp, and the like). Hebrew חקנית*, *Plur.* חקניות, is a non-attested calque from Arab. حقنة, *Plur.* حقن. Do'eg ha-Edomi translates Lat. *clisterizor* as תשומת כלי (see entry תְּשׂוּמָה). Moses ibn Tibbon translates Arab. حقن as קלוחים (cf. BCD 243 (NM 4:183)).

חֹר • **הכניס בחור התחתון** → [כנס].

חֲרָדָה · **tremor**: Lat. *tremor* (Arab. رعشة) · Constantinus Africanus, *Viaticum* · trans. Do'eg ha-Edomi, *Sefer Ya'ir Netiv*, bk. 1, ch. 25: אך אפיסת הכח המניע הלאצרטוש הם ברדונש הוא סבה להתחלת החרדה (But weakness of the faculty that moves the muscles, i.e., [Rom.] BRDWNŠ, causes the beginning of a tremor). Hebr. חֲרָדָה is attested for in the Bible and Rabbinic literature in the sense of 'trembling, quaking' (of terror) (BDB 353), 'excitement, anxiety, fear, reverence' (JD 499), and 'terror' (BM 1740). Moses ibn Tibbon translates Arab. رعشة as רעש.

• **חרדת הישן** · **lucid stupor (i.e., catochus; coma vigil)**: Lat. *expergefactio a somno* (Arab. المنتبه (lit., the awake[135])) · Constantinus Africanus, *Viaticum* · trans. Do'eg ha-

133 מהסמום: السموم a.

134 *Plur.* חקניות is possibly equal to חקנות, and the singular not a theoretical חקנית but חקנה, a calque from Arab. حقنة, which is attested for in BM 1722 in an attestation from Me'ir Aldabi, *Shevilei Emunah*.

135 The disease called 'the awake' (Arab. *muntabih*) was mentioned by Dozy (D 2:638), who quoted from G. Dugat, 'Études sur le traité de médicine d'Abou Djàfar Ah'mad, intitulé: زاد

Edomi, *Sefer Ya'ir Netiv*,[136] bk. 1, ch. 15: מחרדת הישן: אם סוף המוח סובל ⟨מן⟩ בלבנה ומן האדומה שנתערבו יהיה החולה נעזב כמת ועיניו הם פקוחות (Lucid stupor [i.e., coma vigil]: If the posterior part of the brain suffers from phlegm and yellow bile and if they intermingle, the patient is left like a dead man, with his eyes open). Hebr. חרדת הישן does not feature in the current dictionaries. Moses ibn Tibbon renders Arab. المنتبه as מוקץ (see entry [קוץ]) and Abraham ben Isaac as חולי הנקרא בלשון ישמעאל מניה ובלשון יון מניאה.

• **חרדת המחשבה** ‣ **torpor; lethargy**: Lat. *stupor mentis* (Arab. سبات) · Constantinus Africanus, *Viaticum* · trans. Do'eg ha-Edomi, *Sefer Ya'ir Netiv*, bk. 1, ch. 16: חרדת המחשבה היא כמו שינה ועינים סגורות (Torpor is like sleep with the eyes closed). Hebr. חרדת המחשבה does not feature in the current dictionaries. Moses ibn Tibbon renders Arab. سبات as תרדמה (cf. BCD 298 (NM 4:222–223)) and Abraham ben Isaac as חולי הנקרא בלשון ישמעאל אלסבאת ובלש׳ יון ליתרגוס.

חֲרְפָּה ‣ **I. sharpness; pungency; acridity**: Lat. *pungens* (Arab. لذّاع) · Constantinus Africanus, *Viaticum* · trans. Do'eg ha-Edomi, *Sefer Ya'ir Netiv*, bk. 3, ch. 8: הכח הדוחה ינוע מאד בסבת הליחות המחודדות ובחורפתם או מהמלוחות לבנות ובלויות (The expulsive faculty becomes very active because of sharp, acrid humors or salt, phlegmatic or putrid humors). Hebr. חֲרְפָּה features in BM 1778 only in an attestation from Elijah Mizrachi's *Ḥokhmat ha-Mispar* (*On Arithmetics*). For the Aramaic counterpart חורפא, cf. SDA 443. Moses ibn Tibbon translates Arab. لذّاع as עוקץ.

‣ **II. gripe; colic**: Lat. *punctura* (Arab. مغص) · Constantinus Africanus, *Viaticum* · trans. Do'eg ha-Edomi, *Sefer Ya'ir Netiv*, bk. 3, ch. 14: אם הוא עשוי בכל הגוף נראה בכל האברים עיפות וכובד ואם הוא מהאסטומ׳ יתראו תמיד כל היום תמונות לנגד עיניו והרוח הנדחה מהגרון והאיסטניסות והכאב במצח אם הוא מהמעים יהיה כובד ונפח לבעלי השחורה והחורפה לבעלי האדומה (If the whole body is full with [superfluous matter], we observe that all the limbs of [someone suffering from fainting] are tired and heavy; if [only] the stomach is full, he will see images in front of his eyes the whole day long and he will [suffer] from eructation, vomiting, and headache. If the intestines are full

---

المسافر, *Zad al-mocafir*, 'La provision du voyageur',' *Journal asiatique* 5, no. 1 (1853): 341: 'du mal appelé el-mountabih, qui excite, qui tient réveillé.' Ibn al-Jazzār's description comes close to Paul of Aegina's account of the disease called κάτοχος ('catochus, or coma vigil;' cf. F. Adams (ed.), *The Seven Books of Paulus Ægineta: Translated from the Greek with Commentary Embracing a Complete View of the Knowledge Possessed by the Greeks, Romans, and Arabians on all Subjects Connected with Medicine and Surgery*, 3 vols. (London 1844–1847), 1:369ff.) Galen did not strictly differentiate between κάτοχος and κατάληψις ('catalepsy').

136 Cf. the quotation in the anonymous *Sefer ha-Yosher* (Ms Oxford, Bodleian Library, Opp. 180 (cat. Neubauer 2134), fol. 8[b]): מחרדת הישן כתב יצחק אם סוף המוח סובל מן שתי הליחות הלבנה והאדומה (On lucid stupor: Says R. Isaac: If the posterior part of the brain suffers from the two humors, i.e., phlegm and yellow bile ...).

of melancholic matter, he will suffer from heaviness and swellings; if they are full of bilious matter, he will suffer from gripes). Moses ibn Tibbon translates Arab. مغص as עצורים (cf. BCD 207 (NM 1:64)).

חַרְצִין • *Plur.* **חרצינים** ‣ **kernels; pits; stones:** Arab. عَجَم · Ibn al-Jazzār, *Zād al-musāfir wa-qūt al-ḥādir* · trans. Moses ibn Tibbon, *Sefer Ṣedat ha-Derakhim* bk. 3, ch. 12: ואם היה הטבע עצור נשלשל אותו במאנא וקשיא פישטולה מנוקה אחר שימרסהו במים שנתבשל בהם ג׳וג׳ובש פרונש ומעט צמוקים שהוסרו חרציניהם (If [the patient suffering from pleurisy] is constipated, we purge him with manna, purified purging cassia after it has been steeped in water in which common jujube, plums, and some pitless raisins have been cooked). Hebr. *Sing.* חַרְצִין is a variant reading of חַרְצָן and features in BM 1782 in an attestation from Sa'adya Gaon's commentary on tb*Berakhot*.

חָרָשׁ • *Plur.* **חרשים** • **חרשי ברזל** ‣ **metal workers (i.e., blacksmiths):** Arab. حدّادون · Ibn al-Jazzār, *Zād al-musāfir wa-qūt al-ḥādir* · trans. Moses ibn Tibbon, *Sefer Ṣedat ha-Derakhim* bk. 3, ch. 13: וישתה מי בוסר או מי רמונים עם מיראבלנוש ויחבוש האצטו׳ מחוץ בשני מיני השנדלש וקמח שעורים ואפר חרשי ברזל (He [i.e., someone suffering from palpitations] should drink juice from unripe, sour grapes, or from pomegranates with [citrine] myrobalan; on the outside of the stomach he should put a dressing of the two kinds of sandalwood, barley flour, and the ashes [resulting from the work] of the metal workers [i.e., blacksmiths]). Hebr. *Sing.* חרש ברזל is only attested for in biblical literature; cf. BDB 360; BM 1786. In the sense of 'metal worker,' the term חָרָשׁ on its own is attested for in Rabbinic literature (cf. SD 216). Do'eg ha-Edomi translates the parallel Latin term *ciner ferrarii* as דשן פיארירי.

חָשַׁב ‣ **to look at closely; to inspect; to examine:** Lat. *considero* (Arab. نظر) · Constantinus Africanus, *Viaticum* · trans. Do'eg ha-Edomi, *Sefer Ya'ir Netiv*, bk. 2, ch. 19: וכאשר נרצה לעזור אל העניינים האלה נחשב גוף החולה בעבור שנטהר שפעת הליחות ואחרי העזר המחזק והמטהר נשוב לתקן השנים כן: נכתוש גטלא אין נקובה עם עיני ליציא (When we want to treat these things, we should examine the body of the patient in order to purge it from the surplus of humors. Once we have applied a strengthening and a purging drug, we should treat the teeth as follows: pulverize gallnut that has no holes in it with wolfberry buds …). Hebr. חָשַׁב does not feature in this sense in the current dictionaries. Moses ibn Tibbon renders Arab. نظر as עיין.

חֲשֵׁיכוּת • **חשיכות העינים** ‣ **dimsightedness:** Arab. ظلمة البصر (Gr. ἀμβλυωπία) (cf. UW 90) · Ibn al-Jazzār, *Zād al-musāfir wa-qūt al-ḥādir* · trans. Abraham ben Isaac, *Sefer Ṣedah la-Oreḥim*, bk. 1, ch. 10: ועוד ריקוח אחר שתיקן בן מאוסיא והזכירו בספר אל בצירה יועיל מרוחות עבות התוקפות בגוף וגם יועיל לחשיכות העינים ולכובד הגוף מרוחות מרה שחורה ומריבוי הליחה וכל רפשיה הקרים העבים (Another recipe, described by Ibn Māsawayh in the book *al-Baṣīra*, which is good for coarse winds that attack the body and also for dimsightedness, heaviness of the body caused by winds [coming from] the black bile, a surplus of phlegm and all cold, viscous superfluities). Hebr. חשיכות העינים features as חשכות עינים in EM 597 in an attestation from Rashi's commentary on tb*Shabbat* 151.

Moses ibn Tibbon translates Arab. ظلمة البصر as כהות הראות (see entry כֵּהוּת). Do'eg ha-Edomi translates the parallel Latin term *obscuritas visus* as מחשך הראות.

חָתוּם (*Part. Pass.*) → **חָתַם**.

[חתך] • *Part. Nif'al* **נֶחְתָּךְ** • **decisive**: Arab. قطعي · Maimonides, *Medical Aphorisms* 25.72 · trans. Zeraḥyah Ḥen (BMMZ 269): והתבונן מה שיחיבנו האדם לשמוע[137] דעתו וממה שראוי שנתעורר עליו כי אילו היה אמת מה שזכרהו גליאינוס לא היה לו טענה נחתכת יבטל בו דעת אריסטו׳ בשהתחלת החוש והתנועה מן הלב (Consider to what consequences a person is necessarily lead when he wants to support[138] his opinion. One of the things that should be pointed out is that if what Galen says is correct, it would not be a decisive argument for refuting Aristotle's opinion that the principle of sensation and motion comes from the heart). In the sense of 'decisive,' Hebr. נֶחְתָּךְ is a non-attested calque from Arab. قطعي. Nathan ha-Me'ati translates Arab. قطعي as גּוֹזֵר (see entry גָּזַר).

חָתַם • *Part. Pass.* **חָתוּם** • **בול חתום** → **בּוּל**.

• **טיט חתום** → **טִיט**.

---

137 לשמוע: نصرة a.

138 'to support': Trans. after a.

ט

טְבִיעָה · **nature**: Arab. طبيعة · Ibn al-Jazzār, *Zād al-musāfir wa-qūt al-ḥādir* · trans. Abraham ben Isaac, *Sefer Ṣedah la-Oreḥim*, bk. 1, ch. 19: וכבר אמר אחד מן החכמים כי החשק הוא שם[139] חיבה וכמו שהחיבה[140] ריבוי הידידות כמו כן החשק ריבוי האהבה ושמא תהיה עילת החשק צורך הטביעה להוציא רפש הנשתלט בגוף (A philosopher said that lovesickness is a word signifying love.[141] For just as love[142] is an excess of friendship, so lovesickness is an excess of love. Occasionally, lovesickness is caused by a natural need to expel superfluities that dominated the body). In the sense of 'nature,' Hebr. טְבִיעָה is a non-attested loan word from Arab. طبيعة. Moses ibn Tibbon translates Arab. طبيعة as טבע.

טֶבַע · **matter (i.e., bodily fluid)**: Lat. *materia* (Arab. كيموس) · Constantinus Africanus, *Viaticum* · trans. Do'eg ha-Edomi, *Sefer Ya'ir Netiv*, bk. 1, ch. 22: והאיפלמסיא שכינה אל האפופלקשיא כי המקום ההוא עצמו והטבע מאשר נולדת הוא קר וגס אבל האיפופלקשיא תגזול כל הכח הרץ באברים (Epilepsy is closely related to apoplexy because [both originate from] that same place and the matter [i.e., bodily fluid] from which they originate is cold and coarse. The only [difference] is, that apoplexy takes away all the power that flows to the nerves). Hebr. טֶבַע does not feature in this sense in the current dictionaries. Moses ibn Tibbon translates Arab. كيموس as ליחה and Abraham ben Isaac as כימוס. Do'eg ha-Edomi again uses טֶבַע for Lat. *materia* in bk. 1, ch. 22: מאשר אמר גלינוס אפלמסיא הבאה בגדול הלבנה יראה טבעה להיות לחה מאד (As Galen stated: In the case of epilepsy occurring when the moon is waxing, the matter [that causes it] is extremely moist). The original Arabic term is المادّة, which is translated by Moses ibn Tibbon as חומר. Cf. also bk. 3, ch. 6, where Do'eg's טֶבַע stands for Constantine's *materia*, which in turn stands for Arab. رطوبة.

[טהר] • *Pi'el* **טִהֵר** · **1. to administer a cathartic**: Lat. *do catarticum* · Constantinus Africanus, *Viaticum* · trans. Do'eg ha-Edomi, *Sefer Ya'ir Netiv*, bk. 2, ch. 18: ואם ימנעו אלה האותות יאות להקיזו משני המקורות אשר תחת הלשון ויאות לטהרו עם ג'ירא פיגרא קשיא פישתולא (If these symptoms make [a venesection of the cephalic vein] impossible, one should bleed the two veins beneath the tongue and administer a cathartic of hiera picra and purging cassia). Hebr. טִהֵר features in biblical and Rabbinic literature in the sense of 'to cleanse, to purify' (cf. BDB 372; JD 520; BM 1840). Ben-Yehuda also mentions the term in the sense of 'to cleanse [the body from superfluities]' in an attestation from Abraham ibn Ezra's commentary on Ec 12:3.

---

139 שם חיבה: اسم لما فضل عن المحبّة a.

140 שהחיבה: أن النصح a.

141 'love': 'signifying a surplus of affection' a.

142 'love': 'loyalty' a.

‣ II. **to cleanse; to purify**: Lat. *purgo* · Constantinus Africanus, *Viaticum* · trans. Do'eg ha-Edomi, *Sefer Ya'ir Netiv*, bk. 2, ch. 18: וכאב השנים מליחות גסות יורדות מן הראש יאות לטהר עם טאודוריטון ודומיהם (When toothache is caused by coarse superfluities that descend from the head, they should be cleansed with [the hiera called] Theodoretus and the like).

• *Part. Pi'el* **מְטַהֵר • הרפואה המטהרת** → **רְפוּאָה**.

• *Part. Pu'al* **מְטֹהָר** ‣ **purified**: Arab. منقّى · Ibn al-Jazzār, *Zād al-musāfir wa-qūt al-ḥāḍir* · trans. Abraham ben Isaac, *Sefer Ṣedah la-Oreḥim*, bk. 1, ch. 10: כיאר שנבר מטוהר (purified purging cassia). Hebr. מְטֹהָר is not attested for in the current dictionaries in medieval medical literature. Moses ibn Tibbon translates Arab. منقّى as מנוקה.

טָהֳרָה ‣ I. **evacuation**: Arab. استفراغ · Ibn al-Jazzār, *Zād al-musāfir wa-qūt al-ḥāḍir* · trans. Abraham ben Isaac, *Sefer Ṣedah la-Oreḥim*, bk. 1, ch. 10 (Ms Jerusalem, National Library of Israel, Fr. 95, fol. 91[a]): ויוסיף עם אילו הסמים אחרי טהרת הגוף כיאר שנבר וכמומילון בנפסג' ושעורים קלופים (After the evacuation of the body, he should add to these [ingredients] purging cassia, camomile, violet [blossoms], and husked barley). Hebrew טָהֳרָה features in the sense of 'purefying, cleansing, pureness, purification' in the Bible and Rabbinic literature; cf. BDB 372–373; JD 520–521; BM 1849–1850. Moses ibn Tibbon translates Arab. استفراغ as הרקה.

‣ II. **purification**: Lat. *mundificatio* (Arab. إنقاء) · Constantinus Africanus, *Viaticum* · trans. Do'eg ha-Edomi, *Sefer Ya'ir Netiv*, bk. 1, ch. 15: ואחרי טהרת סוף המוח נכון לרחוץ ראשו במים שנתבשל בם קאמומילא ויאולא אניט מילילוד שמבוק ורדים ודומיהם (After the purification of the rear part of the brain, the [patient's] head should be washed with water in which camomile, violets, dill, melilot, marjoram, roses, and the like have been cooked). Moses ibn Tibbon translates the parallel Arabic term إنقاء as נקוי and Abraham ben Isaac as טהרה.

‣ III. **purgation**: Lat. *purgatio* · Constantinus Africanus, *Viaticum* · trans. Do'eg ha-Edomi, *Sefer Ya'ir Netiv*, bk. 3, ch. 3: ואולם דבר מועיל הוא שלא יחתך לפני טהרת הבטן אם העת ראוי לכך (But it is good not to cut [the uvula] before the stomach has been purged at the appropriate time).

טוֹב • האם הטובה → **אֵם**.

טיבשנא ‣ **drink or liquid food (i.e., porridge) made from barley**: Lat. *ptisana* (cf. DMLBS 2912) (Arab. حسو) · Constantinus Africanus, *Viaticum* · trans. Do'eg ha-Edomi, *Sefer Ya'ir Netiv*, bk. 3, ch. 6: ואחר כן יאות לתת לו אישופו ואישרוב העשוי מגוגובש ואחר ג' שעות נתן לו טיבשנא עם שמן שקד גם פניס ודבש ויאולד (Then one should give him [a decoction of] hyssop and syrup made from common jujube, and three hours later we give him a drink or liquid food made from barley with almond oil, sugar candy, or violet preserve). Hebr. טיבשנא is a non-attested loan word from Lat. *ptisana*. Moses ibn Tibbon translates Arab. حسو as דִּיְסָה (see entry). In addition to טיבשנא, Do'eg ha-Edomi (ibid.) uses the standard Hebrew term מרק, when recommending a porridge made from bran: מרק מסובין כמו טיבשנא.

טִיט · **pus**: Lat. *sanies* (cf. DMLBS 3282) (Arab. قيح) · Constantinus Africanus, *Viaticum* · trans. Do'eg ha-Edomi, *Sefer Ya'ir Netiv*, bk. 3, ch. 7: ואם לא יוכל לרוק כאשר יקשה הנפח יאות לתת לו דברים מחממים ומטהרים הדם והטיט ומביאים השעול (If he [i.e., the patient suffering from phtisis] cannot expectorate and the tumor has become hard one should give him ingredients that have a heating effect and that purify the blood and the pus and provoke cough). Hebr. טִיט does not feature in this sense in the current dictionaries. Variant readings are בלוי הטיט and בלוי עב הטיט (cf. also entry בְּלוֹי), featuring in the *Sefer Agur*, i.e., Do'eg ha-Edomi's translation of a Latin version of Hippocrates' *Aphorisms* (cf. BCD 36; NM 3:36–37). Moses ibn Tibbon translates Arab. قيح as מוגלא.
• **טיט חתום** · **sealed earth or clay (i.e., terra sigillata) from the island of Lemnos**:[143] Arab. طين مختوم (cf. MIG 1060) · *Shinnui ha-Shemot ha-Niqra'im Synonimis*, Ms Munich, Bayerische Staatsbibliothek, Cod. hebr. 8, fol. 198^b: טין מכתום הוא טיט חתום ([Arab.] *ṭīn makhtūm*; i.e., [Hebr.] *ṭiṭ ḥatum*). Hebr. טיט חתום is a calque from Arab. طين مختوم. The term also features in Shem Tov ben Isaac's *Sefer ha-Shimmush*, bk. 29, list 1 (cf. SHS 1:239–240 (Ṭet 1)). Instead of טיט, we find טין in Moses ibn Tibbon's translation of Maimonides, *On Poisons* 19 (BMP 77): *ha-ṭin he-ḥatum*.
• **בלויי עב טיט** → **בְּלוֹי**

טִיפְּשִׁי · **phthisis**: Lat. *ptisi* (abl. of *ptisis*: *de ptisi*) (Arab. ذبول) · Constantinus Africanus, *Viaticum* · trans. Do'eg ha-Edomi, *Sefer Ya'ir Netiv*, bk. 3, ch. 7: טיפשי הוא השחתת ליחות הגוף (Phthisis is a corrosion of the humors of the body). Hebr. טיפשי is a non-attested loan word from Lat. *ptisi*. Moses ibn Tibbon renders Arab. ذبول as שדפון.

טישט · **skull**: Lat. *testa* · Guillaume de Congenis, *Treatise on Surgery* · trans. Isaiah, fol. 45^b: כאשר נפח מהמכה בלי שבירת הטישט מגיד שזה התחבושת יועיל להרגיע הכאב (When a swelling [occurs on the head] because of a blow but the skull is not fractured, it indicates that the following poultice is useful for alleviating the pain). Hebr. טישט is a non-attested loan word from Lat. *testa* or Rom. *test*.

טִמְטוּם · **obstruction**: Arab. سدّ · Isḥāq ibn ʿImrān, *Treatise on Melancholy* · trans. Anonymous, fol. 49^a (50^a): וכשאזכור האבלאמסיא אזכור גבולו ואומר שהאבלמסיא לחות עולה ומטמטמת מעברי המוח טמטום חסר (Now that I mention epilepsy, I will give its definition, namely, a moisture that flows to the brain and partly obstructs its channels). Hebr. טִמְטוּם features in Rabbinic literature in the sense of 'becoming a cohesive shapeless mass' (JD 532).

[טמטם] • *Part. Pilpel* **מְטַמְטֵם** · **obstructing; closing up**:[144] Arab. سدّ · Isḥāq ibn ʿImrān, *Treatise on Melancholy* · trans. Anonymous, fol. 49^a (50^a): וכשאזכור האבלאמסיא אזכור

143 'sealed earth or clay (i.e., terra sigillata) from the island of Lemnos': It was called in this way because the pastilles prepared from these kinds of earth or clay were marked with a seal. Maimonides (M 172) mentions three different kinds of terra sigillata, namely from Lemnos, Buḥayra, and Yemen.

144 The same term features (ibid.) in הלחות המטמטמת for Arab. الرطوبة السادّة (the obstructing moisture).

גבולו ואומר שהאבלמסיא לחות עולה ומטמטמת מעברי המוח טמטום חסר (Now that I mention epilepsy, I will give its definition, namely a moisture that flows to the brain and partly obstructs its channels). Hebr. טמטם features in Rabbinic literature in the sense of 'to thicken into a cohesive mass' and 'to thicken, to obstruct, to blunt the understanding;' cf. tb*Pesaḥim* 42ª: מטמטם את הלב 'obstructs the heart' (i.e., makes a person dull); cf. JD 532. In liturgical literature it is attested for in the sense of 'to close [the eyes];' cf. BM 1884. Constantine the African translates Arab. سدّ as *impleo*.

טִפָּה · **gout**: Lat. *gutta* (DMLBS 1399: 'one of several ailments attrib. to 'defluxion' of humors: a) arthritic ailment, gout or sim. (sts. w. *arthritica, erratica, sciatica*); b) (w. *caduca* or *cadiva*) epilepsy; c) (w. *calida*) dysury; d) (w. *festra*) ulcerous disease e) (w. *rosea* or sim.) disease (affecting face) accompanied by rash;' ND 468: 'gout or some other type of arthritis (inflammation of joint), in some texts also sciatica' · Guillaume de Congenis, *Treatise on Surgery* · trans. Isaiah, fol. 60ª: כנגד[145] כל טפה קרה ואחרת שמן האבפורבי העשוי כך ([A remedy] for any gout, but [especially] for cold gout: [Take] resin spurge oil that is prepared as follows ...). In the sense of 'gout,' Hebr. טִפָּה is a non-attested loan translation of Lat. *gutta*.

• **טפה ארטיטיקא** · **arthritic ailment; gout**: Lat. *gutta artetica* · Guillaume de Congenis, *Treatise on Surgery* · trans. Isaiah, fol. 59ᵇ: משיחה אבריאום הנעשה מן אבריאה אלכסנדרינאה[146] ושמן לאברין מעורב יחד יועיל כנגד כל טפה ארטיטיקא (The ointment [called] 'aureum,' which is prepared from a mixture of aurea[147] Alexandrina and bay laurel oil is good for any arthritic ailments). Hebr. טפה ארטיטיקא is a non-attested loan translation of Lat. *gutta artetica*.

• **טפה קרה** · **cold gout or arthritis (also sciatica) due to dropping of 'cold humors' (esp. phlegm) on a joint**: Lat. *gutta frigida* (ND 469) · Guillaume de Congenis, *Treatise on Surgery* · trans. Isaiah, fol. 60ª: כנגד[148] כל טפה קרה ואחרת שמן האבפורבי העשוי כך ([A remedy] for any gout, but [especially] for cold gout: [Take] resin spurge oil that is prepared as follows ...). Hebr. טפה קרה is a non-attested loan translation of Lat. *gutta frigida*.

• **טפה רושה** · **red rash on the face**:[149] Lat. *gutta rosea*; Rom. *gute rose* (DMLBS 1399; ND 471) · Guillaume de Congenis, *Treatise on Surgery* · trans. Isaiah, fol. 60ª: כנגד טפה רושה קח שומן חזיר ישן ושחוק יפה ושים בו כסף חי ושחוק יחד עד שישוב שחור ואחר משח פני הסובל (To treat red rash on the face: Take fat of an old pig, pound it well, put mercury

145 כנגד כל טפה קרה ואחרת: *contra omnem guttam, sed contra frigidam* L.
146 אלכסנדרינאה: emendation editor אלכסנדריאה Ms.
147 'aurea Alexandrina': Cf. DMLBS: 214: 'a sort of a pill.'
148 כנגד כל טפה קרה ואחרת: *contra omnem guttam, sed contra frigidam* L.
149 Cf. ND 471: 'gout involving red swollen joints.'

in it, pound this together until it turns black, then rub it on the face of the patient). Hebr. טפה רושה is a non-attested loan translation of Lat. *gutta rosea* or Rom. *gute rose.*

• זוב טפת הזרע → **זוֹב.**

טַרְפָּשָׁה • צמח בטרפשה → **צֶמַח.**

יאורי → יְאֹרִי.

יְאֹרִי · **of the river; river-**: Arab. نهري · Maimonides, *Medical Aphorisms* 22.45 · trans. Zeraḥyah Ḥen (BMMZ 212): עור סוס הים שרוף יועיל מן המורסות הגסות. הסרטן היאורי כשתשחק אותו ותשים אותו על המורסא הקשה יפזרנה (The skin of a hippopotamus, burnt, is beneficial for hard tumors. If a river crab is pulverized and put on a hard tumor, it dispels it). Hebrew יְאֹרִי is a non-attested adjective coined from יְאֹר, which features in the current dictionaries in the sense of 'the river Nile' and 'stream' in general (cf. KB 381–382; BM 1942–1943). Nathan ha-Me'ati translates Arab. نهري as נהרי.

יָבֵשׁ • **החלי היבש** → חֳלִי.

יגיעות → יְגֵעוּת.

יְגֵעוּת · **exhaustion**: Arab. إعياء · Maimonides, *Medical Aphorisms* 10.18 · trans. Zeraḥyah Ḥen (BMMZ 121): אין להם טוב אלא ההרקה עם החפיפה החזקה עד[150] שתתחדש בהם היגיעות מפני ריצוץ בשרם ברבוי החפיפה הנקרא הערבי דלך (They [i.e., those who suffer from fever while their body contains a very large quantity of crude superfluities] only benefit from an evacuation by means of strong massage, which brings the patient to near-exhaustion[151] because of the bruising of flesh through the intensive massage, that is called *dalk* in Arabic). Hebr. יְגֵעוּת features as a modern term in EM 653. Nathan ha-Me'ati translates Arab. إعياء as יגיעה.

יָד • **חלוב מיד** → חָלַב.

• **נחלב מיד** → חָלַב.

יְדִיעָה • **הקדמת הידיעה** → הַקְדָּמָה.

[ידע] • *Part. Pu'al* **מְיֻדָּע** • **כלי מיודע להעלות זיעתו** → כְּלִי.

יוֹחָנָן • **עשב יוחנן** → עֵשֶׂב.

יוֹם • **יום הגבול** · **a day of prognostic indication**: Lat. *dies prenunciata* (Arab. يوم الإنذار) · Constantinus Africanus, *Viaticum* · trans. Do'eg ha-Edomi, *Sefer Ya'ir Netiv*, bk. 3, ch. 12: ואם הוא רגיל לאכל הרבה בבריאותו וזה המאכל לא יספיק לו ינתן לו קוקורביטא מלבא קרישולוקנא עם שמן שקדים ואם יום הגבול ידוע אליו נמנע ממנו כל המאכלים לבד אבשאנא ומוח הפת (If the patient [suffering from pleurisy] is used to [the consumption of] much food when he was healthy and this food [i.e., that recommended during illness and mentioned before] is not sufficient for him, we give him pumpkin, garden orach, or mallow with almond oil; if the day of prognostic indication is known, we only give him barley gruel and the soft part of bread). Hebr. יום הגבול does not feature in the current dictionaries. The term גְּבוּל on its own in the sense of 'crisis' features in BCD 42 (NM 2:33) in an attestation from Nathan ha-Me'ati's translation of

---

150 עד שתתחדש: الذي يكاد أن يحدث a.

151 'near-exhaustion': Trans. after a.

the introduction of Maimonides, *Medical Aphorisms* (BMMN 20). Moses ibn Tibbon translates Arab. يوم الإنذار as יום ההוראה (see next entry).

• **יום ההוראה · a day of prognostic indication**: Arab. يوم الإنذار · Ibn al-Jazzār, *Zād al-musāfir wa-qūt al-ḥādir* · trans. Moses ibn Tibbon, *Sefer Ṣedat ha-Derakhim* bk. 3, ch. 12: ואם היה החולה מנהגו להרבות מן המזון ולא יספיקהו דיסת השעור ולב הלחם הרחוץ נתן לו קרא או ארמולץ או מלבש בשמן שקדים מתוקים וכשיהיה יום ההוראה נמנענו מהמזון ולא נתן לו כי אם דיסת השעור לבד (If the patient is used to [the consumption of] much food and barley gruel and the soft part of washed bread is not sufficient for him, we give him pumpkin, garden orach, or mallow with sweet almond oil; but on the day of prognostic indication we only give him barley gruel). In the sense of 'a day of prognostic indication,' Hebr. יום הוראה features in BCD 115 (NM 3:104) in an attestation from Moses ibn Tibbon's translation of Maimonides' *Commentary on Hippocrates' Aphorisms* 2.24 (76) (BMHA 1:340). Do'eg ha-Edomi translates the parallel Latin term *dies prenunciata* as יום הגבול (see previous entry).

יַיִן • יין מבושל · syrup: Arab. ميبختج[152] · Ibn al-Jazzār, *Zād al-musāfir wa-qūt al-ḥādir* · trans. Moses ibn Tibbon, *Sefer Ṣedat ha-Derakhim*, bk. 3, ch. 1: או יגרגר במי שעור עם סוכרי או יגרגר בחלב עז חלוב מיד או חלב אתון עם מעט סוכרי או יין מבושל (Or let him gargle with barley gruel with sugar or with fresh goat's milk or donkey's milk with some sugar or syrup). Hebr. יין מבושל is not attested for in the current dictionaries. The same Hebrew term is used by Moses ibn Tibbon to render Arab. ربّ ('rob,' i.e., fruit juice boiled down to syrup) in the combination יין מבושל עד ששב כדבש (cf. BCD 117 (NM 4:77)), cf. also entry בשול יין above. In his glossary to the *Sefer ha-Qanun*, Nathan ha-Me'ati remarks: טלא הוא יין מבושל שלא נתערב וכשנתעבה נקרא מיבכתג׳ כלומר שפא אוקרינו בלשון (ṬL'. This is unmixed boiled wine; when it is thickened it is called MYBKTĞ; i.e., ŠP'[153] or QRYNW in [Latin]); cf. NM 2:114, 140 (Ṭet 6). In addition to יין מבושל, Moses ibn Tibbon translates Arab. ميبختج as רב ענבים (see entry רֹב).

• **בִּשּׁוּל → בשול יין**

יָם • אישפונגא מן הים → אִישְׁפּוּנְגָא.

• **לָשׁוֹן → לשון הים.**

---

152 Arab. ميبختج: From Pers. مى پخته; cf. VL 2:1246: 'syrupus, et sec. al. vinum cum aliis medicamentis bullitum et defaecatum' (syrup, according to others wine boiled and purified with other medications).

153 The Mss read ŠP' [read: ŚP'] 'WQRYNW, the correct reading is ŠP' [read: ŚP'] 'W QRYNW, i.e., *sapa* or *carenum*. Cf. the following passage in A. García González (ed.), *Alphita: Edición crítica y comentario* (Florence 2007), 384b: 'Carenum est vinum coctum in vendemiis, cuius due partes sunt consumpte, tercia residua; sapa e contrario' (*Carenum* is wine that is boiled at the time of the vintage, while two parts are evaporated and one part remains; *sapa* is the reverse [i.e., one part evaporated and two parts remaining]). For further references and sources, see ibid. and Sin 185; for *sapa*, cf. entry שפא below.

• צף הים → צף.
• קֶצֶף הים → קֶצֶף.

יְסוֹד · **superfluity**: Arab. فضل[154] · Ibn al-Jazzār, *Zād al-musāfir wa-qūt al-ḥāḍir* · trans. Abraham ben Isaac, *Sefer Ṣedah la-Oreḥim*, cf. bk. 1, ch. 24: ואם לא תהיה תוספת הדם בגוף כי אם תוספת יסוד אחר ראוי שלא נקיזהו כי אם נשקה אותו הרפואות המשלשלות ומורידות לרפשים העבים הרעים שבגוף (If there is no surplus of blood in the body, but a surplus of another superfluity, we should refrain from venesection but administer [the patient] remedies that evacuate and bring down the coarse, bad superfluities in the body). Moses ibn Tibbon renders Arab. *Plur.* فضول as מותרות; Do'eg ha-Edomi translates Lat. *humores* as ליחות.

• *Plur.* **יסודות** · **humors**: Arab. أخلاط · Ibn al-Jazzār, *Zād al-musāfir wa-qūt al-ḥāḍir* · trans. Abraham ben Isaac, *Sefer Ṣedah la-Oreḥim*,[155] bk. 1, ch. 5 (Ms Jerusalem, National Library of Israel, Fr. 95, fols. 86ᵃ–86ᵇ): השני כאשר יעלה ההבל חד של רפשי ארבע יסודות (The second [cause of dandruff is] a sharp vapor that arises from the residues of the four humors [to the brain]). Hebr. *Sing.* יְסוֹד, *Plur.* יסודות, does not feature in this sense in the current dictionaries. Moses ibn Tibbon renders Arab. أخلاط as ליחות.

[יסף] • *Part. Nifʿal* **נוֹסָף** · **superfluous**: Arab. فضلي · Isḥāq ibn ʿImrān, *Treatise on Melancholy* · trans. Anonymous, fol. 51ᵇ (52ᵇ): והשני שיש בהם רטיבות נוספת נעשה להם מן המים ואין לגוף בה תועלת (The second reason [that patients suffering from melancholy should be careful regarding the consumption of vegetables] is that [their body] contains superfluous moisture that comes from their [watery substance] and that is not beneficial for the body). Hebr. נוֹסָף does not feature in this sense in the current dictionaries, but features in the same sense in Moses ibn Tibbon's translation of Maimonides' *Commentary on Hippocrates' Aphorisms* 4.57 (194) (BMHA 1:370). Do'eg ha-Edomi uses the term הנוסף as a noun in the sense of 'residue' in the *Sefer Agur*, i.e., his translation of a Latin version of Hippocrates, *Aphorisms* 1.2 (cf. BCD 117 (NM 3: 151–152)). Constantine the African translates Arab. فضلي as *accidentalis*.

יעפות · **tiredness; fatigue**: Arab. هزال · Isḥāq ibn ʿImrān, *Treatise on Melancholy* · trans. Anonymous, fol. 44ᵃ (45ᵃ): וכמו שיגיעת הגוף תביא את האדם לחלאים הקשים הקטן שבהן היעפות כך יגיעת הנפש תביאנו בחולי קשה ורע מאד והוא חולי המלאנקוניא (Exertion of a person's body causes severe illnesses, a minor one being fatigue. Similarly, psychical [i.e., mental] fatigue causes a severe and very nasty illness, i.e., melancholy). Hebr. יעפות, coined from the verb יָעַף ('to be tired;' cf. BM 2089) is not attested for in the current dictionaries

154 In addition to יְסוֹד, Abraham ben Isaac translates Arab. فضل as רֶפֶשׁ (see entry).

155 Ms Florence, Biblioteca Medicina Laurenziana, Plut. 88.37, also has *Plur.* יסודים; cf. entry פַּרְנָסָה. Note that the term יְסוֹד also features in the sense of 'humor' in the anonymous abbreviation of *Sefer Ṣedah la-Oreḥim*; cf. entry הַפְסָדָה.

יַעֲרִי • **wild**: Arab. بَرِّي • Ibn al-Jazzār, *Zād al-musāfir wa-qūt al-ḥādir* • trans. Abraham ben Isaac, *Sefer Ṣedah la-Oreḥim*, bk. 1, ch. 23: וזה ריקוח רפואה להעטיש מאשר תיקן בן מאוסיה לעיוות ולפלג ולשיתוק גם יטהר מוח הראש: קח כנדס ג׳ שקל׳ וחצי ופלפלים לבנים ושחורים וקשטוריו מכל אחד חצי שקל ופיגנון יערי וחרדל מכל אחד שקל פחות מעט (Recipe of a remedy inducing sneezing composed by Ibn Māsawayh, [which is beneficial] for facial paresis, hemiplegia, apoplexy, and which cleanses the brain: Take three and a half *shekel*s of sneezewort; half a *shekel* each of white and black pepper and castoreum; and a little bit less than one *shekel* of wild rue [i.e., Syrian rue] and mustard). Hebr. יַעֲרִי only features in the current dictionaries in the sense of 'of the forest, belonging to the forest;' cf. BM 2092; EM 681. Both dictionaries quote the term featuring as דבש היערי in Nathan ha-Meati's translation of Maimonides, *Medical Aphorisms* 23.54 (BMMN 225). However the correct version is דבש היערה (Arab. عسل الشهد). Moses ibn Tibbon translates Arab. بَرِّي as מִדְבָּרִי (see entry).

[יצא] • *Hif'il* **הוֹצִיא** • **to invent**: Arab. وضع • Ibn al-Jazzār, *Zād al-musāfir wa-qūt al-ḥādir* • trans. Abraham ben Isaac, *Sefer Ṣedah la-Oreḥim*, bk. 1, ch. 20 (Ms Florence, Biblioteca Medicina Laurenziana, Plut. 88.37, fol. 95b): וכבר אמרו בעבור יעקב בן יצחק הכינדי כי אמר בעבור ארפייאנוס שהוציא מיני[156] זמר וכל זני זמרא כי היה אומר: המלכים קורין אותי למשתאותיהם כדי שישמחו וישחקו ממני (It is related in the name of Yaʿqūb ibn Isḥāq al-Kindī, that Orpheus, the inventor of all kinds of melodies, said: Kings invite me to their banquets so that they may take pleasure in me and are entertained by me). Hebr. הוֹצִיא does not feature in this sense in the current dictionaries. Moses ibn Tibbon translates Arab. وضع as מצא.

[ירד] • *Hif'il* **הוֹרִיד** • **to evacuate**: Arab. أنزل (Gr. ἀπάγω; cf. UW 115–116) • Ibn al-Jazzār, *Zād al-musāfir wa-qūt al-ḥādir* • trans. Abraham ben Isaac, *Sefer Ṣedah la-Oreḥim*, bk. 1, ch. 18: ואם לא יוכל החולה לשתות הרפואות אז נעשה חקנה הוא קרישטיר להורידו ולשלשלו (If the patient is not able to take orally the drugs [we described above], we prepare for him a clyster, i.e., [Rom.] QRYŠṬYR, that evacuates and purges). Hebr. הוֹרִיד does not feature as a medical term in the current dictionaries. Moses ibn Tibbon translates Arab. أنزل as הוֹרִיד as well.

ירוק → יָרֹק.

יְרוֹקָה • **הירוקה שעל פני המים** • **common duckweed** [*Lemna minor* L.]: Arab. طحلب (cf. MIG 698) • Maimonides, *Medical Aphorisms* 21.79 • trans. Zeraḥyah Ḥen (BMMZ 204): ובמאמר השני מספר אגלוקן בדברו בנמלה המתאכלת אמר מאמר זה לשונו: והזהר מעשות בזה החולי החסא או הוירגא פשטורי או הסיליאו והירוקה שעל פני המים או הנינופר או הפורקקלא או חי לעולם או זולת זה ממה שטבעו הקירור והלחלוח (In the second book of his treatise *Ad Glauconem* [*de medendi methodo*], when speaking about corrosive shingles, he [i.e., Galen] says the following and these are his words: In this illness be careful not to use

156 מיני זמר וכל זני זמרא: اللحون a.

cultivated lettuce, common knotgrass, fleawort, common duckweed, water lily, common purslane, tree aeonium (sempervivum), or similar [ingredients] with cooling, moistening properties). For Hebr. ירוקה שעל פני המים in the sense of 'common duckweed' and featuring in *Mishnah Shabbat* 2.1, cf. LF 1:14ff. Jastrow (JD 595) explains the term as 'grass upon the water, a sort of sea-weed or moss used for wicks.' Ben-Yehuda (BM 2154) remarks that it is 'a sort of green herb that grows on the water.' For the identification of طحلب as הירוקה שעל פני המים in Jewish sources, see LF 1:18 and SHS 1:377–378 (Ayin 2)). Nathan ha-Me'ati translates Arab. طحلب as עדש המים; cf. SHS 1:377 (Ayin 2): עדש המים ב״ה טחלב ובל״ל לינטיליאסה ('DŠ HMYM; Arab. *ṭuḥlub*, vern. LYNṬYLY'SH [i.e., O.Occ. *lentil(h)a/lentilla* and/or O.Cat. *l(l)entilla*]).

יָרֵחַ • **חיסור הירח** → חִסּוּר.

• **חסרון הירח** → חִסּוּר.

יָרֹק · **verdigris:** Lat. *viridis* (cf. DMLBS 4039) · Guillaume de Congenis, *Treatise on Surgery* · trans. Isaiah, fol. 49[a]: כמו כן קחליט׳ שומן חזיר ישן ושלגיימא אוקי׳ ומן ירוק חצי אוקי׳ וירקח ויעשה משיחה ממיתה פישטולה (Likewise, take one pound of fat of an old pig, one ounce of rock salt and half an ounce of verdigris, mix these [ingredients] and prepare a salve from it that mortifies [i.e., closes up] fistulas). In the sense of 'verdigris,' Hebr. יָרֹק is a non-attested loan translation of Lat. *viridis*.

• **ירוק הנחושת** · **verdigris:** Lat. *viridis aeris* · Guillaume de Congenis, *Treatise on Surgery* · trans. Isaiah, fol. 48[b]: הקולוריש אשר יועילו לפישטולאש להמית ולעצור הדמעות ולהסיר הבשר המת ולחכוך העינים יקח אניץ לבן ירוק הנחושת מ״א אוקיא (Collyria, which are good for mortifying [i.e., closing up] fistulas, for stopping tears, for removing dead flesh, for pruritus in the eyes: Take white anise, verdigris, one ounce of each ...). Hebr. ירוק הנחושת is a non-attested loan translation of Lat. *viridis aeris*. Hillel ben Samuel renders the Latin synonym *flos eris* ('verdigris') as פרח הנחשת (cf. BCD 223 (NM 1:36)).

• **גרגרים ירוקים** → גַּרְגַּר.

יֶרֶק • **ירק הסנונית** · **(lit., swallow plant); greater celandine [*Chelidonium majus* L.]:** Arab. بقلة الخطاطيف (cf. MIG 128) · *Shinnui ha-Shemot ha-Niqra'im Synonimis*, Ms Munich, Bayerische Staatsbibliothek, Cod. hebr. 8, fol. 195[b]: בקלא אלכטאטיף כלומר ירק הסנונית הוא צילידוניאה ויקרא מאמיראן בערבי ג״ב ([Arab.] *baqla al-khaṭāṭīf* ['swallow-wort']; i.e., [Hebr.] *yereq ha-senunit*; i.e., [Lat.] *celidonia*; also called in Arab. *māmīrān*). In the sense of 'greater celandine,' Hebr. ירק הסנונית is a non-attested calque from Arab. بقلة الخطاطيف.

• **ירק הנוצריים** · **(lit., vegetable of the Christians); cabbage [*Brassica oleracea* L.]:** Arab. بقلة الأنصار[157] (cf. MIG 112) · *Shinnui ha-Shemot ha-Niqra'im Synonimis*, Ms Munich, Bayerische Staatsbibliothek, Cod. hebr. 8, fol. 195[b]: בקלה אלנצר כלומר ירק

157 الأنصار: emendation editor النصر Ms.

הנוצריים ונקרא הכרוב ונקרא כן באהבתם אותו ([Arab.] *baqla al-anṣār*;[158] i.e., [Hebr.] *yereq ha-Noṣriyim*; also called [Hebr.] *keruv*; it is called by that name because they love it so much). In the sense of 'cabbage,' Hebr. ירק הנוצריים is a non-attested calque from Arab. *baqla al-anṣār*, read as *baqla al-naṣārā*.

[ישן] • *Part Piʿel* **מְיַשֵּׁן** • **דברים מישנים** → דָּבָר.

יָשֵׁן • **חרדת הישן** → חֲרָדָה.

158 *al anṣār* (i.e., the Medinan followers of Mohammed): emendation editor *al-naṣr* Ms.

כ

כְּאֵב • כאב דוקר בלב · **cardialgia[159] (i.e., palpitation or heartburn)**: Arab. نخس في الفؤاد · Ibn al-Jazzār, *Zād al-musāfir wa-qūt al-ḥādir* · trans. Abraham ben Isaac, *Sefer Ṣedah la-Oreḥim*; cf. bk. 1, ch. 10 (Ms Jerusalem, National Library of Israel, Fr. 95, fol. 91[a]): ואם עלילת הכאב מחמת רפש חום חד שנקבץ בפי האצטומכוס וסימן כי ירגיש החולה עם הכאב אל[160] כרב ואל גשי וכאב הדוקר בלב (If [the headache] is caused by a hot, sharp residue that has accumulated in the orifice of the stomach, it has the following symptoms: the patient feels—next to the [headache]—distress, indisposition,[161] and cardialgia [i.e., heartburn]). Hebr. כאב דוקר בלב is not attested for in the current dictionaries. Moses ibn Tibbon renders the parallel Arabic term النخس في الفؤاد as עקיצה בפי האצטומכא; the same term features in Zeraḥyah Ḥen's translation of Maimonides' *Commentary on Hippocrates'* Aphorisms 4.17 (154) (BMHA 1:458; cf. BCD 213 (NM 3:183)), where Moses ibn Tibbon has נשיכה במוראה (BMHA 1:361; cf. BCD 213 (NM 3:164)).

כֹּבֶד • כובד השמע · **hearing loss**: Lat. *gravitas auditus* (Arab. ثقل السمع / Gr. δυσηκοΐα; cf. UW 212) · Constantinus Africanus, *Viaticum* · trans. Do'eg ha-Edomi, *Sefer Ya'ir Netiv*, bk. 2, ch. 8: משיחה זאת טובה לכובד השמע בהברה ובקול בא מרוח גס או מכאב או מקרירות (The following salve is beneficial for hearing loss, ringing and buzzing arising because of a coarse wind or pain [occurring because of] coldness). Hebr. כובד השמע is not attested for in the current dictionaries. Ben-Yehuda (BM 2230) mentions the term כֹּבֶד in different contexts featuring in medieval medical literature. Moses ibn Tibbon translates Arab. ثقل السمع, just like Do'eg, as כובד השמע, but also as כבדות השמע (see next entry כְּבֵדוּת). A Latin synonym of *gravitas auditus*, i.e., *diminutio auditus* is translated by Do'eg ha-Edomi as חסרון השמע (see entry חֶסְרוֹן).

כְּבֵדוּת • כבדות השמע · **hearing loss**: a) Arab. ثقل السمع · Ibn al-Jazzār, *Zād al-musāfir wa-qūt al-ḥādir* · trans. Moses ibn Tibbon, *Sefer Ṣedat ha-Derakhim*, bk. 2, ch. 7: בכבדות השמע (On hearing loss). Hebr. כבדות השמע is not attested for in the current dictionaries. In addition to כבדות השמע, Moses ibn Tibbon translates Arab. ثقل السمع as כובד השמע (see previous entry כֹּבֶד). Do'eg ha-Edomi translates Lat. *diminutio auditus* as חסרון השמע (see entry חֶסְרוֹן).

b) Lat. *gravitas (gravitudo) auditus* · Ms Cambridge, T-S K14.14, fol. 2[b]: שער די גראוויטוטוש אבדיטוש: ראוי שתדע שכבדות השמע יהיה על ב׳ פנים ר״ל טבעי מתחלת

---

159 Cf. Hippocrates, *Aphorisms* 4.17 (Galen, *In Hippocratis Aphorismos commentarius*, ed. Kühn, 17b:676: καρδιωγμός; Hippocrates, *Aphorisms*, trans. Littré, 4:507: 'la cardialgie;' ibid., trans. Jones, 139: 'heartburn;' UW 325: "Herzstechen;" UWS 1:518, s. v. καρδία: 'Herz; Magenmund' (*inna l-qudamā'a kānū yusammūna fama l-ma'idati fu'ādan*)).

160 אל כרב ואל גשי: الكرب والغثي a الكرب الغشي a (variant reading).

161 'indisposition': Trans. after a: الغثي.

היצירה וזה המין אין תוחלת ברפואתו או מקרי (Chapter on DY GR'WWYṬWṬWS [DY *GRWWYṬ'ṬY or DY *GRWWYṬWDYNY] 'BDYṬWS: You should know that that there are two kinds of hearing loss: natural; it is from birth on, and there is no hope that it can be cured; or accidental ...).

כִּבּוּס • *Plur.* **כבוסים** · **purgatives**: Lat. *cathartica* · Constantinus Africanus, *Viaticum* · trans. Do'eg ha-Edomi, *Sefer Ya'ir Netiv*, bk. 1, ch. 17: והכבוסים ראוים להנתן לו לכבות האדומה (... the purgatives that should be given to him to extinguish [the heat] of the yellow bile ...). As a medical term, Hebr. כִּבּוּס features in BM 2241 in an attestation from the *Sefer ha-Kibbusim* [*we-ha-Toharot*], which is possibly an anonymous translation of a treatise on compound medicines, entitled, a.o., *Modus medendi*, by a certain Gerardus (cf. HU 792; and Richler[162]). Ben-Yehuda explains the term as 'a clyster for purging the intestines.' The term also features in the sense of 'evacuation; purgation' in the *Sefer Agur*, i.e., Do'eg ha-Edomi's translation of a Latin version of Hippocrates' *Aphorisms* (cf. BCD 124 (NM 3:115–116)). Cf. also entry [כבס].

[כבס] • *Pi'el* **כִּבֵּס** · **to purge**: Lat. *purgo* · Constantinus Africanus, *Viaticum* · trans. Do'eg ha-Edomi, *Sefer Ya'ir Netiv*, bk. 3, ch. 4: ואם הוא מדם יעיד עליו האודם ומלואת המקורות בפנים ואז יאות להקיזו מן הספליקא ולחסר הדם כפי כחו לסבול ולכבס אותו (If [hoarseness] is caused by blood, which is indicated by redness and fulness of the vessels of the face, one should bleed the cephalic vein and extract blood as much as he can endure and purge him). Hebr. כִּבֵּס features in BM 2247 in an attestation from the *Sefer ha-Kibbusim* [*we-ha-Toharot*], which is possibly an anonymous translation of a treatise on compound medicines, entitled, a.o., *Modus medendi*, by a certain Gerardus (cf. HU 792; and Richler[163]). Ben-Yehuda explains the term as 'cleansing (purging) the intestines with a clyster.' See also entry כִּבּוּס.

• *Part. Pi'el* **מְכֻבָּס** • **הרפואה המכבסת** → רְפוּאָה.

[כבר] • *Hif'il* **הִכְבִּיר** · **to sieve**: Arab. نخل · Ibn al-Jazzār, *Zād al-musāfir wa-qūt al-ḥādir* · trans. Abraham ben Isaac, *Sefer Ṣedah la-Oreḥim*, bk. 1, ch. 23: תכתוש הכל ותכביר ולוש במיצוי כרישים ותעשה פולים ותיבשם בצל (Pound all [these ingredients], sieve them, and knead them together with garden leek juice. Mould this into pills and dry them in the shadow). In the sense of 'to sieve,' Hebrew הִכְבִּיר is attested for in medieval medical literature in BM 2248 in a quotation from Shabbetai Donnolo, *Sefer ha-Yakar*, also known as *Sefer ha-Merqaḥot*.

---

162 B. Richler, 'On the Existing Manuscripts of Marpé la-Ezem by ibn Waqar,' *Korot* 19 (2007–2008), 132. Note that a *Sefer ha-Kibbusim we-ha-Toharot* also features as *Sefer ha-Kibbusim we-ha-Toharot ha-Gufaniyyot* in the list of translations prepared by Do'eg ha-Edomi; cf. G. Freudenthal, 'The Father of the Latin-into-Hebrew Translations: 'Do'eg the Edomite,' the Twelfth-Century Repentant Convert,' in *Latin-into-Hebrew: Texts and Studies*, vol. 1: *Studies*, ed. R. Fontaine and G. Freudenthal (Leiden 2013), 119, no. 8.

163 See previous note.

• *Part. Hofʿal* מְכֻבָּר · **sieved**: Arab. منخول · Ibn al-Jazzār, *Zād al-musāfir wa-qūt al-ḥādir* · trans. Abraham ben Isaac, *Sefer Ṣedah la-Oreḥim*, bk. 1, ch. 23: תקבץ הכל שחוקים ומוכברים וישרה מהם הראוי לשרות במיצוי הכרישים (Mix all [these remedies] together after pounding and sieving them and soak the required quantity in garden leek juice). In the sense of 'to be sieved,' Hebr. *Hofʿal* הֻכְבַּר is attested for in medieval medical literature in BM 2248 in a quotation from Shabbetai Donnolo, *Sefer ha-Yakar*, also known as *Sefer ha-Merqaḥot*. Moses ibn Tibbon translates Arab. منخول as מנופה.

כָּבַשׁ • **כבש בידו על** · **to palpate**: Arab. غمز · Maimonides, *Medical Aphorisms* 4.36 · trans. Nathan ha-Me'ati (BMMN 61): המנוחה הנכנסת אי אפשר שתדענה באמת בעת מן העתים אך תושג אם יהיה הדפק חזק מאד ותכבוש עליו בידך כבישה חזקה. (Internal rest [of the artery] can never be known for certain, but it is possible to perceive it by means of firm palpation when the pulse is very strong). Hebr. כבש בידו על is not attested for in the current dictionaries. Zeraḥyah Ḥen translates Arab. غمز as לחץ אצבעותיו על.

כֵּהוּת • **כהות הראות** · **dimsightedness**: Arab. ظلمة البصر (Gr. ἀμβλυωπία; cf. UW 90) · Ibn al-Jazzār, *Zād al-musāfir wa-qūt al-ḥādir* · trans. Moses ibn Tibbon, *Sefer Ṣedat ha-Derakhim*, bk. 1, ch. 10: ומהם תאר רפואה חברה בן מאסויה בספר האצטומכא מועיל מן הרוחות העבות וכהות הראות וכובד הגוף הבא בסבת רוחות המרה השחורה ולמותרות ליחה לבנה קרה דביקה (Another recipe described by Ibn Māsawayh in the *Book on the Stomach* for coarse winds, dimsightedness, heaviness of the body caused by winds [coming from] the black bile, and superfluities of cold, viscous phlegm). The unattested Hebr. כהות הראות also features in the anonymous translation of Hippocrates' *Aphorisms* 3.31 (cf. NM 3:28, s.v. אפיסת המראה). A synonymous כהות עיניים is attested for in Rabbinic literature (cf. JD 614; BM 2271) and also in Joseph Delmedigo's translation of Hippocrates' *Aphorisms* 3.31 (cf. NM 3:28, s.v. אפיסת המראה). Abraham ben Isaac translates Arab. ظلمة البصر as חשיכות העינים (see entry חֲשֵׁיכוּת). Do'eg ha-Edomi translates the parallel Latin term *obscuritas visus* as מחשך הראות (see entry מַחְשָׁךְ).

[כון] • *Part. Nifʿal* נָכוֹן · **susceptable**: Arab. مستعدّ · Isḥāq ibn ʿImrān, *Treatise on Melancholy* · trans. Anonymous, fol. 43ᵇ (44ᵇ): ויש לנו לחקור הסבות של ששה דברים שהגוף צריך אליהם והיאך[164] תהיה המלאנקוניא בין חליים מחוסר טוב תהיינה מן המאכלים או הם לא יעשוהו כהוגן יביא לידי חולי זה במיהור בכל מי שהוא נכון לקבלו (We need to look into the six [fundamental things] which are necessary for the body and how melancholy is among the illnesses that arise from a lack of a proper regimen regarding food, and how these [fundamental things], if they are not observed, quickly cause illness in every one who is susceptable to be affected [by such an illness]). Hebr. נָכוֹן does not feature in this sense in the current dictionaries.

כותל → כֹּתֶל.

164 והיאך: emendation editor והאך Ms.

כַּזְבָנִי · **untruthful; false**: Arab. كاذب · Isḥāq ibn ʿImrān, *Treatise on Melancholy* · trans. Anonymous, fol. 50[a] (51[a]): ומפני שהיה בחולי המלאנקוניא מקריו הנפשיים קשים וכבר בארנום בנקדם במאמר מבואר יתכן להיות מגמתך לאותן המקרים הנפשיים להסיר אותן המחשבות הכזבניות והדמיונים המופסדים והמראות[165] הכזבניות הרעות (Since the psychical symptoms of the illness of melancholy are severe, as we clearly explained in a previous [part of this treatise], we should now pay attention to [the treatment of] those psychical symptoms; i.e., [how] to remove those false beliefs, corrupt phantasies, and false,[166] bad visions). Hebr. כַּזְבָנִי only features as a modern term in EM 727. Constantine the African translates Arab. كاذب as *falsus*.

כֹּחַ • **הכח האוחז** · **retentive faculty**: Arab. القوة الماسكة · Isḥāq ibn ʿImrān, *Treatise on Melancholy* · trans. Anonymous, fol. 46[b] (47[b]): ואין כח המזון עושה שום דבר בגוף אלא בארבע הכחות הטבעיים והם הכח המושך והכח האוחז והמעכל והדוחה (The nutritive faculty does not effect anything in the body except through the four natural faculties; i.e., the attractive faculty, the retentive faculty, the digestive [faculty], the excretory [faculty]). Constantine the African translates Arab. القوة الماسكة as *virtus contentiva*. Hebr. הכח האוחז is not attested for in the current dictionaries. The term current in medieval philosophical literature is הכח המחזיק (cf. KTP 2:74; BM 2317).

• **הכח ההודף** · **excretory faculty**: Arab. القوة الدافعة · Isḥāq ibn ʿImrān, *Treatise on Melancholy* · trans. Anonymous, fol. 46[b] (47[b]): וה(כח) ההודף אינו אלא הודף מותרי המזון ופסולתו כל מה שאין בהם צורך לכח המעכל (The excretory faculty excretes the food residues and remainders; everything that the digestive faculty has no need for). Hebr. הכח ההודף is not attested for in the current dictionaries. The standard term, i.e., הכח הדוחה, is also used by the anonymous translator, cf. entry הכח האוחז above. Constantine the African translates Arab. القوة الدافعة as *virtus expulsiva*.

• **כח קרוב אליו** · **specific property**: Lat. *proprium* · Constantinus Africanus, *Viaticum* · trans. Do'eg ha-Edomi, *Sefer Ya'ir Netiv*, bk. 1, ch. 19:[167] ויאות לחזק השכור ההוא עם דברים עשוים במחבת וצלוים בכרובות עם בשר עבה או עם כרובות מבושלים במים עם אופשומגרו ושמן כי כח קרוב הוא אל הכרובות להסיר השכרות בעבור כי לא יניחו העשן הגס מן היין לעלות אל המוח (One should strengthen people who are drunk with ingredients prepared and roasted with cabbage in a frying pan with fat meat or with cabbage boiled in water with ʾWPŠWMGRW [Lat. *opsumugarum/obsumugarum*] and oil, for cabbage has the specific property to undo [i.e., cure] inebriety because it prevents the coarse vapors from arising to the brain). Hebr. כח הקרוב אליו does not feature in the current dictionaries. Abraham ben Isaac translates the original Arabic term خاصّية as מִדָּה (see entry); Moses ibn Tibbon renders Arab. خاصّية with the standard term סגולה.

---

165 והמראות הכזבניות הרעות: والخطرات الردية a.

166 'false, bad visions': 'bad ideas' a.

167 Do'eg ha-Edomi uses the same term in bk. 1, ch. 21, for Lat. *proprietas*.

כַּכָּא (*Aram.*) · **gums**: Arab. لثة · Ibn al-Jazzār, *Zād al-musāfir wa-qūt al-ḥādir* · trans. Moses ibn Tibbon, *Sefer Ṣedat ha-Derakhim*, bk. 2, ch. 22:[168] השער השנים ועשרים בככא הוא בשר השנים (Ch. 22: On the gums [Aram. KK']; i.e., [Hebr.] *besar ha-shinnayim*). As an anatomical term, Aram. כַּכָּא only features in the current dictionaries in the sense of 'molar tooth' (cf. SDA 580).[169] Hebr. *Plur.* ככים in the sense of 'gums' features in *Sefer Ṣedat ha-Derakhim*, bk. 2, ch. 18 (cf. BCD 127 (NM 4:81)). Do'eg ha-Edomi translates Lat. *gingivae* as בשר השינים (see entry בָּשָׂר).

כֶּלֶב • הורג הכלב → הָרַג.

כַּלָּחוּת · **old age**: Arab. هرم · Shem Tov ben Isaac, *Sefer ha-Shimmush*, bk. 29, list 1 (SHS 1:281 (Kaf 32)): כלחות ב"ה הרם (*kallaḥut*; Arab. *haram*). In the sense of 'old age,' Hebr. כַּלָּחוּת is a non-attested variant of Hebr. כלח featuring in the Bible (Job 5:26) (KB 478; BM 2387).

כְּלִי • כלי מיודע להעלות זיעתו · **alembic**: Arab. إنبيق · Ibn al-Jazzār, *Zād al-musāfir wa-qūt al-ḥādir* · trans. Abraham ben Isaac, *Sefer Ṣedah la-Oreḥim*, bk. 1, ch. 4 (Ms Jerusalem, National Library of Israel, Fr. 95, fol. 85[b]): כלי מיודע להעלות זיעתו כאשר עושים אומנים ארס טמא (An alembic as is used by the artisans [i.e., manufacturers] of unclean poison [i.e., drugs?]). Hebr. כלי מיודע להעלות זיעתו does not feature in the current dictionaries. Moses ibn Tibbon translates Arab. إنبيق as כלי שעושים ⟨בו⟩ מי ורדים (cf. BCD 128 (NM 4:82)).

• *Plur.* **כלים • כלי הרוח** · **respiratory organs**: Lat. *instrumenta spiritus* (Arab. آلات النفس) · Constantinus Africanus · *Viaticum*, trans. Do'eg ha-Edomi, *Sefer Ya'ir Netiv*, bk. 3, ch. 6: והשעול שאינו רע כזה הוא יוצא מהחבור הרע מכלי הרוח או מניחור הגרון או מצנורות הריאה (Cough that is not that bad originates from a bad temperament of the respiratory organs or roughness of the throat or trachea). Hebr. כלי הרוח is not attested for in the current dictionaries. Moses Ibn Tibbon translates Arab. آلات النفس as כלי הנשימה.

כְּמִישׁוּת · **emaciation**: Arab. ضُمْر · Ibn al-Jazzār, *Zād al-musāfir wa-qūt al-ḥādir* · trans. Moses ibn Tibbon, *Sefer Ṣedat ha-Derakhim*, bk. 3, ch. 6: תואר בשול מועיל למי שהיה בו שעול או כמישות והיה עם זה מתרעם מן הכבד (Recipe of a decoction that is good for someone suffering from cough or emaciation while he also suffers from an illness of the liver). Hebr. כְּמִישׁוּת features in EM 748 in an attestation from medieval Rabbinic literature (R. Asher ben Yehiel) and from modern literature.

[כנס] • *Part. Nif'al* **נִכְנָס** · **internal**: Arab. داخل · Maimonides, *Medical Aphorisms* 4.36 · trans. Nathan ha-Me'ati (BMMN 61): המנוחה הנכנסת אי אפשר שתדענה באמת בעת מן העתים אך תושג אם יהיה הדפק חזק מאד ותכבוש עליו בידך כבישה חזקה (Internal rest [of the artery] can never be known for certain, but it is possible to perceive it by means

---

168 בככא: בחנכים Ms Oxford, Bodleian Library, Poc. 353, Uri Heb. 314.

169 The regular Hebrew term for 'gums,' i.e., חנכים, features in Ms Oxford, Bodleian Library, Poc. 353, Uri Heb. 314.

of firm palpation when the pulse is very strong). Hebr. נִכְנָס is not attested for in this sense in the current dictionaries. Zeraḥyah Ḥen translates Arab. داخل as פנימי.

• *Hif'il* הִכְנִיס • הכניס בחור התחתון · **to insert into the rectum** (Arab. احتمل من أسفل) · Ibn al-Jazzār, *Zād al-musāfir wa-qūt al-ḥādir* · trans. Abraham ben Isaac, *Sefer Ṣedah la-Oreḥim*, bk. 1, ch. 17: ואמר דיאסקורידוס: אם יעשו מן האופיו פתילה עם שמן ויאולטו ויכניסנה בחור התחתון תביא שינה מיושרת (Dioscurides stated that suppositories made from opium with violet oil induce well-balanced sleep, when inserted into the rectum). Hebr. הכניס בחור התחתון is not attested for in the current dictionaries. Moses ibn Tibbon translates Arab. احتمل من أسفل as הכניס מלמטה (see entry below). Do'eg ha-Edomi translates Lat. *facio suppposituram* as לעשות לו אחת מן ההנחות העשויות למטה.

• **הכניס מלמטה** · **to insert into the rectum** (Arab. احتمل من أسفل) · Ibn al-Jazzār, *Zād al-musāfir wa-qūt al-ḥādir* · trans. Moses ibn Tibbon, *Sefer Ṣedat ha-Derakhim*, bk. 1, ch. 17: ואמר דיאסקורידש שאם יעשה מן האופי פתילה ויכניסוה מלמטה תביא שינה שוה (Dioscurides stated that suppositories made from opium induce well-balanced sleep, when inserted into the rectum). Hebr. הכניס מלמטה does not feature in the current dictionaries. Abraham ben Isaac translates Arab. احتمل من أسفل as הכניס בחור התחתון (see entry above).

כֶּסֶף • דשן הכסף → דֶּשֶׁן.

כַּרְכֻּמּוּת · **yellow color**: Arab. صفرة · Ibn al-Jazzār, *Zād al-musāfir wa-qūt al-ḥādir* · trans. Moses ibn Tibbon, *Sefer Ṣedat ha-Derakhim*, bk. 3, ch. 6: ואם היה חזה החולה חם וסיפר שהוא ימצא בו דומה לעשן עם נחירות ושיקרה לו צמא ולא ירוק הרבה ויהיה מראה רוקו נוטה לכהות או לכרכמות וטעמו מלוח ידענו אז כי החומר דק מימי חד ונשתדל לעבותו ברפואה (If the chest of the patient is hot and he relates that he feels as if it contains something that is rough and similar to smoke, and that he suffers from thirst but not not expectorate a lot, and that the color of the sputum tends to be livid or yellow and tastes salty, we know that the matter is thin, watery, and sharp, and we should try to thicken it with a medicine). Hebr. כַּרְכֻּמּוּת only features in BM 2521 in a later attestation from the *Sefer ha-Qanun*. Do'eg ha-Edomi translates Constantine the African's parallel Latin term *color citrinus* as צבע מכורכם.

כשפנות · **magic**: Arab. سِحْر · Maimonides, *Medical Aphorisms* 22.17 · trans. Zeraḥyah Ḥen (BMMZ 209): אבן המרקישיטא כשתלבנהו באור ותזה עליו חומץ והושם האבר אשר בו מורסא קשה על העשן העולה ממנו תראה בהתרתו נפלאות וכאילו הוא פעולת הכשפנות. בשני מאגלוקן (If one heats the marcasite stone on a fire and sprinkles vinegar on it and then places the limb that has a hard tumor above the vapor that arises from it, you will see it dissolve in an amazing way, as if it is an act of magic. *Ad Glauconem* [*de medendi methodo*] 2). Hebrew כשפנות is not attested for in the current dictionaries. Nathan ha-Me'ati translates Arab. سِحْر as כשפים.

כתונת → כֻּתֹּנֶת.

כָּתוּשׁ (*Part. Pass.*) → כָּתַשׁ.

כְּתִישָׁה • כתש כתישה עבה › כָּתַשׁ.

כֹּתֶל · **skin**: Lat. *cutis* · Guillaume de Congenis, *Treatise on Surgery* · trans. Isaiah, fol. 46[a]: אם הכותל מוכה בלא שבירת העצם קודם התפירה יושם אבק לבונה ואחר יתפר (When the skin is injured but the bone is not broken one should put frankincense powder on it and then suture the spot). Hebr. כֹּתֶל does not feature in this sense in the current dictionaries.

כֻּתֹּנֶת • הכתונת החוברת · **conjunctiva**: Lat. *coniunctiva* (Arab. ملتحم / Gr. ἡ περιοστίου κάταφυσις) · Constantinus Africanus, *Viaticum* · trans. Do'eg ha-Edomi, *Sefer Ya'ir Netiv*,[170] bk. 2, ch. 3: הקליפה[171] היא דם היורד אל הכתונת החוברת זהו קונגוקטיבא ואל[172] הארטיריאש שלה בהבקעם ונעשה משני ענינים מהכאת העין ומבקיעת החוברת או בעבור הנפח הנולד בחוברת (Hyposphagma[173] is blood that streams to the conjunctiva, i.e., [Lat.] QWNGWQṬYB', [from][174] blood vessels torn in it. It is caused either by a blow to the eye or by a tear in the conjunctiva or by a tumor originating in the conjunctiva). Hebr. הכתונת החוברת does not feature in the current dictionaries. Moses ibn Tibbon translates Arab. ملتحم as לובן (cf. BCD 134 (NM 4:88)).

כָּתַשׁ • כתש כתישה עבה · **to crush**: Arab. رضّ · Ibn al-Jazzār, *Zād al-musāfir wa-qūt al-ḥāḍir* · trans. Abraham ben Isaac, *Sefer Ṣedah la-Oreḥim*, bk. 1, ch. 23: תכתוש הכל כתישה עבה ותשים על השמן וישים על האש וירתיח עד שיצא כח הסמים בשמן ותורידהו מן האש ולא תצלילהו (Crush all this and add it to the oil. Put it on a fire and boil it until the oil absorbs the power of the drugs. Then, remove it from the fire and do not filter it). Hebr. כתש כתישה עבה is not attested for in the current dictionaries. Moses ibn Tibbon translates Arab. رضّ as רצץ.

• *Part. Pass.* **כָּתוּשׁ • בשר כתוש** → **בָּשָׂר**.

170 As synonyms of הכתונת החוברת (Lat. *coniunctiva*), we find החלק הדבק and החלק החוברת (see entry חֵלֶק) and חוֹבֶרֶת (see entry חָבֵר).

171 הקליפה: *crustula* L طرفة a.

172 ואל הארטיריאש: *a suis arteriis* L.

173 'Hyposphagma': See entry קְלִפָּה.

174 '[from]': Trans. according to Lat. *a*.

ל

לֵב • **the inside; the inner part; pulp:** Arab. لباب • Ibn al-Jazzār, *Zād al-musāfir wa-qūt al-ḥādir* • trans. Moses ibn Tibbon, *Sefer Ṣedat ha-Derakhim*, bk. 3, ch. 6: ויעשה דיסא מן לב לחם עם דבש ושקדים (He should make porridge prepared from the inner part of bread with honey and almonds). In the sense of 'the inside; inner part; pulp,' Hebr. לֵב features in BM 2596, a.o., in an attestation from Maimonides' commentary on *Mishnah Ukzin*, and in later attestations from the *Sefer ha-Qanun*. Moses ibn Tibbon's ויעשה דיסא מן לב לחם עם דבש ושקדים is quoted verbatim by Me'ir Aldabi, *Shevilei Emunah* (see BM 2596).

• **הדפים הסובבים הלב** → דַּף.

• **כאב דוקר בלב** → כְּאֵב.

• **המכסה המקיף הלב** → מִכְסֶה.

• **פלצות הלב** → פַּלָּצוּת.

לְבָבִי • **רפואה לבבית** → רְפוּאָה.

לָבָן • **בהרת לבנה** → בַּהֶרֶת.

לֹבֶן • **צמח בלובן העין** → צֶמַח.

לְבָנָה[1] • **גדול הלבנה** → גִּדּוּל.

• **חיסור הלבנה** → חִסּוּר.

לְבֻנָה[2] • **בעלי הלבנה** → בַּעַל.

[להב] • *Hitpaʿel* הִתְלַהֵב • **to become inflamed** • Ibn al-Jazzār, *Zād al-musāfir wa-qūt al-ḥādir* • trans. Abraham ben Isaac, *Sefer Ṣedah la-Oreḥim*, bk. 1, ch. 18: והב' מחמת הרתחת הדם שבתוך הלב כי דם זה שבלב כאשר ירתח ויתלהב מחמת מרירה האדומה אז יעלה מן הדם בהרתחתו עשן אל הראש ואז יולד במוח הראש צמח חד מרירי (The second [cause of phrenitis] is the boiling of the blood within the heart. When this blood seethes and becomes inflamed because of the yellow bile vapors arise to the head and cause a sharp bilious swelling in the brain). Hebr. הִתְלַהֵב features as *Part. Hitpaʿel* מִתְלַהֵב ('inflamed') in BCD 135 (NM 2:13); BMZ 62 (Ayin 4) in an attestation from Shem Tov ben Isaac, *Sefer Almansur*, i.e., his translation of al-Rāzī's *K. al-Manṣūrī*. Moses ibn Tibbon translates Arab. التهب as התלהב as well.

• *Hifʿil* הִלְהִיב • **to inflame; to cause an inflammation:** Arab. ألهب • Isḥāq ibn ʿImrān, *Treatise on Melancholy* • trans. Anonymous, fol. 43^{a} (44^{a}): וכן ראינו ביין החם הישן כשיתמידהו ולהשתכר ממנו יפסיד השכל וילהיב המוח ומוליד בגוף להב חזק (I have also observed that if one frequently drinks hot old wine until one gets drunk, it corrupts the mind, inflames the brain, and produces a severe heat in the body). Hebr. הִלְהִיב is attested for in medieval literature in EM 797 in an attestation from Elʿazar ha-Kallir in the sense of 'to kindle, to fan the fire.' For *Piʿel* לִהֵב in the sense of 'to cause an inflammation;' cf. BCD 135 (NM 4:89).

לְהִיבָה • **inflammation:** Arab. التهاب • Ibn al-Jazzār, *Zād al-musāfir wa-qūt al-ḥādir* • trans. Abraham ben Isaac, *Sefer Ṣedah la-Oreḥim*, bk. 1, ch. 18 (Ms Florence, Biblioteca Medicina Laurenziana, Plut. 88.37, fol. 94[a]): ויולד צמח זה מא׳ מב׳ עניינים: הא׳ מפני להיבת מרה אדומה ובעירתה במקום המוח (This swelling originates from one of two causes; the first is an inflammation and burning of the yellow bile within the brain). Hebr. לְהִיבָה features in EM 798 as a modern term in the sense of 'fire, burning.' It is possibly a variant reading of לֶהָבָה, which features as a translation of Arab. التهاب in the sense of 'inflammation' in Shem Tov ben Isaac's *Sefer Almansur* (cf. BCD 135 (NM 2:13); BMZ 60 (Ayin 1)). Moses ibn Tibbon translates Arab. التهاب as התלהבות (cf. BCD 76 (NM 1:55; 3:73)). Do'eg ha-Edomi translates the parallel Latin term *incensio* as שלהבת. The latter term features in Do'eg ha Edomi's translation of Hippocrates' *Aphorisms* (i.e., *Sefer Agur*) 4.65 in the sense of 'heat' (cf. BCD 275 (NM 3:227)).

לוז • *Plur.* **לוזים** · **tonsils**: Ms Cambridge, T-S K14.48, P.8 (recto): האגוזים הרטובים הירוקים חצר בערבי וירד בלעז אם יעצרו מימיהם ויבושלו עד היותם כדבש מעור[בים] [ב]מיבכתג׳ ויגרגר בהם יועיל ממורסות הלוזים (If one extracts the moisture from green (Arab. *khaḍir*; Rom. *verde*), fresh almonds, boils them until they become like honey, mixes [this substance] with *maybakhtaj* [i.e., syrup, Arab. ميبختج; cf. entry יַיִן: יין מבושל above] and uses this as a gargle, it is beneficial for swollen tonsils). In the sense of 'tonsils,' Hebr. לוזים features in MD 724, s.v. 'tonsil,' without any further reference.

• **לוזים הודיים** · **betel nuts** [***Areca catechu*** **L.**]: Arab. الفوفل or البندق الهندي (cf. MIG 776) · Shem Tov ben Isaac, *Sefer ha-Shimmush*, bk. 29, list 1 (SHS 1:300 (Lamed 30)): לוזים הודיים ב״ה פופל ובי״ל אבילאנה אינדיגא (*luzim hodiyim*; Arab. *fawfal*; O.Occ. *avelana *indiga* or **endega* [occitanized form of L.Lat. *abellana indica*]). In the sense of 'betel nut,' Hebr. *Sing.* לוז הודי is a non-attested calque of Arab. البندق الهندي.

לומבריק • *Plur.* **לומבריקש** · **earthworms**: Rom. *lumbrics* · Guillaume de Congenis, *Treatise on Surgery* · trans. Isaiah, fol. 55[a]: ושים בזה המקום וכיוצא בו התולעים הנקראים לומבריקש מבושלים במחבת וימלאו היטב המכה ויעזבו שם ב׳ ימים או ג׳ (Put earthworms called LWMBRYQŠ, once they been boiled in a pot, on this spot and similar ones. One should carefully fill the spot of the injury with them and leave them for two or three days). Hebr. *Sing.* לומבריק, *Plur.* לומבריקש, is a non-attested loan word from Rom. Sing. *lumbric*, Plur. *lumbrics* (and var.).

[לזג] • *Pass. Part.* **לָזוּג** · **viscous**: Arab. لزج · Ibn al-Jazzār, *Zād al-musāfir wa-qūt al-ḥādir* · trans. Abraham ben Isaac, *Sefer Ṣedah la-Oreḥim*, bk. 1, ch. 7 (Ms Jerusalem, National Library of Israel, Fr. 95, fol. 87[b]): חולי זה יקרה בעור הראש והיא שחינים ויהיה בהם נקבים דקים קטנים ויצא מהם לחלוחית עבה לזוגה (This illness [i.e., honeycomb] occurs in the scalp and consists of ulcers with fine, small openings from which a thick, viscous moisture exudes). Hebr. לָזוּג is a non-attested loan word from Arab. لزج. Moses ibn Tibbon translates Arab. لزج as דבק.

לָזוּג (*Pass. Part.*) → [**לזג**].

לְחִיכָה · **linctus**: Arab. لعوق · Ibn al-Jazzār, *Zād al-musāfir wa-qūt al-ḥādir* · trans. Moses ibn Tibbon, *Sefer Ṣedat ha-Derakhim*, bk. 3, ch. 7: ואם יקשה להשליך החומר מן הריאה נצוה החולה לשתות בשול איזוף עם סוכר ויאולד או יעשה הלחיכה הזאת (If the patient finds it difficult to expel the [superfluous] matter from the lungs, we tell him to take a hyssop potion with violet preserve or to use the following linctus …). Hebr. לְחִיכָה is attested for in medical literature in BM 2653 in a quotation from *Perush Ibn Rushd ʿal Ḥaruzei Ibn Sina* (Ibn Rushd's commentary on Ibn Sīnā's *ʿUrjūza*) in the Hebrew translation prepared by Solomon ibn Ayyub in the year 1261. Ben-Yehuda defines the term as כנוי לסמי רפואה יבשים ('term used for a dry remedy'). Do'eg ha-Edomi translates the parallel Latin term *electuarium* as מרקחת.

לֶחֶם • לחם חזירי · sowbread (i.e., European cyclamen [*Cyclamen purpurascens* Mill.]): Arab. *ādharyūn* (آذريون) (from Pers. *ādhargūn*)[175] / Lat. *panis porcinus* / Rom. *pan porcine* · *Shinnui ha-Shemot ha-Niqra'im Synonimis*, Ms Munich, Bayerische Staatsbibliothek, Cod. hebr. 8, fol. 192ᵇ: אַדְהוּנָא הוא מין מְצִיקְלַמִין בספרי׳ אחרים נקר׳ אַדַרְבוּנַא הוא לחם חזירי ('aDəHWuNa' [read: 'DRYWN]; a kind of cyclamen; in other books it is called 'aDaRəBWuNa'; i.e., *leḥem ḥaziri*). In the sense of 'cyclamen,' Hebr. לחם חזירי is a non-attested calque from Lat. *panis porcinus* or Rom. *pan porcine*.[176]

לֵחָנִי · phlegmatic; suffering from a surplus of phlegm: Lat. *flegmaticus* · Ibn al-Jazzār, *Zād al-musāfir wa-qūt al-ḥādir* · trans. Abraham ben Isaac, *Sefer Ṣedah la-Oreḥim*, Adaptation, bk. 1, ch. 10 (Ms Berlin, Staatsbibliothek Preußischer Kulturbesitz, Or. fol. 1058, fol. 94ᵇ): ואם האיש ליחני הוסף שם באותו השיעור שרוצה לתפוש שקמוניאה ומלח הודו קולוקינטידה אגריקו טורביטי לבן מכל אחד חלק שוה (If the patient suffers from a surplus of phlegm, add to the [recipe] equal parts [in the desired quantity] of scammony, Indian salt, pulp of colocynth, agarikon, and white St. Thomas lidpod …). Hebr. לֵחָנִי is not attested for in the current dictionaries. Moses ibn Tibbon translates the parallel Arabic term كثير الرطوبات as רב הלחויות and Abraham ben Isaac as בעל רטיבות וליחה. Do'eg ha-Edomi translates Lat. *flegmaticus* as סובלי הלבנה.

ליחני → לֵחָנִי.

לִכְלוּךְ · sordes (i.e., earwax): Arab. وسخ (Gr. ῥυπος)[177] · Ibn al-Jazzār, *Zād al-musāfir wa-qūt al-ḥādir* · trans. Moses ibn Tibbon, *Sefer Ṣedat ha-Derakhim*, bk. 2, ch. 7: ואם נראה בה נגע או מורסא או שחין או יבלת או לכלוך רב או דבר שנפל בו מחוץ (And if we [look inside the ear] and see an ulcer or tumor or swelling or pustule, or [see] that it is full with sordes [i.e., earwax] or something that fell into it from the outside …). In the sense of 'sordes,' Hebr. לִכְלוּךְ is a non-attested indirect semantic borrowing from Gr. ῥυπος

---

175 *Ādharyūn* refers to yet another plant, namely marigold (Calendula officinalis L.); cf. MIG 702.

176 The Hebrew term features as לחם חזיר next to the Rom. פאן פורצין in Pseudo-Ibn Ezra's *Sefer Hanisyonot: The Book of Medical Experiences Attributed to Abraham ibn Ezra*, ed. and trans. J.O. Leibowitz and S. Marcus (Jerusalem 1984), 228: לחם חזיר ר״ל פאן פורצין.

177 Cf. Ḥunayn's translation of Galen's *De simplicium medicamentorum temperamentis ac facultatibus* 10.2.17, ed. Kühn, 12:290 l. 14: ὁ ἐν τοῖς ὠσὶ ῥύπος; Arab. Ms Escurial 793, fol. 165ᵇ, l. 16: *al-wasakhu l-khāriju mina l-udhni*.

via Arab. وسخ. Do'eg ha-Edomi translates the parallel Latin term *res mucidae* as גְּעוּל (see entry). Hebr. לִכְלוּךְ features as לכלוך האוזן in Ibn Tibbon's translation of Arab. وسخ الأذن in *Sefer Ṣedat ha-Derakhim*, bk. 7, ch. 27.3 (cf. IJZ 169).

לְמוּדִי · **theoretical**: Arab. علمي · Ibn al-Jazzār, *Zād al-musāfir wa-qūt al-ḥādir* · trans. Moses ibn Tibbon, *Sefer Ṣedat ha-Derakhim*, bk. 3, ch. 12: ואם לא תצא הרקיקה עם זה כי אם בצער ושעול חזק יורה על חולשת הכח ולאותו ואין לבטוח בו אם לא שיהיה בו יכולת לקבל[178] החולי ומלחמתו ובמה שהבאנו מן הדברים הלמודיים די ספוק וראוי לנו שנזכור עתה רפואות החולי הזה (If next to this, the sputum only comes out with strong painful coughing, it indicates that the strength [of the patient] is weak and cannot be relied upon, let alone that it can endure the illness and fight against it. The theoretical matters that I have mentioned so far are sufficient [for our current discussion]; [it is now time] to mention the remedies for this illness). In the sense of 'theoretical,' Hebr. לְמוּדִי features in KT 2:121 and HCD 39.

לָקַח • לקח עצה · **to contrive**: Lat. *ingenio* (Arab. احتال) · Constantinus Africanus, *Viaticum* · trans. Do'eg ha-Edomi, *Sefer Ya'ir Netiv*, bk. 1, ch. 19: והרופא יקח עצה לישנו בעבור העשות בשול היין ואחר כך יכינו לו מרחץ מזוג ונגרד רגליו (And the physician should contrive [i.e., exercise his skill] to let him sleep so that the wine can be digested, then a moderately hot bath should be prepared for him and his feet should be rubbed). Hebr. לקח עצה does not feature in the current dictionaries. Both Moses ibn Tibbon and Abraham ben Isaac translate Arab. احتال as התחבל. The latter term also features in Zeraḥyah Ḥen's translation of Maimonides' *Medical Aphorisms* 15.17 (BMMZ 155), whereas Nathan ha-Me'ati has הערים (BMMN 156; cf. BCD 88 (NM 1:145)).

לָשׁוֹן • לשון איל · **hart's-tongue fern (Ger. *Hirschzunge*) [*Asplenium scolopendrium* L.]**: Lat. *lingua cervina* · *Shinnui ha-Shemot ha-Niqra'im Synonimi*, Ms Florence, Biblioteca Laurenziana, Or. 17, fol. 69ᵇ: איספילינון ה' לשון איל ה' לינגוא צירבונא ('YSPYLYNWN [i.e., a corruption of 'YSPLYNYWN; i.e., Gr. ἄσπληνον/Lat. *asplenium*]; i.e., [Hebr.] *leshon ayyil*; i.e., [Lat.] LYNGW' ṢYRBWN' [read: LYNGW' ṢYRBYN'; i.e., *lingua cervina*]). In the sense of 'hart's-tongue fern,' Hebr. לשון איל is a non-attested calque of Lat. *lingua cervina*.

• **לשון הים** · **cuttlebone (of a cuttlefish)**; Arab. شيبيا (from Gr. σηπία; cf. LSG 1594); cf. MIG 500 · Shem Tov ben Isaac, *Sefer ha-Shimmush*, bk. 29, list 1 (SHS 1:298 (Lamed 27)): לשון הים ב"ה שביא ובל"ל סיפיא (*leshon ha-yam*; Arab. *shībiyā*; vern. SYPY' [i.e., O.Occ. or O.Cat. *sepia* or *sipia*]). In the sense of 'cuttlebone,' Hebr. לשון הים is a non-attested calque of Arab. لسان البحر, a synonym of شيبيا.

• **לשון הצפור** · **(lit., sparrow's tongue); fruit of the ash tree [*Fraxinus excelsior* L.]**: Arab. لسان العصفر (cf. MIG 505, s.v. لسان العصافير) · Shem Tov ben Isaac, *Sefer ha-Shimmush*, bk. 29, list 1 (SHS 1:286–287 (Lamed 3)): לשון הצפור ב"ה לסאן אלעצפור ובל"ל לנגא אויש (*leshon ha-ṣippor*; Arab. *lisān al-ʿuṣfūr*; vern. LNG' 'WYŠ [i.e., O.Occ.-Lat.

178 לקבל: לסבול Ms London, British Library, Ar. Or. 26, fol. 107ᵇ.

linga/lenga avis, from L. *lingua avis*). In the sense of 'fruit of the ash tree,' Hebr. לשון הצפור is attested as לשון הצפורים in BCD 139 (NM 4:93).

- **נחור הלשון** → **נְחוֹר**.
- **צמח מתחת הלשון** → **צֶמַח**.

מְאֻבָּק (*Part. Pu'al*) → [אבק].
מאובק → מְאֻבָּק.
מְאַוֶּה (*Part. Pi'el*) → [אוה].
מַאֲכָל • *Plur.* **מאכלים** • **חמוץ המאכלים** → חִמּוּץ.
מַאֲמָר • *Plur.* **מאמרות** ‣ **aphorisms:** Arab. فصول · Ibn al-Jazzār, *Zād al-musāfir wa-qūt al-ḥādir* · trans. Abraham ben Isaac, *Sefer Ṣedah la-Oreḥim*, bk. 1, ch. 24: ועל זה אמר איפוקרט בספר המאמרות שלו: כל מי שיבוא לו חולי זה הנקר׳ תשנג׳ או תמדד הנקר׳ בלשון יון טיטנוש ולאחר כן יבוא לו קדחת אז תמיס הקדחת לאותו חולי (Accordingly, Hippocrates said in his *Book of Aphorisms*: If someone is afflicted by this illness [i.e., spasms] that is called [in Arab.] *tashannuj* [lit., cramps] or *tamaddud* [lit., stretching] and that is called in Greek *tetanos* [i.e., tetanus], and if fever occurs after this, the fever will dissolve his disease.) Hebr. מאמרות does not feature in this sense in the current dictionaries. Moses ibn Tibbon translates Arab. فصول as פרקים. Do'eg ha-Edomi transcribes Lat. abl. *aphorismis* as אפורשמש.

• **עשרה מאמרות** → עֶשֶׂר

מְאֹרָע • *Plur.* **מאורעים/מאורעות** ‣ I. **symptoms:** Arab. عوارض · Isḥāq ibn 'Imrān, *Treatise on Melancholy* · trans. Anonymous, fol. 41ª (42ª): וגם זה האיש אע״פ שחבר בו ספר וחלקיו לשני חלקים השתדל בו כל מאודו ודרש וחקר עליו ועל מאורעיו ואיך יאות לרפאתם לא כלל בספרו זה מכל מיניו כי אם מין אחד (Although this man [i.e., Rufus] composed a treatise [on melancholy] and divided it into two parts and studied [the disease], its symptoms, and treatment to the best of his ability, he only included in his treatise one of its [different] kinds). Hebr. *Sing.* מְאֹרָע, *Plur.* מאורעים/מאורעות, does not feature in this sense in the current dictionaries. Constantine the African translates Arab. عوارض as *accidentia*.

‣ II. **afflictions:** Arab. آفات · Isḥāq ibn 'Imrān, *Treatise on Melancholy* · trans. Anonymous, fol. 42ª (43ª): אע״פ שמא יהיה חולשת האבר מחמת הנהגתו או מחמת הרכבתו בתחלת בריתו או מחמת החולי וגוברו והתמדתו עליו עד שיפסיד מזונו ויחלשו כוחותיו ויביאהו[179] לקבל המאורעות במיהור (The weakness of the organ may also be caused by its [bad] regimen or by its composition at the time it was created or by an illness that has such a strong, lasting effect on it that it corrupts its nourishment, weakens its strength, and makes it quickly predisposed for afflictions). Ben-Yehuda (s.v. מְאוֹרָע) mentions the term in the sense of 'afflictions' affecting the body in a quotation from Maimonides, *Mishneh Torah, Hilkhot Yesode ha-Torah* (BM 2758–2759). Nathan ha-Me'ati translates Arab. آفات as פגעים in his translation of Maimonides, *Medical Aphorisms* and Zeraḥyah Ḥen as חולי, חולי(י)ם, or רעות. Constantine the African translates Arab. آفات as *morbi*.

179 ויביאהו: emendation editor ויבא⟨.⟩הו Ms.

מַבְדִּיל (*Part. Hifʿil*) → [**בדל**].
מבושל → **מְבֻשָּׁל**.
מְבַכֶּרֶת (*Part. Piʿel f.*) → [**בכר**].
מְבֻשָּׁל (*Part. Puʿal*) → [**בשל**].
מַגִּיד (*Part. Hifʿil*) → [**נגד**].
מגרי • **הדפק המגרי** → **דֹּפֶק**.
מַדְבִּיק (*Part. Hifʿil*) → [**דבק**].
מִדְבָּרִי ‣ **wild:** Arab. بَرّي · Ibn al-Jazzār, *Zād al-musāfir wa-qūt al-ḥāḍir* · trans. Moses ibn Tibbon, *Sefer Ṣedat ha-Derakhim*, bk. 1, ch. 23: תאר רפואה מעטשת חברה בן מאסויה לעקום הפה והפלג והשתוק והפחד ונקוי המוח יקח כנדיס ז׳ דר׳ פלפל לבן ושחור וקשטורן מ״א דרהם רודא מדברית ושניבי מ״א ב׳ דרהם (Recipe of a remedy inducing sneezing composed by ibn Māsawayh, [which is beneficial] for facial paresis, hemiplegia, apoplexy as well as fear, and which cleanses the brain: Take seven *dirhams* of sneezewort, one *dirham* each of white and black pepper and castoreum, two *dirhams* each of wild rue [i.e., Syrian rue] and mustard). In the sense of 'wild,' Hebr. מִדְבָּרִי features in BM 2796 in an attestation from Maimonides' *Commentary on the Mishnah*. Ben-Yehuda explains the term as ההפך מן גני ('the opposite of 'cultivated''). Abraham ben Isaac translates Arab. بَرّي as יַעֲרִי (see entry).
• **שום מדברי** → **שׁוּם**.
• **שרף רוטא מדברית** → **שְׂרָף**.

מִדָּה ‣ **I. temperament**: Arab. مزاج · Ibn al-Jazzār, *Zād al-musāfir wa-qūt al-ḥāḍir* · trans. Abraham ben Isaac, *Sefer Ṣedah la-Oreḥim*, bk. 1, ch. 9 (Ms Jerusalem, National Library of Israel, Fr. 95, fol. 88ᵇ): ואם יארעו הכינים בראש שיש מדתו חום הנק׳ אגתאה אז ראוי להטיח הראש (If lice appear on a head having a hot temperament, called ʾGTʾH(?), it is necessary to rub the head …). Hebr. מִדָּה does not feature in this sense in the current dictionaries. A regular term for 'temperament' used by Abraham ben Isaac is a loan word from Gr. κρᾶσις, i.e., קראסיס (see entry). Moses ibn Tibbon translates Arab. مزاج as מזג.
‣ **II. specific property**: Arab. خاصّية · Ibn al-Jazzār, *Zād al-musāfir wa-qūt al-ḥāḍir* · trans. Abraham ben Isaac, *Sefer Ṣedah la-Oreḥim*, bk. 1, ch. 19: ויותר שיועיל לשיכורי היין אם ישתה אפסינתיאה כי יש מידת העשב הזה להעביר חמת היין ושכרותו (The best thing to recover for people who are drunk from wine is to take absinth wormwood, since one of its specific properties is to undo the heating and inebrieting effect of wine). Hebr. מִדָּה does not feature in this sense in the current dictionaries. Moses ibn Tibbon renders Arab. خاصّية with the standard term סגולה. Doʾeg ha-Edomi translates the parallel Latin term *proprietas* as כח קרוב אליו (see entry כֹּחַ).
• **למדת** ‣ **I. like; resembling**: Lat. *sicut* (Arab. أمثال) · Constantinus Africanus, *Viaticum* · trans. Doʾeg ha-Edomi, *Sefer Yaʾir Netiv*,[180] bk. 1, ch. 10: ותמזוג עם מיץ מראטרי ותעשה

180 For a synonym used by Doʾeg ha-Edomi, cf. entry לדמות :דְּמוּת.

גרגרים למדת פלפל ותתן ג׳ דרכמ׳ עם מים חמים (Mix [these ingredients] with fennel juice and mould this into pills resembling peppercorns [in weight] and administer three *dirhams* with hot water). Hebr. למדת does not feature in the current dictionaries. Moses ibn Tibbon renders Arab. أمثال as כמו and Abraham ben Isaac as כמין (see entry מִין).

‣ II. **the amount of**: Lat. *in modum* (Arab. مقدار) · Constantinus Africanus, *Viaticum* · trans. Do'eg ha-Edomi, *Sefer Ya'ir Netiv*, bk. 3, ch. 1: ותכתוש לאבק ותחבר עם דבש די ספקו ויקבל למדת לוז (Pulverize [these ingredients], mix them with sufficient honey, and take the amount of one hazelnut). Moses ibn Tibbon translates Arab. مقدار as שעור.

מדוכה → מְדֹכָה.

מְדוֹר • *Plur.* **מדורים** ‣ **ventricles**: Lat. *ventriculi* (Arab. أوعية) · Constantinus Africanus, *Viaticum* · trans. Do'eg ha-Edomi, *Sefer Ya'ir Netiv*, bk. 1, ch. 11: המוח נחלק באורך אל הימין ואל השמאל ושם קו אמצעי מפריד את מדוריו ובעלות עשן אחת הליחות ונדח בתולדתו אל הימין או אל השמאל יחול שם כאב ונקרא מיקראניאה (The brain is divided lengthwise in a right and left [part], and there is a line [i.e., groove] in the middle that divides the ventricles; when vapors from one of the humors arise [to the head] and nature pushes them to the right or left, [head]ache called [in Lat.] MYQR'NY'H [i.e., migraine] occurs there). In the sense of 'ventricle,' Hebr. *Sing.* מָדוֹר (for Arab. وعى) features in BCD 142 (NM 4:95) in a later attestation from Moses ibn Tibbon's *Sefer Ṣedat ha-Derakhim*, bk. 1, ch. 11.

מְדֹכָה • **מדוכה** ‣ **mortar**: Lat. *mortarium* · Guillaume de Congenis, *Treatise on Surgery* · trans. Isaiah, fol. 47^b: לעפעפים ההפוכות או הגסות לפעמים לזקנים ביותר תעשה משיחה בזאת: קח אלואין סיטרין צירושא ב׳ דרכמו׳ מ״א שומן[181] חזיר חדש בלי מלח אוקי׳ ירקח ביחד בכלי זך וחזק ואחר שחוק במדוכה וישאר לעת הצורך בכלי זכוכית (For eyelids that are folded inwards [i.e., entropion] or rough and that sometimes [affect] especially old people one should prepare the following salve: Take two *dirhams* each of aloe, citron, ceruse, one ounce of the unsalted fat of a young pig, mix [these ingredients] in a strong clean vessel, pound [the mixture] in a mortar and [put it] in a glass and leave it there until you need it). In the sense of 'mortar,' Hebr. מְדֹכָה is attested for the Bible and Rabbinic literature only (cf. BDB 189; JD 733, s.v. מדוכה; BM 2812).

[מהר] • *Pi'el* מִהֵר ‣ **to urge; to instigate; to induce**: Arab. حفز · Ibn al-Jazzār, *Zād al-musāfir wa-qūt al-ḥādir* · trans. Moses ibn Tibbon, bk. 1, ch. 21: ופעמים יהיה העטוש כשימהר החולי לטבע שיתנועע בזולת העת אשר ראוי שיתנועע כמו המתהוה ממנו הזוכאם או בחולי הריאה (Sometimes sneezing occurs because a disease induces nature to move [the brain] at inappropriate times—such as in the case of the illness called *al-zukām* [i.e., rheum] and pneumonia). Hebr. מִהֵר features in biblical literature as a transit-

181 שומן: Ms[1].

ive verb in the sense of 'to prepare quickly, to bring quickly' (BDB 554–555); but cf. EM 870: להאיץ, לזרז ('to urge, to press, to stimulate'). Abraham ben Isaac translates Arab. حفز as הִנְחִיץ (see entry [נחץ]).

מוח → מֹחַ.

מוֹךְ · **a piece of cotton**: Arab. قطنة · Ibn al-Jazzār, *Zād al-musāfir wa-qūt al-ḥādir* · trans. Abraham ben Isaac, *Sefer Ṣedah la-Oreḥim*, bk. 1, ch. 17: מרקחת אחר להרדים ולישן בטוב: קח אופיו ובנג׳ וזרע יברוחין בד בבד כתוש הכל ונפה ולוש במים ושים בשמש ה׳ ימים וכשתצטרך לו תקח ממנו במעט מוך ומשח בו המצח וגם בין העינים (Another remedy to fall asleep and sleep well: Take one part each of opium, henbane, and mandrake seeds. Pulverize this, sieve it, knead it with water, and let it stand in the sun for five days. When you need it, take some of it in a small piece of cotton and rub it on the forehead and between the eyes). Hebr. מוֹךְ is not attested for in medieval Hebrew medical literature. It features in Rabbinic literature (cf. JD 741: 'a soft, spongy substance, hackled wool, rag, lint etc.') and medieval halakhic literature (cf. ShMM 488–489). In his commentary on tb*Shabbat* 47, Rashi remarks that the term applies to anything soft, as, e.g., cotton (כל דבר רך קרוי מוכין כגון צמר גפן) (cf. KA 5:132). Moses ibn Tibbon translates Arab. قطنة as מוֹךְ as well.

מוכבר → מַכְבָּר.

מונח → מֻנָּח.

מופשט → מֻפְשָׁט.

מוֹפֵת · **evidence; proof; symptom**: Arab. برهان · Ibn al-Jazzār, *Zād al-musāfir wa-qūt al-ḥādir* · trans. Moses ibn Tibbon, *Sefer Ṣedat ha-Derakhim*, bk. 3, ch. 1 (fol. 74[a]): וכשנרצה לרפאת החולה מן החולי הזה נעיין ואם היה התילדות החולי מדם והורה על זה המופת אשר זכרנו (If we want to heal the patient from this illness, we should consider: if the illness originates from blood, which is indicated by the symptoms that I mentioned …). Hebr. מוֹפֵת does not feature in a medical context in the current dictionaries.

מוֹקֵד · **fire; heat**: Lat. *ardor* (Arab. الحرارة الشديدة) · Constantinus Africanus, *Viaticum* · trans. Do'eg ha-Edomi, *Sefer Ya'ir Netiv*, bk. 2, ch. 4: אחר זה טוב ליבש הדמעות ולמחשך ולחכוך ולמוקד (Another [remedy] that is good for drying tears, loss [lit., darkness] [of vision], itching, and heat). Hebr. מוֹקֵד features in the current dictionaries in the sense of 'burning mass' (BDB 428) and 'fire-place, hearth' (JD 747; BM 2800). Ben-Yehuda refers to the term featuring in medical literature as מוקד הקדחת (for Arab. مستوقد الحمّى ('the hearth of fever')) in Maimonides, *Pirkei Moshe* 23, i.e., Zerahyah Ḥen's translation of Maimonides' *Medical Aphorisms* 23.20 (BMMZ 218). Moses ibn Tibbon translates Arab. الحرارة الشديدة as החום החזק.

מוקץ → מֻקָּץ.

מוֹרָד · **abatement (i.e., receding) (of an illness)**: Lat. *declinatio* (Arab. هبوط) · Constantinus Africanus, *Viaticum* · trans. Do'eg ha-Edomi, *Sefer Ya'ir Netiv*, bk. 3, ch. 12: ואם החולי יהיה במורד נתן לו שפא ומילקרט ונמשח אותו עם שמן קמומילא ושמן אניט ונאכילהו מרק זרעונים עם שמן שקדים (When the illness recedes, we give [the patient] [a drink of] boiled down wine and melicrate and we rub him with Roman camomile oil and dill oil and we feed him a broth of chickpeas with almond oil). Hebrew מוֹרָד does not feature in a medical sense in the current dictionaries. Moses ibn Tibbon translates Arab. هبوط as ירידה (see BCD 120 (NM 3:110)).

מורסן • **קמח שחוסר המורסן ממנו** → קֶמַח.

מָזַג • *Pass. Part.* מָזוּג · **moderate**: Lat. *temperatus* · Constantinus Africanus, *Viaticum* · trans. Do'eg ha-Edomi, *Sefer Ya'ir Netiv*, bk, 1, ch. 2: בבאו בסבת צום יתכן להכניסו במרחץ מזוג (If it [i.e., hair loss] is caused by abstention from food it is possible to let [the patient] visit the bathhouse with a moderate [atmosphere]). In the sense of moderate (more specifically, 'balanced,' for Lat. *moderatus*), Hebr. מָזוּג features in BCD 144 (NM 3:126) in a later attestation from Hillel ben Samuel's translation of Hippocrates' *Aphorisms* 5.62.

מֶזֶג • **במזג** · **moderately**: Lat. *temperate* (Arab. باعتدال) · Constantinus Africanus, *Viaticum* · trans. Do'eg ha-Edomi, *Sefer Ya'ir Netiv*, bk, 1, ch. 20: עוד אמר רופין: אין היין לבדו בהיותו שתוי במזג מסיר הדאגה אך דברים אחרים הדומים אליו (Rufus also said: Not only wine—when consumed moderately—takes away anxiety, but other similar things as well). Hebr. מֶזֶג does not feature in the sense of 'moderateness' in the current dictionaries. Moses ibn Tibbon translates Arab. باعتدال as בשווי.

מָזוּג (*Pass. Part.*) → מָזַג.

מזמר • **מזמר הרועה** · **European water plantain [*Alisma plantago-aquatica* L.]**: Arab: زمارة الراعي or مزمار الرالي (cf. StH 948; IBF 2126; DT 3:144 (505–506)) · *Shinnui ha-Shemot ha-Niqra'im Synonimis*, Ms Munich, Bayerische Staatsbibliothek, Cod. hebr. 8, fol. 197[b]: זמארה אלרעי כלומר מזמר הרועה ובלשונינו אבובא דרעיא ([Arab.] *zammāra al-rāʿī*; i.e., [Hebr.] *MZMR ha-roʿeh*; and in our language [i.e., Aram.] *abbuba de-raʿya*). In the sense of 'European water plantain,' Hebr. מזמר הרועה is a non-attested calque from Arab. زمارة الراعي or مزمار الرالي. For Aram. אבובא דרעיא, see entry אֲבוּבָא.

מֹחַ · **pulp**: Arab. دماغ · Ibn al-Jazzār, *Zād al-musāfir wa-qūt al-ḥādir* · trans. Moses ibn Tibbon, *Sefer Ṣedat ha-Derakhim*, bk. 3, ch. 6: ומי שירצה שיהיה פעולתו לחזה יותר גדולה ויותר חזקה יקח לב זרע קשואים הנקראים קתא ולב זרע קשואים הנקראים כיאר ולב זרע אבטיח ולב זרע קרא וזרע חבושים ודרגגן לבן וזרע פפאויר מ״א י׳ דר׳ יודק עד שישוב כמוח (If you want that its effect on the chest is greater and stronger, you should take the core of the seeds of [the kind of] cucumber called *qiththā*, and core of [the kind of] cucumber called *khiyār* [i.e., possibly a small variety of cucumber[182]], and the core of watermelon seeds, and of pumpkin seeds, and quince seed, and white gum tragacanth, and poppy seed; one *dirham* of each, [and] pound these until it turns into pulp). Hebr. מֹחַ features in BM 2891, a.o., in attestations from Rashi's commentary on the Talmud in the sense of 'pith' of plants and in one attestation from Elijah de Vidas,

182 Cf. DT 4:173 (692, n. 14).

Reshit Hokhmah, in the sense of 'kernel' of nuts. In the sense of 'pulp,' Hebr. מֹחַ is a non-attested semantic borrowing from Arab. دماغ. In Ms London, British Library, Add. 27542, fol. 43[a], Arab. دماغ is rendered as עִסָּה (see entry).
• **סוף המוח → סוֹף.**
• **צמח המוח → צֶמַח.**
• **ראש המוח → רֹאשׁ.**
[מחה] • *Hifʿil* **הִמְחָה** ‧ **to dissolve:** Arab. حلّ ‧ Ibn al-Jazzār, *Zād al-musāfir wa-qūt al-ḥāḍir* ‧ trans. Moses ibn Tibbon, *Sefer Ṣedat ha-Derakhim*, bk. 3, ch. 6: וישתה בשול אישוף או משקה ג׳וג׳ובש ושבשתן או משקה שליום וישתה אחר שתית מה שספרנו בשלש שעות דיסת שעור בשמן שקדים ומעט פניס או סוכר או ימחה בו אחר שישלם בשולו סוכר ויאולדו (Let him take a decoction of hyssop or a potion of common jujube and sebesten, or of fleawort, and three hours later he should take porridge made from barley with almond oil and a small amount of sugar candy or sugar. Once it has been cooked he may also dissolve violet preserve in it). In the sense of 'to dissolve,' Hebr. הִמְחָה is only attested for in Rabbinic literature; cf. JD 759. For the Aramaic counterpart מחי in the same sense in the Pe'al conjugation, cf. JD ibid., and in the Af'el conjugation, cf. SDA 656 ('to liquefy'). See also KA 5:104.
[מחט] • *Nifʿal* **נִמְחַט** ‧ **to be operated:** Arab. قُدِح ‧ Maimonides, *Medical Aphorisms* 15.31 ‧ trans. Zeraḥyah Ḥen (BMMZ 157): כשתהיה קורע הקרום הקרני יהיה תחלת מה שיפגושך הלחות הדק הרקיק ויהיה ניגר וזב והוא הלחות אשר הרבה פעמים אנו רואים שיגר ויצא מן הנקב אשר ינקב בעין אשר ימחט המים (If you dissect the horn-like tunic, the first thing you find is a fine and thin liquid streaming and pouring out. It is the moisture that we often see flowing out from the opening made in the eye that is being operated [on] for a cataract). A denominative verb מָחַט coined from מַחַט ('needle') features in Rabbinic literature in the sense of 'to snuff, to trim' (JD 758–759). Ben-Yehuda (BM 2907–2908) quotes the term in the sense of 'to abort,' based on KA 5:108. Nathan ha-Me'ati translates Arab. قُدِح as הוקדח.
מַחַט • **מחט הרועה** ‧ **(lit., shepherd's needle); a term used for a group of thistle species:** Arab. إبرة الراعي (cf. MIG 12) ‧ *Shinnui ha-Shemot ha-Niqra Ṣinonimas*, Ms Leiden, Universiteitsbibliotheek, Or. 4719, fol. 31[a]: אברה אלרעי כלו׳ מחט הרועה והוא אל שוכאע ('BRH 'LR'Y [i.e., Arab. *ibra al-rāʿī*]; 'shepherd's needle;' i.e., 'L ŠWK'' [Arab. *al-shukāʿā*]). To indicate different thistle species, Hebr. מחט הרועה is a non-attested loan translation of Arab. *ibrat al-rāʿī*, which is used as a synonym of Arab. *shukāʿā* (i.e., شكاعا) (cf. MIG 12).
מַחְלִיק (*Part. Hifʿil*) → [חלק].
מַחֲנָק ‧ **angina:** Arab. ذبحة ‧ Ibn al-Jazzār, *Zād al-musāfir wa-qūt al-ḥāḍir* ‧ trans. Moses ibn Tibbon, *Sefer Ṣedat ha-Derakhim*, bk. 3, ch. 1 (Ms London, British Library, Add. 27542): וכבר זכר גליינוס כי כל מה שיקרה בגרון שיעצור הנשימה יקרא אסכרה והוא מחנק (Galen has said that all that occurs to the throat and stops breathing is called 'angina;' i.e., [Hebr.] *maḥanaq*). In the sense of 'angina,' Hebr. מַחֲנָק features in

BM 2921 in attestations from Pseudo-Ibn Ezra's *Sefer ha-Nisyonot*, from the *Sefer ha-Qanun* (cf. MD 39), and from Judah al-Ḥarizi's *Sefer Tahkemoni*. See also entry חֶנֶק.

מַחְשָׁבָה • חרדת המחשבה → חֲרָדָה.

• זרות המחשבה → זָרוּת.

מַחְשָׁךְ • מחשך העינים ‣ **dimsightedness (i.e., amblyopia)**: Lat. *obscuritas oculorum* (Arab. الظلمة التي تكون في العين) · Constantinus Africanus, *Viaticum* · trans. Do'eg ha-Edomi, *Sefer Ya'ir Netiv*, bk. 2, ch. 6: פוך טוב אל מחשך העינים ולדמעות ולטהר הבלוי משם (A collyrium that is beneficial for dimsightedness, tears, and for cleansing the [eyes] from the putrefied matter). Hebr. מחשך העינים does not feature in the current dictionaries. Moses ibn Tibbon translates Arab. الظلمة التي تكون في العين as אֹפֶל (cf. BCD 26 (NM 4:20): 'dullness [of sight] (Gr. ἀμαύρωσις[183])').

• מחשך הראות ‣ **dimsightedness**: Lat. *obscuritas visus* (Arab. ظلمة البصر) (Gr. ἀμβλυωπία; cf. UW 90) · Constantinus Africanus, *Viaticum* · trans. Do'eg ha-Edomi, *Sefer Ya'ir Netiv*, bk. 1, ch. 10: רקוח אחר אל יוחנן מדמשק עשוי כנגד הרוח הגס ולמחשך הראות ולכובד הגוף הבא בסבת הרוח הבא מן הלבנה ומן השחורה (Another recipe by Iohannes Damascenus [i.e., Ibn Māsawayh] for coarse winds, dimsightedness, heaviness of the body caused by winds that come from phlegm and black bile). Hebr. מחשך הראות does not feature in the current dictionaries. A synonymous אפיסת המראה features in the *Sefer Agur*, i.e., Do'eg ha Edomi's translation of a Latin version of Hippocrates' *Aphorisms* 3.31 (cf. BCD 25 (NM 3:28)). Moses ibn Tibbon translates Arab. ظلمة البصر as כהות הראות (see entry כֵּהוּת) and Abraham ben Isaac as חשיכות העינים (see entry חֲשֵׁיכוּת). See also BCD 25–26 (NM 3:28; 4:20).

מַטָּה • הכניס מלמטה → [כנס].

• ההנחות העשויות למטה → הֲנָחָה.

מַטֶּה ‣ **penis**: Lat. *virga virilis* · Guillaume de Congenis, *Treatise on Surgery* · trans. Isaiah, fol. 56b: מן מכה בגיד הערוה נקרא מטה: כנגד פיק[184] במטה תחלה תקשרנו בחוט משי או בחוט[185] הבהמה (On an injury of the penis, which is called *maṭṭeh*: If there is a tumor on the penis, one should first of all tie it off with a thread from silver or with the hair of a horse[186] ...). Hebr. מַטֶּה does not feature in the sense of 'penis' in the current dictionaries. See also entry גִּיד: גיד הערוה.

מְטַהֵר (*Part. Pi'el*) → [טהר].

מְטֹהָר (*Part. Pu'al*) → [טהר].

מטוהר → מְטֹהָר.

---

183 Gr. ἀμαύρωσις ('amaurosis') should be corrected as: Gr. ἀμβλυωπία ('amblyopia'). For the confusion of both terms, cf. Ibn al-Jazzār *Zād al-musāfir wa-qūt al-ḥāḍir*, bk. 2, ch. 6 (forthcoming ed. Bos and Käs).

184 פיק: *ficus* L.

185 הבהמה: *equus* L.

186 'horse': Trans. after L.

מְטַמְטֵם (*Part. Pilpel*) → [**טמטם**].
מידה → מִדָּה.
מְיֻדָּע (*Part. Puʿal*) → [**ידע**].
מיודע → מְיֻדָּע.
מיצוי → מִצּוּי.

מַיִם • **מי דבש** · **hydromel; mead**: Arab. ماء العسل · Ibn al-Jazzār, *Zād al-musāfir wa-qūt al-ḥādir* · trans. Moses ibn Tibbon, *Sefer Ṣedat ha-Derakhim*, bk. 3, ch. 7: ויתמיד להריח ריחות טובות ויתמיד לכנס במרחץ ויזון במזונות מולידות ליחה טובה וישתה מי דבש (They [i.e., those suffering from a lung tumor] should frequently smell fragrant ingredients, and visit the bathhouse, and feed themselves with foods that produce good humors, and drink hydromel). Hebr. מי דבש features in BM 2969 without any explanation, in attestations from the translation of Hippocrates' *Aphorisms* by the otherwise unknown Jacob bar Joseph ibn Zabara (cf. NM 3:11), and from Me'ir Aldabi's *Shevilei Emunah*. Do'eg ha-Edomi renders the parallel Latin term *mellicratum* as מליקראט.

• **מי הדשן** · **(lit., ash water); lye**: Arab. رأس الصابون or ماء أوّل or ماء الرماد or ماء الصابون (cf. D 2:625, s.v. ماء أوّل: 'l'eau tiède qui a passé pour la première fois à travers une couche de cendres de bois'; see also KM 1:592–593; 2:751) · Shem Tov ben Isaac, *Sefer ha-Shimmush*, bk. 29, list 1 (SHS 1:309–310 (Mem 12)): מי הדשן ב"ה מא אלצאבון וב"ל לשיב (*mey ha-deshen*; Arab. *mā al-ṣābūn*; vern. LŠYB [i.e., O.Occ. *lissiu, lesiu, leis(s)iu*, a.o.]). In the sense of 'lye,' Hebr. מי הדשן is a non-attested calque of Arab. ماء الرماد. Subsequently, the same Hebrew term recurs in Zerahyah Ḥen's translation of Maimonides' *Medical Aphorisms* 15.45 (BMMZ 159; cf. NM 2:59, s.v. מי האפר).

• **מי שאור** · **broth; soup**: Arab. حسو[187] · Ibn al-Jazzār, *Zād al-musāfir wa-qūt al-ḥādir* · trans. Moses ibn Tibbon, *Sefer Ṣedat ha-Derakhim*, bk. 3, ch. 1: או יגרגר מי שאור מותך במי רמונים ממוצעים (Or let him gargle with broth mixed with sweet-sour pomegranate juice [i.e., juice of unripe pomegranates]). Hebr. מי שאור does not feature in the current dictionaries. Shem Tov ben Isaac, *Sefer ha-Shimmush*, bk. 27, translates Arab. حسو as שרף (cf. BCD 286 (NM 4:213)). In his glossary to the *Sefer ha-Qanun*, Nathan ha-Me'ati defines Arab. حسو as חסו הוא שם לחביץ קדרה כלומר איזה קמח או פתיתות מבושל בקדרה (ḤSW: This is the name for ḤBYṢ QDRH [i.e., a type of soup]; i.e., flour or bread-crumbs boiled in a pot) (cf. NM 2:114, 139 (Ḥet 17)).

• **זיתי המים** → זַיִת.

• **הירוקה שעל פני המים** → יְרוֹקָה.

187 Cf. NA 607: 'light, smooth, and thin soup made with water, flour, or fine bread crumbs, and fat ... In fact, it may apply to any thin and light soups, which can be sipped;' cf. Lane 572, s.v. حساء: 'A well-known kind of food; soup; i.e., what is supped or sipped; thin cooked food, that is supped or sipped, made of flour and water and oil or grease, and sometimes sweetened: also called حَسُوٌ and حَسِيَّةٌ and حَسًا and حَسْوٌ.'

מִין • כמין · **like; resembling**: Arab. أمثال · Ibn al-Jazzār, *Zād al-musāfir wa-qūt al-ḥādir* · trans. Abraham ben Isaac, *Sefer Ṣedah la-Oreḥim*, bk. 1, ch. 10: ולושם במי שומר לח הנקרא מלינרי ועשה גרגרים כמין פלפלין ושיעור השתייה ב׳ שקל׳ במים חמין (Mix [these ingredients] with fresh fennel juice called MLYNRY and mould this into pills resembling peppercorns [in weight] and administer two *shekels* with hot water). In the sense of 'like, resembling,' Hebr. כמין is only attested for in Rabbinic (cf. JD 776; BM 2972–2973; EM 926) and modern literature (EM 926). Do'eg ha-Edomi translates the parallel Latin term *sicut* as למדת (see entry מִדָּה). Moses ibn Tibbon translates Arab. أمثال as כמו.

מְיַשֵּׁן (*Part Pi'el*) → [ישן].

מְכַבֵּס (*Part. Pi'el*) → [כבס].

מֻכְבָּר (*Part. Hof'al*) → [כבר].

מִכְסֶה · **roof**: Lat. *tectum* (Arab. سقف) · Constantinus Africanus, *Viaticum* · trans. Do'eg ha-Edomi, *Sefer Ya'ir Netiv*, bk. 3, ch. 12: ברבות הדם וירתח עם החום הפנימי מהגוף שולח העשן העולה אל הראש ובמצאו נקבי הראש סתומים לא יוכל לצאת ובהתעכבו בראש נתחמם עם חום המוח ובהיותו נתר ישוב בתחתית הגוף למטה כמו שנראה בלחלוח עשן המרחץ כאשר לא יוכל לנקוב המכסה ישוב למטה ואם יזל מן הראש אל הקרב יולד הנפח החם ומשם נעשה פליורשין אמיתי (When the blood (of a pleurisy patient) increases and boils through the internal heat of the body, vapors are emitted and then ascend to the head. When these vapors find the pores of [the skin of] the head closed and cannot exit and are detained in the head they are heated by the heat of the brain. And when they dissolve, they return to the lower parts of the body. This is similar to what we see in the case of the moist vapors in the bathhouse when they cannot exit through the roof. When it [i.e., the moisture of the vapors] streams from the head to the diaphragm, it causes an inflammation and results in true pleurisy). In the sense of 'roof,' Hebr. מִכְסֶה is a non-attested semantic borrowing from Lat. *tectum*. Moses ibn Tibbon translates Arab. سقف with the standard term גג.

• **המכסה המקיף הלב** · **pericardium**: Arab. الطبقة المحيطة بالقلب · Ibn al-Jazzār, *Zād al-musāfir wa-qūt al-ḥādir* · trans. Moses ibn Tibbon, *Sefer Ṣedat ha-Derakhim*, bk. 3, ch. 13: דפיקת הלב פעמים שתקרה מפני לחות שיתקבץ במכסה המקיף הלב (Sometimes palpitation occurs because of moisture that collects in the pericardium). Hebr. המכסה המקיף הלב does not feature in the current dictionaries. Hebrew synonyms are (1) כיס הלב, featuring in Nathan ha-Me'ati's translation of Ibn Sīnā, *K. al-Qānūn fī al-ṭibb* (for Arab. غلاف القلب (cf. BCD 126 (NM 4:80))); (2) מכסה הלב, featuring in Joshua Lorki's translation of Ibn Sīnā, *K. al-Qānūn fī al-ṭibb* (cf. BCD 150 (NM 4:100)); and (3) קרום הלב, featuring in Judah al-Ḥarizi's translation of Pseudo-Galen, *Prohibition of Burial* (cf. BCD 249 (NM 4:189)). Do'eg ha-Edomi translates Lat. *circumdantes et cor pellicula* as הדפים הסובבים הלב (see entry דַּף).

מֶלַח • מלח מחצבי · **(lit., mineral salt); rock salt**: Arab. ملح أندراني, syn. ملح معدني (cf. KM 2:1036–1040) · Shem Tov ben Isaac, *Sefer ha-Shimmush*, bk. 29, list 1 (SHS 1:

331 (Mem 60)): מלח מחצבי ב״ה מלח אנדראני וב״ל שאל ג׳ימא (*melaḥ maḥṣavi*; Arab. *milḥ andarānī*; vern. š'L ǦYM' [i.e., O.Occ./O.Cat. or L.Lat. *salgema/sal gema/salgemma*[188]]). In the sense of 'rock salt,' Hebr. מלח מחצבי is a non-attested calque of Arab. ملح معدني.

• **פרח המלח** → **פֶּרַח**.

• **קצף המלח** → **קֶצֶף**.

[מלל] • *Part. Piʿel* **מְמַלֵּל** • **נפש ממללת** → **נֶפֶשׁ**.

• **נפשות חכמות ממללות** → **נֶפֶשׁ**.

ממוצע → **מְמֻצָּע**.

מְמַלֵּל (*Part. Piʿel*) → **[מלל]**.

מְמֻצָּע (*Part. Puʿal*) → **[מיצע]**.

מְמָרֵק (*Part. Piʿel*) → **[מרק]**.

מֻנָּח (*Part. Hofʿal*) → **[נוח]**.

[מנע] • *Part. Nifʿal* **נִמְנָע** • **נמנע מן** · **free from:** Arab. معرّى من · Maimonides, *Medical Aphorisms* 3.4 · trans. Nathan ha-Me'ati (BMMN 40): גוף האיש יתנפש נפישה טובה והוא נקי ונמנע מהמותרים ומהחליצה (The body of a man breathes well when it is clean and free from superfluities and pressure). Hebr. נִמְנָע features in medieval philosophical literature in the sense of 'impossible' (cf. EF 85; HCD 58; KT 3:40). In addition to נמנע מן, Nathan ha-Me'ati translates Arab. معرّى من as משולל מן. Zeraḥyah Ḥen translates the Arabic term as מופשט מן (BMMZ 32; see entry [פשט]).

מַנְעִים (*Part. Hifʿil*) → **[נעם]**.

מנשב • *Plur.* **מנשבים** · **fans:** Lat. *flabellum* (Arab. مراوح) · Constantinus Africanus, *Viaticum* · trans. Do'eg ha-Edomi, *Sefer Ya'ir Netiv*, bk. 3, ch. 14: ואם השינקופיש היא מרוב חמום או מרוב התעכבו במרחץ או מן האויר הסגור שם יאות לטבול אותו במים קרים ולתת לו גונגובש במים קרים ויין חלק ודק ומזוג במים קרים ולסוב פניו אל העבר אשר הרוח מנשבת משם גם לפניו נעורר רוח עם המנשבים הם וינטלש (If fainting is caused by intense heat, or by staying in the bathhouse for a long time, or by the air over there that is not being refreshed, we should immerse the patient in cold water and give him common jujube with cold water and thin, fine wine mixed with cold water; we should let him face the wind and refresh the air by means of fans, i.e. [Rom.] WYNṬLŠ [cf. RL 5:500, s.v. *ventalh, ventaylh, ventilateur*]). Hebr. מנשב is not attested for in the current dictionaries. Moses ibn Tibbon translates Arab. مراوح as מנשבים as well.

מִסְגֶּרֶת • *Plur.* **מסגרות** · **vertebrae:** Lat. *spondili* (Arab. فقارات) · Constantinus Africanus, *Viaticum* · trans. Do'eg ha-Edomi, *Sefer Ya'ir Netiv*, bk. 1, ch. 23: ותרחץ הראש והצואר והמסגרות אם סובלים מאומה במים שנתבשלו בם קמומילא אניט מלילוד שמבוק ייניברי ונעשה לו עטוש בענין שינוע המוח (If the head, neck, or vertebrae [of a patient suffering from

188 Cf. entry שלגיימה.

apoplexy] are in any way affected, they should be washed with water in which camomile, dill, melilot, marjoram, and savin juniper have been cooked. A sternutatory should be applied so that the brain gets stimulated). Hebr. *Sing.* מִסְגֶּרֶת, *Plur.* מסגרות, does not feature in this sense in the current dictionaries. Moses ibn Tibbon and Abraham ben Isaac translate Arab. فقارات as חוליות.

מָסָךְ · **diaphragm**: Arab. حجاب · Ibn al-Jazzār, *Zād al-musāfir wa-qūt al-ḥādir* · trans. Moses ibn Tibbon, *Sefer Ṣedat ha-Derakhim*, bk. 3, ch. 11: ואם ראינו שהתחדש החולי מפני שתוף האברים הקרובים מכלי הנשימה כמו שזכרנו למעלה יהיה השרש ברפואתו ההשתדלות לרפאת האבר אשר מדבקותו ושתופו עם המסך או שאר כלי הנשימה התחדש החולי (When we observe that illness [i.e., of difficulty of breathing] occurs because of the connection between the respiratory organs and the organs that are close to them, as I mentioned above, one should start the treatment by attempting to treat the organ that caused the illness because of its connection with the diaphragm or with the other respiratory organs). In the sense of 'diaphragm,' Hebr. מָסָךְ features in BM 3119, a.o., in a later attestation from the *Sefer ha-Qanun*. The term also features in MD 221, s.v. 'diaphragma.'

[מסס] • *Inf.* **מְסוֹס** · **to dissolve (*transitive*)**: Arab. تحليل · Isḥāq ibn 'Imrān, *Treatise on Melancholy* · trans. Anonymous, fol. 50^b (51^b): ואזכור הרפואות ⟨...⟩[189] שחורה שבגופם אם תתערב עמה המרה האדומה והבלגם תעזרם על העכול ולמסוס הרוחות השראסיף (I will mention the remedies that purge[190] the black bile in their bodies when it is mixed with yellow bile and phlegm. They are good for the digestion and for the dissolution of the epigastric winds). Hebr. מסס does not feature, in its different conjugations, in a medical context in the current dictionaries. Constantine the African translates Arab. تحليل as *dissolutivus*.

• *Hif'il* **הֵמֵס** · **to dissolve (*transitive*)**: Arab. حلّل · Ibn al-Jazzār, *Zād al-musāfir wa-qūt al-ḥādir* · trans. Abraham ben Isaac, *Sefer Ṣedah la-Oreḥim*, bk. 1, ch. 24: ואם יקרה החולי הזה הנקר׳ אלכוזאז בתחילה בלא קדחת אז יש לו תקוה כל שכן אם תבוא לו אחרי כן הקדחת על כי קדחת מחממת הרפש והכימוס הרע אשר נתמלאו ממנו אותם הגידים ותמיס אותם ותאפיסם (If this illness called [in Arab.] *al-kuzāz* [i.e., spasms] occurs at the very beginning without a fever [before it], there is hope [that the patient will recover], especially if fever befalls him after this. For the fever heats the superfluity and bad chyme that fill the nerves; it dissolves and annihilates it). Moses ibn Tibbon translates Arab. حلّل as התיך. Do'eg ha-Edomi renders Lat. *dissolvitur* as ניתר.

• *Inf. Hitpa'el* **הִתְמַסֵּס** · **to dissolve (*intransitive*)**: Arab. تحليل · Isḥāq ibn 'Imrān, *Treatise on Melancholy* · trans. Anonymous, fol. 42^b (43^b): לפי שהמקומות ימנעו לשוכנים בם מלהתמסס מגופותם הליחות הרעות (... for these places prevent the bad humors to dis-

189 ⟨...⟩: المسهلة a.

190 'purge': Trans. after a.

solve from the bodies of their inhabitants). Constantine the African translates Arab. تحليل as *solutio*.

מַעֲבִיד (*Part. Hifʿil*) → [עבד].

מַעֲבָר • *Plur.* **מעברים** • **passages; channels (in the body)** · Ms Cambridge, T-S K14.48, P7 (recto): התאנים היבשים יפתח<ו> מעברי המזון אם יאכלם (The consumption of dried figs opens the passages of the food [in the body]). In the sense of 'passage in the body,' Hebr. *Sing.* מַעֲבָר features as part of the term מעבר השתן ('urethra') in BCD 153 (NM 1:103–104) in an attestation from Shem Tov ben Isaac, *Sefer ha-Shimmush*, bk. 30. The term also features as *Plur.* מעברות in Do'eg ha-Edomi's *Sefer Agur* (BCD 153 (NM 3:134)).

מְעִי • **המעי החלול** • **colon**: Arab. المعا الأجوف · Isḥāq ibn ʿImrān, *Treatise on Melancholy* · trans. Anonymous, fol. 46ᵇ–47ᵃ (47ᵇ–48ᵃ): האחד שרוב המזון שלא נתעכל יפה יולדו[191] ממנו רוחות עבים ונפח רב אינם מתמססים במהרה עד שינפחו ויתמלאו אותן האיברים והמקומות שתחת השראסיף בשני צדדין יחד וירד מהם רוח אל המעי החלול הנק׳ קולון (One [kind of harm] is that most of the food is not well digested so that thick winds and much flatulence originate from it that are not quickly dissolved. Consequently those organs and places that are beneath the hypochondria at both sides are blown up and filled and a wind descends from them into the colon, which is called [in Lat.] *colon*). Hebr. המעי החלול does not feature in the current dictionaries. Constantine the African translates Arab. المعا الأجوف as *colon*.

[מעך] • *Hitpaʿel* **הִתְמַעֵךְ** • **to rub oneself**: Arab. تمرّخ · Ibn al-Jazzār, *Zād al-musāfir wa-qūt al-ḥādir* · trans. Abraham ben Isaac, *Sefer Ṣedah la-Oreḥim*, bk. 1, ch. 9 (Ms Jerusalem, National Library of Israel, Fr. 95, fol. 88ᵇ): דוק הכל ושחוק בשמן ויתמעך בהם במרחץ (Pulverize all these [ingredients], ground it together with oil, and rub [the head] with this in the bathhouse). Hebr. הִתְמַעֵךְ features in Rabbinic literature in the sense of 'to be crushed, squashed, rubbed off' (JD 816). Ben-Yehuda (BM 3171) mentions the term in the Nitpaʿel in a medical context in an attestation from Shabbetai Donnolo's, *Sefer ha-Yakar*, also known as *Sefer ha-Merqaḥot*, in the sense of 'to be crushed': ויכתוש את המרקחת עד אשר תמעך. Moses ibn Tibbon translates Arab. تمرّخ as חפף.

מַעֲלֶה (*Part. Hifʿil*) → עָלָה.

מַעֲשֶׂה • **recipe; composition**: Arab. صفة[192] · Ibn al-Jazzār, *Zād al-musāfir wa-qūt al-ḥādir* · trans. Abraham ben Isaac, *Sefer Ṣedah la-Oreḥim*, bk. 1, ch. 23: וזה מעשה שמן יועיל לכל בעלי חולי הפלג ולכל מי שיבש חצי גופו ולכל מי שנתקרר גופו ולא ישיט ידו ולא ירים רגלו (Recipe of an oil beneficial for all persons suffering from hemiplegia, dryness of one side of the body, coldness of the body—so that they can neither extend a hand nor lift a leg …). Hebr. מַעֲשֶׂה does not feature in this sense in the current dictionaries. Moses ibn Tibbon translates Arab. صفة as תאר.

---

191 יולדו: emendation editor יולידו Ms.

192 In addition to מַעֲשֶׂה, Abraham ben Isaac translates Arab. صفة as רִקּוּחַ (see entry).

מַפְלִיג (*Part. Hif'il*) → [פלג].
מַפְסִיד (*Part. Hif'il*) → [פסד].
מֻפְשָׁט (*Part. Hof'al*) → [פשט].
מִצּוּי • **extract:** Arab. عصير • Ibn al-Jazzār, *Zād al-musāfir wa-qūt al-ḥādir* • trans. Abraham ben Isaac, *Sefer Ṣedah la-Oreḥim*, bk. 1, ch. 10: ועם יהיה עם אותו כאב נידוד שינה אז יעטישהו בשמן ויאולטו או בשמן אופיו או שמן פפברו עם מיצוי עלי לטוקא וימשח רגליו בשמן בנפסג׳ ומלח (If the [headache] is accompanied by sleeplessness, one should administer the patient a snuff made from violet oil, opium oil, or poppy oil, and extract of cultivated lettuce leaves. The feet [of the patient] should be anointed with oil of violets and salt). In the sense of 'extract,' Hebr. מִצּוּי is attested for in medieval medical literature in BM 3243 in a quotation from Shabbetai Donnolo, *Sefer ha-Yakar*, also called *Sefer ha-Merqaḥot*. Moses ibn Tibbon translates Arab. عصير as סחיטה.
מצולל → מְצֻלָּל.
מָצוֹק • **I. obstruction:** Lat. *constipatio* (Arab. انسداد) • Constantinus Africanus, *Viaticum* • trans. Do'eg ha-Edomi, *Sefer Ya'ir Netiv*, bk. 1, ch. 23: ואם המצוק ההוא ירד בגיד אחד לבדו נעשה הליחות[193] באותו אבר לאשר אותו הגיד משרת (If the obstruction occurs only in one nerve, the softness[194] [i.e., looseness] occurs only in the organ that is served by that nerve). Hebr. מָצוֹק features in the current dictionaries in the sense of 'straitness, straits, stress' (BDB 848), and 'anguish' (BM 3246). Abraham ben Isaac translates Arab. انسداد as סְתִימָה (see entry) and Moses ibn Tibbon as סתום (cf. BCD 195 (NM 4:140)).

• **II. narrowness:** Lat. *angustia* (cf. DMLBS 113) (Arab. ضيق) • Constantinus Africanus, *Viaticum* • trans. Do'eg ha-Edomi, *Sefer Ya'ir Netiv*, bk. 3, ch. 11: והחולה מתחזק להניע תמיד כל החזה בגובה הנשימה והתנועה ההיא נקראת אורטומיא ונעשה מארבעה ענינים או מרוב צורך הנשימה כמו שנראה בבריאים המיגעים עצמם מאד או בקוצר החזה כמו בסובלי צמחים הם אפושטימש או נגעים בחזה או במצוק בראשי מעברות הרוח (The patient is[195] forced always to move his whole chest, because breathing is difficult for him [lit., breathing occurs high in the chest]. This movement is called 'orthopnea.' It is caused by [one of] four [read: three] things: Because of a intense need to breath as we see in the case of healthy people who exert themselves, or because of the narrowness of the chest cavity in the case of those who suffer from tumors, i.e., [Lat.] *apostemas*, or because of the narrowness of the top ends of the respiratorial passages). Moses ibn Tibbon translates the parallel Arabic term ضيق as צרות.
מְצוּקָה • **מצוקת הנשימה** • **hardness (i.e., difficulty) of breathing (i.e., dyspnea):** Arab. عسر النفس • Ibn al-Jazzār, *Zād al-musāfir wa-qūt al-ḥādir* • trans. Moses ibn Tibbon,

---

193 הליחות: *mollities* L.
194 'softness [i.e., looseness]': Trans. after L.
195 'is forced': Cf. entry [חזק]: הִתְחַזֵּק.

Sefer Ṣedat ha-Derakhim, bk. 3, ch. 6: ואמ׳ ג״כ: כשישתה שעור פול ממירא אדומה יועיל משעול נושן וממצוקת נשימה אשר יצטרך בה אל הזקיפה (He [i.e., Dioscorides] also said: If one drinks the quantity of one bean of red myrrh it is good for chronic cough and for hardness [i.e., difficulty] of breathing [i.e., dyspnea] in which case one should stand straight). Hebr. מצוקת נשימה does not feature in the current dictionaries. Arab. عسر النفس is translated as עוצר הניפוש by Zeraḥyah Ḥen in his translation of Maimonides, *Medical Aphorisms* 23.79 (BMMZ 227; cf. BCD 212 (NM 1:178)). Shem Tov ben Isaac uses the synonym קושי הנשום in the *Sefer Almansur* (cf. BMZ 64–65 (Pe 5)).

מִצְטַעֵר (*Part. Hitpa'el*) → [**צער**].

מְצֻלָּל (*Part. Pu'al*) → **צָלַל**.

[**מיצע**] • *Part. Pu'al* **מְמֻצָּע** · **having a taste between sweet and sour; sweet-sour**: Arab. مزّ · Ibn al-Jazzār, *Zād al-musāfir wa-qūt al-ḥāḍir* · trans. Moses ibn Tibbon, *Sefer Ṣedat ha-Derakhim*, bk. 3, ch. 1 (fol. 74b): או יעשה גרגור מי שאור מותך במי רמונים ממוצעים (Or let him gargle with broth mixed with sweet-sour pomegranate juice [i.e., juice of unripe pomegranates]). Hebr. מְמֻצָּע does not feature in this sense in the current dictionaries.

מקוצף → **מְקֻצָּף**.

מָקוֹר · **vein**: Lat. *vena* · Constantinus Africanus, *Viaticum* · trans. Do'eg ha-Edomi, *Sefer Ya'ir Netiv*, bk. 1, ch. 1: ואז אם יוכל הסובל לסבול נקיזהו מן המקור כפי שניו וכחו הנקרא ספליקא (Then, if the patient can endure it, we bleed the vein[196] called 'cephalic' according to his age and strength). In the sense of 'vessel, vein, artery,' Hebr. מָקוֹר features in BCD 159 (NM 3:141) in an attestation from the *Sefer Agur*, i.e., Do'eg ha Edomi's translation of a Latin version of Hippocrates' *Aphorisms* 1.2.

• **המקור האמצעי** · **the median vein**: Lat. [*vena*] *media* (Arab. الأكحل) · Constantinus Africanus, *Viaticum* · trans. Do'eg ha-Edomi, *Sefer Ya'ir Netiv*, bk. 2, ch. 17: וכל הדברים האלה כאשר נסדר אותם לעזור בכל מלואת הגוף יאות לנו לחסר דם מן המקור האמצעי או מן הספאליקא אם אין דבר אחר מונע (When we [look at] all these things with regard to a treatment when the body is full, we should bleed from the median or cephalic vein if there is no impediment). Hebr. המקור האמצעי does not feature in the current dictionaries. Moses ibn Tibbon translates Arab. الأكحل as הגיד האמצעי (cf. BCD 44 (NM 1:54)).

• **המקור אשר בין האצבע הקטן לאחיהו** · **(lit., the vein that is between the little toe and the next one); saphenous vein**: Lat. *vena inter auricularem et medicum* (Arab. الصافن) · Constantinus Africanus, *Viaticum* · trans. Do'eg ha-Edomi, *Sefer Ya'ir Netiv*, bk. 3, ch. 8: וכאשר נרפא אותו אשר ירוק דם יאות לתת לו מנוחה ושירגע מאד ושלא יוציא הנשימה בכח. ואם הוא חזק והעת מזוג וכפי שניו יוכל לסבול יאות לחסר המקור הבאשליקא ולהוציא הדם ב׳ פעמים או ג׳ עד שיכיר שיצא כל השפע גם יאות לחסר הדם מצד הכאב מן המקור אשר בין האצבע הקטן לאחיהו (If we [want to] cure someone who spits blood, we should [first

196 The standard term for 'vein,' i.e., עורק, features as a gloss in the margin.

of all] let him rest so that he becomes very calm and does not exhale forcefully. If he is strong and the weather is moderate and it fits his age, we should bleed from the basilic vein twice ot three times until it is clear that all the superfluous matter has come out. It is also fitting to bleed [the patient] from the saphenous vein that is on the same side as the pain). In the sense of 'saphenous vein,' Hebr. המקור אשר בין האצבע הקטן לאחיהו is a non-attested loan translation from Lat. *vena inter auricularem et medicum*. Moses ibn Tibbon translates Arab. الصافن as העורק אשר אצל העקב (see entry עוֹרֶק). For מָקוֹר in the sense of 'vein,' see entry above.

• **המקור העומד בין האצבע הקטון לחבירו · (lit., the vein that is between the little finger and the next one); vena salvatella**: Lat. *vena que inter auricularem et medicum extat* (Arab. الأسيلم) · Constantinus Africanus, *Viaticum* · trans. Do'eg ha-Edomi, *Sefer Ya'ir Netiv*, bk. 3, ch. 7: העזר יאות לחפש מאין נעשה החולי ואם הוא מליחה חמה יאות לחסר דם הבשליקה או מן המקור העומד בין האצבע הקטון לחבירו (Its treatment: Examine the cause of the disease: If it is caused by a hot humor one should bleed the basilic vein or the vena salvatella). In the sense of 'vena salvatella,' Hebr. המקור העומד בין האצבע הקטון לחבירו is a non-attested loan translation from Lat. *vena que inter auricularem et medicum extat*. Moses ibn Tibbon translates Arab. الأسيلم as העורק אשר בין האצבע הקטן וחברו הנקרא אסילם (see entry עוֹרֶק). For מָקוֹר in the sense of 'vein,' see entry above.

מַקִּיף (*Part. Hif'il*) → [**נקף**].

מֻקָּץ (*Part. Hof'al*) → [**קוץ**].

מְקֻצָּף (*Part. Pu'al*) → **קָצַף**.

מִקְרֶה • *Plur.* **מקראות** · I. **symptoms; afflictions**: Arab. أعراض · Ibn al-Jazzār, *Zād al-musāfir wa-qūt al-ḥādir* · trans. Abraham ben Isaac, *Sefer Ṣedah la-Oreḥim*, bk. 1, ch. 18: וכאשר יתגדל החולי ויגיע לתוקפו יקרה לחולה מקראות רעות כגון צמא גדולה ויובש הפה ועובי הלשון ושחרותו ... ושינוי מראות פניו מפיסי שלו (When the illness increases and becomes more severe, the patient suffers from bad symptoms such as severe thirst, dryness of the mouth, thickness and blackness of the tongue [...] His face loses its natural color). Hebr. מקראות only features in the current dictionaries as a plural of מִקְרָא (cf. BM 3289–3291). Moses ibn Tibbon translates Arab. أعراض as the standard plural מקרים. The same term is used by Do'eg ha-Edomi for the parallel Latin term *accidentia*.

· II. **afflictions; pains**: Arab. أوجاع · Ibn al-Jazzār, *Zād al-musāfir wa-qūt al-ḥādir* · trans. Abraham ben Isaac, *Sefer Ṣedah la-Oreḥim*, bk. 1, ch. 20: החשק הוא מן החלאים הנולדים במוח הראש והוא רוב איווי עם הירהור ותאוה ועל זה יקרה לכל מי שיארע לו חולי זה מקצת מקראות הנפש המה נדידת השינה גם ההירהור (Lovesickness belongs to the diseases that originate in the brain. It is an excess of desire accompanied by brooding and longing. Therefore, anyone affected by this illness, will suffer from some afflictions of the soul, i.e., sleeplessness and brooding). Moses ibn Tibbon translates Arab. أوجاع as the standard כאבים.

‣ III. **afflictions:** a) Arab. أحداث · Ibn al-Jazzār, *Zād al-musāfir wa-qūt al-ḥādir* · trans. Abraham ben Isaac, *Sefer Ṣedah la-Oreḥim*, bk. 1, ch. 20: ואם תעמיק הנפש ברוב ההירהור אז יפסידו פעליה וכל מעשיה גם כל מעשה הגוף כמו כן בעבור כי הגוף טפל לנפש והולך אחר פעליה וכמו כן הנפש הולכת אחר פעלי הגוף במקראותיו (If the soul sinks into excessive brooding both the activities of the soul and the activities of the body deteriorate. For the body follows the soul as regards its activities. Likewise, the soul follows the body as regards its afflictions). Moses ibn Tibbon translates Arab. أحداث as התחדש.

b) Arab. عوارض · Ibn al-Jazzār, *Zād al-musāfir wa-qūt al-ḥādir* · trans. Abraham ben Isaac, *Sefer Ṣedah la-Oreḥim*, bk. 1, ch. 20: כל אילו כח[197] הנעימות ושתיית היין לתקן מקראות הנפש (All this is the effect of [listening to] melodious singing and drinking wine on healing the afflictions of the soul). Moses ibn Tibbon translates Arab. عوارض as מקרים.

מַרְאֶה • מראה עור הפנים ‣ **external skin; complexion:** Arab. بشرة · Ibn al-Jazzār, *Zād al-musāfir wa-qūt al-ḥādir* · trans. Moses ibn Tibbon, *Sefer Ṣedat ha-Derakhim*, bk. 2, ch. 25: וכאשר יצטרך אליהם יתקן[198] מהם אחת ויטוח בו השחין וכאשר יתנגב ירטיבהו במים פושרים כי הוא יסיר השחין וינקה מראה עור הפנים (And if he needs one of these, he should dissolve[199] [a pastille] and put it on the ulcer. And if the ulcer is dry he should moisten it with lukewarm water for this will make the ulcer go away and cleanse the complexion). Hebr. מראה עור הפנים does not feature in the current dictionaries. Arab. سحنة, a synonym for بشرة in the sense of 'complexion,' is translated by Moses ibn Tibbon as תמונת הפנים (cf. BCD 296 (NM 4:221)).

מָרָה • מרת הפיל ‣ **(lit., elephant's gall); buckthorn [*Rhamnus* sp. L.] sap:** Arab. فيلزهرج (from Pers. *pīl* ('elephant') and *zahrah* ('gall-bladder; bile'); cf. MIG 787: 'Ibn al-Bayṭār gave an interesting explanation of the term *fīlzahraj*. According to him inspissated buckthorn sap is collected and traded in animal stomachs. Since these resemble gall-bladders of elephants they were called *marārat al-fīl*.') · *Shinnui ha-Shemot ha-Niqra'im Synonimis*, Ms Munich, Bayerische Staatsbibliothek, Cod. hebr. 8, fol. 198ᵃ: חצץ הוא ליציאו והוא סחיטת עשב הנקרא פיל זהרג כלומר מרת הפיל שם עשב נקרא כן ([Arab.] *ḥuḍaḍ* is LYṢY'W [i.e., boxthorn, *Lycium* sp. L.]; it is an extract of a plant called [in Arab.] *fīlzahraj*; i.e., [Hebr.] *marat ha-pil*; it is the name of a plant with that name). In the sense of 'buckthorn sap,' Hebr. מרת הפיל is a non-attested calque from Arab. فيلزهرج.

מֻרְבֶּה (*Part. Pu'al*) → [רבה].

מרובה → מֻרְבֶּה.

מרוקח → מְרֻקָּח.

---

197 כֹּחַ הנעימות: مبلغ أوزان النغم a.
198 יתקן: أذيبت a.
199 'dissolve': Trans. after a.

מַרְחִיב (*Part. Hifʿil*) → **[רחב]**.

מֶרְחָץ · **fomentation; application of a poultice:** Lat. *fomentatio* · Guillaume de Congenis, *Treatise on Surgery* · trans. Isaiah, fol. 58ᵇ: פרח הקמאליאונקה מעורב עם מי מטר ועם אישרוף רושאט שתוי עוצר דם התחתוניות ומרחץ עלי העשבים עצמם מן הטבור ולמטה (A potion of camomile blossom mixed with rain water and juice of roses stops the bleeding of hemorrhoids, next to the application from the navel downwards of a poultice of the leaves of the herbs themselves). Hebr. מֶרְחָץ does not feature in this sense in the current dictionaries.

מרינא • **צף מרינא** → **צף**.

מְרִירִי · **bilious:** Arab. صفراوي · Ibn al-Jazzār, *Zād al-musāfir wa-qūt al-ḥādir* · trans. Abraham ben Isaac, *Sefer Ṣedah la-Oreḥim*, bk. 1, ch. 18: והב׳ מחמת הרתחת הדם שבתוך הלב כי דם זה שבלב כאשר ירתח ויתלהב מחמת מרירה האדומה אז יעלה מן הדם בהרתחתו עשן אל הראש ואז יולד במוח הראש צמח חד מרירי (The second [cause of phrenitis] is the boiling of the blood within the heart. When this blood seethes and becomes inflamed because of the yellow bile, vapors arise to the head and cause a sharp bilious swelling in the brain). Hebr. מְרִירִי is not attested for in medieval medical literature. The term features in the Bible in the sense of 'bitter' (cf. BDB 601). Ben-Yehuda (BM 3332) mentions the term as featuring in Joseph Schönhak's *Toledot ha-Areṣ* in the sense of 'somewhat bitter' in the context of the taste of plants. Moses ibn Tibbon translates Arab. صفراوي as כרכומי.

מָרַךְ • *or Piʿel* **מֵרֵךְ** · **to rub:** Arab. لطخ · Ibn al-Jazzār, *Zād al-musāfir wa-qūt al-ḥādir* · trans. Abraham ben Isaac, *Sefer Ṣedah la-Oreḥim*, bk. 1, ch. 3 (Ms Jerusalem, National Library of Israel, Fr. 95, fol. 85ᵇ): וכאשר יתבאר לך כי תוספת יסוד החמימות כלתה וחדותה נכנעה אז נחזור למשוח בו משיחות למרך בהם כדי לקרר החמימות ולרטב השיער כגון הגיר של זרע איפשיליאו הוא בזר קוטוני שתערב אותו בשמן ויאולטו ותמרך בו עור השיער (When it is clear that the element of heat does not increase any more and that its sharpness has gone, we should turn to rubbing salves on it [i.e., the head] in order to cool the heat and to moisten the hair with [ingredients] such as mucilage of fleawort seed, i.e., [Arab.] *bizr quṭūnī* [read: *bizrqaṭūnā*], mixed with violet oil, and rub the skin below the hair with it). Hebr. מרך features in the current dictionaries in the Nitpaʿel and Hofʿal in the sense of 'to be softened,' and in the Hifʿil in the sense of 'to soften;' cf. JD 844; BM 3333; EM 1060. Moses ibn Tibbon translates Arab. لطخ as משח.

[מרק] • *Part. Piʿel* **מְמָרֵק** • **סם הממרק** → **סַם**.

מְרֻקָּח (*Part. Puʿal*) → **[רקח]**.

מִשְׁחֶזֶת · **whetstone:** Arab. مسنّ · Ibn al-Jazzār, *Zād al-musāfir wa-qūt al-ḥādir* · trans. Moses ibn Tibbon, *Sefer Ṣedat ha-Derakhim*, bk. 3, ch. 15: או יקח מה שיפל ממשחזת המים ויטוח בו המורסא (... or take [in the case of a tumor in the breasts] what falls down [i.e., grindings] from a whetstone that is [found in] water and rub it on the tumor). Hebr. מִשְׁחֶזֶת features in Rabbinic literature and modern Hebrew ethical literature; cf. JD 851; KT 2:307; BM 3367; EM 1075, and entry אֶבֶן: אבן משחזת above. Do'eg ha-Edomi translates the parallel Latin term *ferramenta molendini* as כלי ברזל אשר בבית הרחים. The Arabic source of משחזת המים, namely مسنّ الماء, is explained by Dozy (D 1:689) as being called by this name because it is found in big rivers.

• **אבן משחזת** → אֶבֶן.

מְשִׁיחָה • **משיחה ירוקה** · **an ointment made from verdigris**: Lat. *unguentum viridis aeris* · Guillaume de Congenis, *Treatise on Surgery* · trans. Isaiah, fol. 49[a]: משיחה לפישטולא: קח שלגיימה ומלח ושוגה בשוה וירקח עם חומץ ויפעל יותר ממשיחה ירוקה (A salve that is [good] for fistulas: Take equal amounts of rock salt, salt, and soot,[200] mix this with vinegar; it will have a stronger effect than an ointment made from verdigris). Hebr. משיחה ירוקה is a non-attested loan translation of Lat. *unguentum viridis* [*aeris*].

מְשַׂכֵּךְ (*Part. Pi'el*) → [שכך].

מְשַׁמֶּשֶׁת (*Part. Pi'el f.*) → [שמש].

מִשְׁתֶּה • **הבדלת האוכל והמשתה** → הַבְדָּלָה.

מִתְגַּבֵּן (*Part. Hitpa'el*) → [גבן].

מִתְגַּדֵּל (*Part. Hitpa'el*) → [גדל].

מִתְהַפֵּךְ (*Part. Hitpa'el*) → [הפך].

מָתוֹק • **גרגרים מתוקים** → גַּרְגֵּר.

מתוקן → מְתֻקָּן.

מתכונת → מַתְכֹּנֶת.

מַתְכֹּנֶת · **consistency**: Arab. قوام · Ibn al-Jazzār, *Zād al-musāfir wa-qūt al-ḥādir* · trans. Moses ibn Tibbon, *Sefer Ṣedat ha-Derakhim*, bk. 3, ch. 6: ואם ישים בו ליט׳ פניס ויבשלהו עד שישוב במתכונת המשקים ויצניעהו בכלי שוע וילוש בו רפואות השעול או ישתה אותו באחת מן המימות המועילות לשעול יהיה יותר מועיל ויותר שלם (If one adds to [this remedy for cough] one liter of sugar candy, cooks it until it assumes the consistency of syrups, and puts it in a glazed vessel [and takes it out] and kneads it with cough remedies or drinks it with one of the potions that are good for cough, it is most beneficial and best). Hebr. מַתְכֹּנֶת features in BM 3446–3447 in the sense of 'quantity, composition, proportion, normal state.' Arab. قوام in the sense of 'consistency' is translated as ממשות by the anonymous translator of Ibn Sīnā, *K. al-adwiya al-qalbiya*; cf. BCD 151 (NM 4:100).

מִתְנוֹעֵעַ (*Part. Hitpolel*) → [נוע].

מְתֻקָּן (*Part. Pu'al*) → [תקן].

מִתְרַעֵד (*Part Hitpa'el*) → [רעד].

מִתְרַעֵם (*Part. Hitpa'el*) → [רעם].

---

200 'soot' (ŠWGH) (O.Occ. *suia, sueia, suga*; cf. RL 5:288a): I thank Guido Mensching for this identification.

נֶאֱכָל (*Part. Nif'al*) → [**אכל**].
נֶאֱפָס (*Part. Nif'al*) → [**אפס**].
נַבְלוּת · **avarice**: Arab. بخل · Ibn al-Jazzār, *Zād al-musāfir wa-qūt al-ḥādir* · trans. Abraham ben Isaac, *Sefer Ṣedah la-Oreḥim*, bk. 1, ch. 20: כי יש לי יכולת להכניע אפם ולהפכו לרצון ואהפכם מן הדאגה לשמחה ומהאבילות לששון ומהיגון לחדוה ומן העצלות אל הזריזות ומן הנבלות אל הנדיבות (For I have the ability to subdue their anger and to turn it into goodwill, I turn their sadness into joy, their mourning into delight, their grief into happiness, their indolence to diligence, and their avarice to generosity). In the sense of 'avarice,' Hebr. נַבְלוּת features in BM 3490–3491 (s.v. נבלת) in an attestation from Samuel ha-Nagid, *Ben Mishlei*. Moses ibn Tibbon translates Arab. بخل as כילות. The latter term is also used by Do'eg ha-Edomi for Lat. *auaritia*.
[נגד] • *Part. Hif'il* **מַגִּיד** • **מגיד ש-** · **note that; pay attention that**: Lat. *nota quod* · Guillaume de Congenis, *Treatise on Surgery* · trans. Isaiah, fol. 44b: מגיד שלעת בריאות המכה שלא יוכל ליגע בה השרורגיאה תעשה משקה וזה מעשהו (Note that when the injury is such that it cannot be touched upon [i.e., treated] by a surgeon, one should prepare the following potion. Its recipe is ...). Hebr. מגיד ש- featuring in this sense throughout the treatise does not feature as such in the current dictionaries.[201]
נָגַע • **אל תיגע בי** → **אַל**.
נֶגַע • *Plur.* **נגעים** • **נגעי הריאה** · **pneumonia**: Lat. *vulnera pulmonis* (Arab. قرحة الرئة) (Gr. φλεγμονή ἐν τῷ πνεύμονι) · Constantinus Africanus, *Viaticum* · trans. Do'eg ha-Edomi, *Sefer Ya'ir Netiv*, bk. 3, ch. 7: והרופאים נחלקו בנגעי[202] הריאה כי האחרים אומרים שאין להם עזר והעיר גיאלינוס ואמר: אם איזה רופא יעזור אל ⟨בעל⟩ פריפליומוניא קודם שהנפח יתעכב שם ויבלה יתרפא הנפח (The physicians disagree [in the matter of] pneumonia. Some of them say that it cannot be cured. Galen remarks and says that if a physician treats a pneumonia [patient] before a tumor settles and putrefies, he can be cured). In the sense of 'pneumonia,' Hebr. נגעי הריאה is a non-attested loan translation from Lat. *vulnera pulmonis*. In addition to נגעי הריאה, Do'eg ha-Edomi uses the standard Latin term for 'pneumonia,' i.e., פריפליומוניא (*peripleumonia*); see entry פריפליומוניא and gloss to נגעי הריאה. Moses ibn Tibbon translates Arab. قرحة as נגע. For this term in the sense of 'fistula, ulcer, wound;' cf. BCD 170 (NM 1:31–32, 62).
נְדוּד • **נידוד השינה** · **sleeplessness**: Lat. *vigiliae* (Arab. سهر) · Ibn al-Jazzār, *Zād al-musāfir wa-qūt al-ḥādir* · trans. Abraham ben Isaac, *Sefer Ṣedah la-Oreḥim*, Adaptation, bk. 1, ch. 10 (Ms Berlin, Staatsbibliothek Preußischer Kulturbesitz, Or. fol. 1058, fol. 92a):

201 Cf. ibid.: מגיד שאלו האבקים צריך לשים במקום אפושטוליקון (Note that the following powders should be applied instead of apostolicon).

202 בנגעי הריאה: פריפליומוניא Ms Oxford, Bodleian Library, Can. Or. 26, fol. 289b.

ואם ממרה שחורה הכאב בשמאל עם כובד וקרירות ונידוד השינה (If [the headache] on the left side is caused by black bile, [it comes] with heavyness, cold, and sleeplessness). Hebr. נידוד השינה features in EM 1122 as a modern term in an attestation from Samuel Joseph Agnon. The variant נְדוּד features as נדודי שנה in Job 7:4. Do'eg ha-Edomi translates Latin *vigiliae* as תעורה. The same term is used by Moses ibn Tibbon for the parallel Arabic term سهر. Abraham ben Isaac (ibid., Ms Jerusalem, National Library of Israel, Fr. 95, fol. 89[a]) translates the Arabic term as נידנוד, which is possibly a scribal error for נדידה, featuring in the same section as נדידת שינה (see next entry נְדִידָה).

נְדִידָה • נדידת שינה · **sleeplessness**: Arab. سهر · Ibn al-Jazzār, *Zād al-musāfir wa-qūt al-ḥāḍir* · trans. Abraham ben Isaac, *Sefer Ṣedah la-Oreḥim*, cf. bk. 1, ch. 10 (Ms Jerusalem, National Library of Israel, Fr. 95, fol. 89[a]): אם יהיה מחמת ריבוי דם אז ירגיש החולה חמות בראשו וכובד במצחו ואדמות בגידי עיניו ובפנים ומילאוי הגידים בשתי הצדעין ואם יהיה מחמת מרירה האדומה אז ירגיש חמות חדה ויובש באפיו ובלשונו ונדידת שינה וצמאה (If [headache] originates from a surplus of blood, the patient feels heat in his head, heaviness in his forehead, reddening of the blood vessels of the eyes and face, repletion of the veins of the temples. If it originates from yellow bile, he feels a sharp heat and dryness of his nostrils and his tongue, and suffers from sleeplessness and thirst). Hebr. נדידת שינה only features in BM 3540 in an attestation from Simeon ben Zemach Duran. Moses ibn Tibbon translates Arab. سهر as תעורה.

נִהוּג · **regimen; therapy**: Arab. تدبير · Ibn al-Jazzār, *Zād al-musāfir wa-qūt al-ḥāḍir* · trans. Abraham ben Isaac, *Sefer Ṣedah la-Oreḥim*, Adaptation, bk. 1, ch. 10: וראוי שיכנס במרחץ תמיד ויאכל מן העוף הנקרא קנביר והוא עוף חם מאד או יאכל מרק אפונים זה הניהוג צריך למי שיש לו כאב הראש מחמת רוח חזקה ועבה (The patient should frequently visit the bathhouse and his nourishment should consist of larks—a bird that is very hot—or soup of chickpeas. This kind of therapy is necessary for people suffering from headaches caused by strong, coarse winds). Hebr. נִהוּג does not feature as a medical term in the current dictionaries; cf. JD 903: 'leading;' KTP 3:21: 'Leitung;' BM 3553. Moses ibn Tibbon translates Arab. تدبير as הנהגה, and Abraham ben Isaac as נִהוּל (see next entry). Do'eg ha-Edomi translates the parallel Latin term *hoc modo medicandi sunt* as ובמדה הזאת יאותו להעזר.

נִהוּל · **regimen; therapy**: Arab. تدبير · Ibn al-Jazzār, *Zād al-musāfir wa-qūt al-ḥāḍir* · trans. Abraham ben Isaac, *Sefer Ṣedah la-Oreḥim*, bk. 1, ch. 10 (Ms Jerusalem, National Library of Israel, Fr. 95, fol. 90[b]): וראוי שיכנס במרחץ תמיד ויאכל עוף הנקרא קנאביר או אל דראג׳ או מי אפונים וכגון זה הניהול ראוי לרופא לרפא כל מי שיש לו ⟨כאב[203] ראש⟩ מחמת רוח חזקה (The patient should frequently visit the bathhouse and his nourishment should consist of larks or francolins or soup of chickpeas. This kind of therapy should be

203 ⟨כאב ראש⟩: صداع a.

applied by the physician to treat anyone suffering from headaches caused by strong winds). In the sense of 'therapy, regimen,' Hebr. נִהוּל is attested for in BM 3553 in an attestation from *Sefer Refu'ot*, Ms Florence.

[נהל] • *Pi'el* **נִהֵל** · **to prescribe a regimen, therapy; to treat**: Arab. دبّر · Ibn al-Jazzār, *Zād al-musāfir wa-qūt al-ḥāḍir* · trans. Abraham ben Isaac, *Sefer Ṣedah la-Oreḥim*, bk. 1, ch. 18: וינהלהו בכל הרפואות שהזכרנו בנידוד השינה (He may treat him with all the remedies that we mentioned for sleeplessness). Hebr. נִהֵל features as a biblical term in the sense of, a.o., 'to refresh with food' (cf. BDB 625; BM 3555). Moses ibn Tibbon translates Arab. دبّر as התנהג.

נֶהְפָּךְ (*Part. Nif'al*) → [**הפך**].

[נוח] • *Part. Hof'al* **מֻנָּח** · **soaked**: Lat. *infusus* (Arab. نقع) · Constantinus Africanus, *Viaticum* · trans. Do'eg ha-Edomi, *Sefer Ya'ir Netiv*, bk. 2, ch. 1: ואם הכאב רב מאד נערב שם קמח שעורה וכן בורטולייגא עם שמן ורד או שילי מונח במי ורדים (If the pain is very strong, we mix [the remedy] with barley meal and also common purslane with rose oil or fleawort soaked in rose water). Hebr. מֻנָּח does not feature in this sense in the current dictionaries. Moses ibn Tibbon translates Arab. نقع as השרה.

נוֹסָף (*Part. Nif'al*) → [**יסף**].

[נוע] • **נָע** · **to be loose (re: teeth)**: Lat. *moveor* (Arab. تحرّك) · Constantinus Africanus, *Viaticum* · trans. Do'eg ha-Edomi, *Sefer Ya'ir Netiv*, bk. 2, ch. 20: לפעמים ינועו השינים בסבת הליחות אשר בשרשיהם ואם הליחות חדות הכרח הוא שיתנקבו ותאספו שם בלויי עב טיט (The teeth may become loose because of the moistures in their roots. If those moistures are sharp, the teeth are affected by holes and accumulation of putrid matters). Hebr. נוע does not feature in a medical context in the current dictionaries. Moses ibn Tibbon translates Arab. تحرّك as הִתְנוֹעֵעַ (see entry below).

• *Hitpolel* **הִתְנוֹעֵעַ** · **to be loose (re: teeth)**: Arab. تحرّك (Gr. σείομαι)[204] · Ibn al-Jazzār, *Zād al-musāfir wa-qūt al-ḥāḍir* · trans. Moses ibn Tibbon, *Sefer Ṣedat ha-Derakhim*, bk. 2, ch. 20: פעמים יתנועעו השנים ויהיה ממנו הזק גדול (Teeth may become loose and cause great harm). Hebr. הִתְנוֹעֵעַ does not feature in a medical context in the current dictionaries. Do'eg ha-Edomi translates the parallel Latin term *moveor* as נָע (see entry above).

• *Part. Hitpolel* **מִתְנוֹעֵעַ** · **disturbed**: Arab. مضطرب (Gr. θορυβώδης) · Maimonides, *Medical Aphorisms* 6.37 · trans. Nathan ha-Me'ati (BMMN 70): אותות פרנשין הם ששה עשר אותות והוא התעורה או השינה המתנועעת ערבוב השכל ומתחיל[205] מעט מעט. קדחת חדה לא תשקוט בעת מן העתים. השכחה מהדברים ההוים לפניו מיעוט הצמא (The signs of phrenitis are sixteen: sleeplessness or disturbed sleep, delirium manifesting[206] itself gradu-

---

204 Cf. Galen, *De compositione medicamentorum secundum locos* 5.4, ed. Kühn, 12:871.

205 ומתחיל (= ويبدأ): ويبدو a.

206 'manifesting': Trans. after a.

ally, acute fever that never subsides, short-term memory loss, lack of thirst ...). Hebr. מִתְנוֹעֵעַ does not feature in this sense in the current dictionaries. Zeraḥyah Ḥen translates Arab. مضطرب as מְצְטַעֵר (see entry [צער]).

נוֹצְרִי • *Plur.* נוצריים • ירק הנוצריים → יֶרֶק.

נֶזֶלֶת • נזלת דם הנחירים • **nosebleed**: Lat. *fluxus sanguis ex naribus* (Arab. رعاف) · Constantinus Africanus, *Viaticum* · trans. Do'eg ha-Edomi, *Sefer Ya'ir Netiv*, bk. 2, ch. 15: נזלת דם הנחירים אשר לפעמים מועיל ולפעמים לא ⟨המועיל⟩ יקרה בקבשון ובפרינישין ובהזלת הפרחים נזלת דם הנחירים אשר לפעמים מועיל ולפעמים לא יקרה בקבשון ובפרינישין ובהזלת הפרחים ובארובות חמות בתנועת התולדת והדם (A nosebleed is sometimes beneficial and sometimes not; the beneficial one occurs during hectic fever, phrenesis, menstruation, and hot catarrhs moved by nature and blood). Hebr. נזלת דם הנחירים does not feature in the current dictionaries. Derived from the same root נזל, we find הזלת דם הנחירים in Judah Shalom's translation of Hippocrates' *Aphorisms* 5.33 (see BCD 65 (NM 3:62)). Moses ibn Tibbon renders Arab. رعاف as עריפת דם החוטם (cf. BCD 214 (NM 4:160)).

נָחוֹר • **rough**: Lat. *asper* · Constantinus Africanus, *Viaticum* · trans. Do'eg ha-Edomi, *Sefer Ya'ir Netiv*, bk. 3, ch. 12: ואם הטבע מהאדומה יהיה הגוף ברזון והשעול יבש וצמאון רב ואם הוא מהשחורה יהיה הגוף נחור והדפק דק ומאוחר (If the matter [that is expectorated] consists of yellow bile, the body [of the patient suffering from pleuritis] will be slim, his cough will be dry, and he will suffer from severe thirst; if it consists of black bile, his body will be [i.e., feel] rough and his pulse will be thin and slow). Hebr. נָחוֹר features in BM 3599 in later attestations from the *Sefer ha-Qanun* and from Isaac Israeli, *Sefer ha-Mis'adim*.

נְחוֹר • נחור הלשון • **roughness of the tongue**: Lat. *lingue asperitas* (Arab. خشونة اللسان) · Constantinus Africanus, *Viaticum* · trans. Do'eg ha-Edomi, *Sefer Ya'ir Netiv*, bk. 1, ch. 18: ובעלות החולי עד מעלתו העליונה יסבול החולה מקרים נרעדים כמו צמאון רב ויבשות גם שחרות הפה נחור הלשון (And when the illness [i.e., phrenitis] reaches its climax, the patient suffers from terrible afflictions such as severe thirst, dryness and blackness of the mouth, and roughness of the tongue). Hebr. נחור הלשון features as נחור לשונם in BM 3599 in a later attestation from the *Sefer ha-Qanun*. Moses ibn Tibbon renders Arab. خشونة اللسان as שעירות לשון (cf. BCD 280–281 (NM 4:209)).

• נחור הקול • **roughness of the voice**: Lat. *vocis asperitas* · Constantinus Africanus, *Viaticum* · trans. Do'eg ha-Edomi, *Sefer Ya'ir Netiv*, bk. 3, ch. 5: ה׳ מנחור הקול (Ch. 5: On roughness of the voice). Hebr. ניחור הקול features in BCD 173 (NM 4:111) in a later attestation from Moses ibn Tibbon, *Sefer Ṣedat ha-Derakhim*.

נחושת → נְחֹשֶׁת.

נְחִיר • *Dual* נְחִירַיִם • נזלת דם הנחירים → נֶזֶלֶת.

• נשימת האויר על הנחירים והפה → נְשִׁימָה.

• צנורות הנחירים → צִנּוֹר.

נֶחֱלָב (*Part. Nif'al*) → חָלַב.

[נחץ] • *Hifʿil* הֵנְחִיץ ‣ **I. to hasten**: Arab. بادر · Ibn al-Jazzār, *Zād al-musāfir wa-qūt al-ḥādir* · trans. Abraham ben Isaac, *Sefer Ṣedah la-Oreḥim*, bk. 1, ch. 17: וראוי להנחיץ רפואת חולי זה כי קשה הוא (One should hasten to treat this illness [i.e., insomnia] because it is a severe one). Hebr. הֵנְחִיץ is not attested for in medical literature. Ben-Yehuda (BM 3610–3611) quotes the term, a.o., from the commentary on Daniel attributed to Saʿadya Gaon; however, Ben-Yehuda does not define its specific meaning. Moses ibn Tibbon translates Arab. بادر as השתדל. Do'eg ha-Edomi translates the parallel Latin term *festino* as מיהר.

‣ **II. to urge; to instigate; to induce**: Arab. حفز · Ibn al-Jazzār, *Zād al-musāfir wa-qūt al-ḥādir* · trans. Abraham ben Isaac, *Sefer Ṣedah la-Oreḥim*, bk. 1, ch. 21: ויש שיבוא העיטוש כי מנחיץ החולי לפיסי שינענע המוח שלא בעת הראוי כמו שיארע לחולי הנקרא אל זכאם או החולי הנקרא דאת אלריה (Sometimes sneezing occurs because a disease induces nature to move the brain at inappropriate times—such as in the case of the illness called *al-zukām* [i.e., rheum] and *dhāt al-riʾah* [i.e., pneumonia]). Moses ibn Tibbon translates the Arab. حفز as מיהר (see entry).

נְחֹשֶׁת • ירוק הנחושת → יָרֹק.

• פרח הנחושת → פֶּרַח.

נֶחְתָּךְ (*Part. Nifʿal*) → [חתך].

נְטִיָּה • מפסיד הראות בנטית השמש → [פסד].

נידוד → נְדוּד.

ניהוג → נִהוּג.

ניהול → נִהוּל.

ניפוח → נִפּוּחַ.

נָכוֹן (*Part. Nifʿal*) → [כון].

נָכוּת ‣ **invalidity**: Arab. زمانة (cf. Lane 1254: 'disease, or an evil affection; a disease of long continuance: such as cripples, or deprives of the power to move or to stand or to walk') · Shem Tov ben Isaac, *Sefer ha-Shimmush*, bk. 29, list 1 (SHS 1:348 (Nun 24)): נכות ב״ה זמאנה וב״ל קונטרייט (*nakhut*; Arab. *zamāna*; vern. QWNṬRYYṬ [i.e., O.Occ. or O.Cat. [adjective] *contreyt*/*contrait* ('paralyzed, mutilated')]). Hebr. נָכוּת is only attested for in modern literature (cf. EM 1671).

[נכל] • *Inf. Hitpaʿel* הִתְנַכֵּל ‣ **to exercise one's skill (i.e., to do one's utmost)**: Arab. احتيال · Isḥāq ibn ʿImrān, *Treatise on Melancholy* · trans. Anonymous, fol. 50^b (51^b): והענין השני להשתדל בסבות העכול והתנכל בכל תחבולה להיות המזון שלם מכל נזק באסטומכה (The second thing [a physician treating epigastric melancholy] should do, is to pay attention to the causes of digestion and to exercise all one's skills [i.e., to do one's utmost] so that the food is healthy [and does not cause] any harm to the stomach). Hebr. הִתְנַכֵּל features in the current dictionaries only in the negative sense of 'to conspire, devise against, plan evil;' cf. BDB 647; BM 3665–3666. The Arabic verb احتال is translated as התחבל by Zeraḥyah Ḥen in his translation of Maimonides, *Medical Aphorisms* 15.17 (BMMZ 155; cf. BCD 88 (NM 1:145)).

נִכְנָס (*Part. Nif'al*) → [כנס].
נמלי • הדפק הנמלי → דֹּפֶק.
נִמְנָע (*Part. Nif'al*) → [מנע].
נֶעֱזָר (*Part. Nif'al*) → [עזר].
[נעם] *Part. Hif'il* מַנְעִים · **mitigating; alleviating (re: pain)** (DMLBS 2166): Lat. *mitigans* (Arab. مخدّر, 'stupefying, benumbing, narcotic,' cf. MMT 184–185) · Constantinus Africanus, *Viaticum* · trans. Do'eg ha-Edomi, *Sefer Ya'ir Netiv*, bk. 3, ch. 8: אחר מן הפאולי זה מקיים[207] ומדביק ומנעים (Another [remedy], composed by Paul [of Aegina]; [a remedy] that has a strengthening, glutinizing, and alleviating [effect]). Hebr. מַנְעִים does not feature in a medical context in the current dictionaries. Moses ibn Tibbon translates Arab. مخدّر as מרדים (cf. BCD 258, NM 4:104–105)).

נִעְנַע • נענע בפיו · **to rinse one's mouth**: Arab. تمضمض · Ibn al-Jazzār, *Zād al-musāfir wa-qūt al-ḥāḍir* · trans. Moses ibn Tibbon, *Sefer Ṣedat ha-Derakhim*, bk. 2, ch. 20: ונצוהו עם זה שיקח אכאסיא והוא קאקיא בערבי מעט ממנו ויודק ויתמיד אותו בשרשי השנים או יבשל עפצים בחומץ יין ויגרגר בו או יבשל קלפת רמונים או סומאק או בלבשטיאש בחומץ וינענע המים בפיו (We also order him to take some acacia, i.e., [*a*]*qāqiyā* in Arabic, to pound it and apply it regularly to the roots of the teeth, or to cook gallnut with wine vinegar and use this as a gargle, or to cook pomegranate peels or tanner's sumach or flowers of the wild pomegranate with vinegar and rinse the mouth with it). Hebr. נענע בפיו is not attested for in the current dictionaries. In *Sefer Ṣedat ha-Derakhim*, bk. 2, ch. 18, Moses ibn Tibbon renders Arab. تمضمض as גמע (or גמא), which has the standard meaning of 'to quaff' (cf. BM 793, 803); cf. IJZ 141.
• בלל ונענע → בָּלַל.
• ערבב ונענע → עִרְבֵּב.

נִפּוּחַ • *Plur.* ניפוחים · **sternutatories**: Arab. نفوخات · Ibn al-Jazzār, *Zād al-musāfir wa-qūt al-ḥāḍir* · trans. Abraham ben Isaac, *Sefer Ṣedah la-Oreḥim*, bk. 1, ch. 24: ויעטישהו בדברים הפותחין הסתומות אשר המה בראש גם הניפוחים (Sneezing should be induced with ingredients that open obstructions occurring in the head, likewise sternutatories). As a medical term, Hebrew נִפּוּחַ only features in the current dictionaries in the sense of 'swelling;' cf. BM 3716. Moses ibn Tibbon translates Arab. نفوخات as נחירות; in bk. 1, ch. 23, he uses the latter term for the Arabic synonym سعوطات (cf. BCD 111 (NM 4:111)).

נֹפַח • עלה בנפח → עָלָה.
נִפְלָג (*Part. Nif'al*) → [פלג].
נֶפֶשׁ • הנפש החיית · **vital soul**: Arab. النفس الحيوانية · Isḥāq ibn 'Imrān, *Treatise on Melancholy* · trans. Anonymous, fol. 43ᵇ (44ᵇ): וכל אלה הם מקרי[208] הנפש החיית לבד (All these are afflictions that are especially symptomatic for the vital soul). Hebr. הנפש

207 מקיים ומדביק: *solidans* L قابض a.
208 מקרי: emendation editor מקרה Ms.

החיית does not feature in the current dictionaries. For synonyms featuring in medieval (philosophical) literature see KTP 3:59. Constantine the African translates Arab. النفس الحيوانية as *anima vitalis*.

• **נפש ממללת** · **rational soul**: Arab. النفس النطقية · Isḥāq ibn ʿImrān, *Treatise on Melancholy* · trans. Anonymous, fol. 48ᵇ (49ᵇ): דע שהפועל לשחוק היא הנפש ה⟨מ⟩מללת (Know that laughing is activated by the rational soul). Hebr. נפש ממללת is a non-attested loan translation from Arab. النفس النطقية. Constantine the African translates the Arabic term as *anima rationalis*.

• **חדוש הנפש** → חִדּוּשׁ.

• **רוח הנפש** → רוּחַ.

• **שיחת הנפש** → שִׂיחָה.

• *Plur.* **נפשות** • **נפשות חכמות ממללות** · **rational souls**: Arab. النفس الناطقة · Isḥāq ibn ʿImrān, *Treatise on Melancholy* · trans. Anonymous, fol. 42ᵇ (43ᵇ): אלא שנפשותם החכמות הממללות יראו הדברים האהובים[209] כגון האחים והקרובים כשונאים (Their rational soul [i.e., of those suffering from melancholy] considers [beings] who love [them] such as brothers and [other] relatives as beings who hate [them]). Hebr. *Sing.* נפש חכמה ממללת,[210] *Plur.* נפשות חכמות ממללות, does not feature in the current dictionaries. Cf. KTP 3:58.

נָקַב · **to penetrate**: Lat. *penetro* (Arab. نفذ) · Constantinus Africanus, *Viaticum* · trans. Do'eg ha-Edomi, *Sefer Ya'ir Netiv*, bk. 1, ch. 25 (fol. 26ᵃ): ותרדמת האברים מחוברת בין התולדת והחולי והסבה היא קרירות שיקבוץ עצום[211] הגידים ויקרר ויעצור שלא יוכל הכח המרגיש לנקוב שם (Numbness is a combination of nature and illness. Its cause is coldness, which coagulates the substance of the nerves, cools and restrains [them] so that the power of sensory perception cannot penetrate them). Hebr. נָקַב features in the current dictionaries in the sense of 'to pierce, bore through' (BDB 666), 'to bore, perforate' (JD 930; cf. BM 930). Moses ibn Tibbon translates Arab. نفذ as עבר and Abraham ben Isaac as נכנס.

• *Hitpaʿel* **הִתְנַקֵּב** · **to be affected by holes**: Lat. *foramina effici* (Arab. كان ثقب) · Constantinus Africanus, *Viaticum* · trans. Do'eg ha-Edomi, *Sefer Ya'ir Netiv*, bk. 2, ch. 20: לפעמים ינועו השינים בסבת הליחות אשר בשרשיהם ואם הליחות חדות הכרח הוא שיתנקבו ותאספו שם בלויי עב טיט (The teeth may become loose because of the moistures in their roots. If those moistures are sharp, the teeth are unavoidably affected by holes and accumulation of putrid matters). Hebr. הִתְנַקֵּב does not feature in a medical context in the current dictionaries. Moses ibn Tibbon translates Arab. كان ثقب as היה נקב.

נֶקֶב • **בדק נקביו** → בָּדַק.

---

209 האהובים: emendation editor האוהבים Ms.

210 For the singular term הנפש החכמה הממללת, cf. fol. 44ᵇ: אבל מקרי פחד הנפש החכמה הממללת (The afflictions affecting the kind of soul that is rational).

211 עצום: *substantiam* L, cf. entry עִצּוּם.

נָקִי · husked (re: barley): Lat. *mundatus* (Arab. مقشور) · Constantinus Africanus, *Viaticum* · trans. Do'eg ha-Edomi, *Sefer Ya'ir Netiv*, bk. 1, ch. 18: אם לא יוכל לשתות משקה נעשה לו תשומת כלי הוא קרישטרי מן ויאולש שעור נקי גוגובש סובין (If he cannot drink the potion [we prescribed], we prepare for him a clyster from violets, husked barley, common jujubes, and bran). Hebr. נָקִי does not feature in this sense in the current dictionaries. Moses ibn Tibbon and Abraham ben Isaac translate Arab. مقشور as קלוף.

נְקִיבָה · hole: Lat. *perforatio* (Arab. تثقّب) · Constantinus Africanus, *Viaticum* · trans. Do'eg ha-Edomi, *Sefer Ya'ir Netiv*, bk. 2, ch. 18 (Ms Oxford, Bodleian Library, Can. Or. 26, fol. 268ª): והחולי משתנה והחלק השנוי נגלה[212] בתולדתו כמו הדברים הבלוים והבואשה והעקירה[213] והנקיבה והתנועה ושאר דברים דומים לאלה (There are different clearly[214] visible symptoms [in the case of toothache] such as putrefaction, bad smell, fractures, holes, movement, and other similar things). Hebr. נְקִיבָה only features in the current dictionaries in the general sense of 'perforation' (cf. BM 3795–3796), and its Aramaic counterpart נקבא/ניקבא/נוקבא in the sense of 'hole, perforation, incision' (cf. JD 930), or 'perforation, body orifice' (SDA 753). Moses ibn Tibbon translates Arab. تثقّب as נקוב (cf. BCD 180 (NM 4:116)).

[נקף] • *Part. Hif'il* **מַקִּיף** • **המכסה המקיף הלב** → **מִכְסֶה**.

נִרְעָד (*Part Nif'al*) → **[רעד]**.

נִרְפָּא (*Part. Nif'al*) → **[רפא]**.

נְשׁוּם · breathing: Arab. تنفّس · Ibn al-Jazzār, *Zād al-musāfir wa-qūt al-ḥādir* · trans. Moses ibn Tibbon, *Sefer Ṣedat ha-Derakhim*, bk. 3, ch. 11: ומה שהיה מן הנשום קטן מתאחר יורה על קרוב החום מן הכבוי (Shallow and slow breathing indicates that the [innate] heat is nearly extinguished). Hebrew נְשׁוּם features in BM 3823 in a later attestation from the *Sefer ha-Qanun*. Do'eg ha-Edomi translates the parallel Latin term *anhelitus* as נשימה.

נְשִׁימָה • נשימת האויר על הנחירים והפה · inhalation of air:[215] Arab. استنشاق الهواء · Isḥāq ibn 'Imrān, *Treatise on Melancholy* · trans. Anonymous, fol. 51ª (52ª): ותהיה הנהגתם מצד המזון כמו שאמר גאלינו' בפרו' בספר בוקרט שהמזון על שלשה מינין עב ורקיק וממוצע ביניהם העב הוא המאכל הזך הוא נשימת האויר על הנחירים והפה והממוצע הוא המשקה (Regarding food, their regimen [i.e., of those who suffer from melancholy] should be according to what Galen said in his commentary on Hippocrates' [*Aphorisms*], namely that there are three kinds of food: coarse, fine, and moderate [i.e., balanced]. Coarse is the [consumption of] food, fine is the inhalation of air, moderate is drink). Hebr. נשימת האויר על הנחירים והפה does not feature in the current dictionaries. Constantine the African translates Arab. استنشاق الهواء as *aer*.

---

212 נגלה בתולדתו: *palam est visui* L.

213 והעקירה: *rupture* L.

214 'clearly visible': Trans. after L.

215 See also entry אֲוִיר: האויר הבא על הנחירים.

• **נשימת הזקיפה** · **orthopnea**: Arab. نفس الانتصاب (Lat. *orthomia*) · Ibn al-Jazzār, *Zād al-musāfir wa-qūt al-ḥādir* · trans. Moses ibn Tibbon, *Sefer Ṣedat ha-Derakhim*, bk. 3, ch. 11: ואולם הנשימה הגבוהה היא אשר יצטרך האדם להניע החזה שלו כלו תנועה תכופה והנשימה הזאת היא הנקראת רבו ר״ל גוייש ונשימת הזקיפה (However, [the condition of] difficult breathing [lit., breathing high (in the chest)] during which someone has to move the whole chest frequently is called 'asthma,' i.e., [Rom.] GWYYŠ[216] or 'orthopnea'). Hebr. נשימת הזקיפה is not attested for in the current dictionaries. Zeraḥyah Ḥen translates Arab. انتصاب as מצב in his translation of Maimonides, *Medical Aphorisms* 24.38 (BMMZ 238; cf. BCD 156 (NM 1:165)) and Nathan ha-Me'ati as התיצבות (BMMN 239; cf. BCD 75 (NM 2:42)). The Arabic synonym ضيق النفس is translated by Zeraḥyah Ḥen as צרות הניפוש in ibid. 3.76 (BMMZ 44; cf. BCD 233 (NM 1:182)). The same Arabic term is rendered as צרות הנשימה by Shem Tov ben Isaac in the *Sefer ha-Shimmush*, bk. 27 (BCD 233–234 (NM 4:176)). Do'eg has-Edomi renders the parallel Latin term *orthomia* as אורטומיא.

• **מצוקת הנשימה** → **מְצוּקָה**.

• **צרות הנשימה** → **צָרוּת**.

• **קצף המלח** → **קֶצֶר**.

נֶתֶק · **scurfy or scabby disease of the scalp; 'scald head'**: Lat. *tinea* (DMLBS 3792) · Guillaume de Congenis, *Treatise on Surgery* · trans. Isaiah, fol. 56b: הבן כי אלה הדברים מועילים להסיר הכותל והנתק (Note that these things are good for removing the skin and for scald head). Hebr. נֶתֶק features in Nathan ha-Me'ati's translation of Arab. سعفة ('cradle cap') in Maimonides, *Medical Aphorisms* 24.53 (BMMN 241; cf. BCD 182 (NM 2:69)).

• **נתק הסלע** · **rock lichen**: Arab. حزاز الصخر (cf. M 152 (118)) / Gr. λειχὴν ὁ ἐπὶ τῶν πετρῶν ('the lichen growing on stones (rocks)') · *Shinnui ha-Shemot ha-Niqra'im Synonimis*, Ms Munich, Bayerische Staatsbibliothek, Cod. hebr. 8, fol. 198b: טחלב[217] הוא עדשי המים ויש מין ממנו סלעיי נקרא נתק הסלע ובלשונם איפטיקה ובערבי חזאז[218] אלצכר ([Arab.] *ṭuḥlub* [i.e., common duckweed (*Lemna minor* L.)]; [Hebr.] *'adashei ha-mayim* (cf. BCD 197 (NM 1:71–72)); there is a variety [that grows on] rocks that is called [in Hebr.] *neteq ha-sel'a* and in Latin 'YPṬYQH, and in Arabic *ḥazāz al-sakhr*). Hebr. נתק הסלע is a non-attested calque of Arab. حزاز الصخر.

---

216 'GWYYŠ': See entry גוייש.

217 טחלב: emendation editor חטלה Ms.

218 חזאז: הזאז Ms.

ס

סבב • *Part.* **סוֹבֵב** • הדפים הסובבים הלב → דַּף.

סָבַל • *Part.* **סוֹבֵל** · **sick person; patient:** Lat. *infirmus*[219] (Arab. عليل) · Constantinus Africanus, *Viaticum* · trans. Do'eg ha-Edomi, *Sefer Ya'ir Netiv*, bk. 2, ch. 23 (Ms Oxford, Bodleian Library, Can. Or. 26, fol. 273^{b}): ריח הפה נולד מבלוי בשר השינים כי אם הסובל בנגעו באצבעותיו ולא ימצא שום בואשה אז נתבובן שהריח הוא מבלוי הליחה הלבנה באיסטמכא (Bad breath arises from putrid gums; if the patient touches them with his fingers and does not [smell] any stench [on them], we know that the [bad breath] comes from the putrefaction of the phlegm in the stomach). Hebr. סָבַל features in the Bible in the sense of 'to bear' (BDB 687), in Rabbinic literature in the sense of 'to carry, to sustain, to endure' (JD 950), and in medieval literature in the sense of 'to endure' (cf. BM 3927: היה לו כח לעשות איזה פעולה). Moses ibn Tibbon renders Arab. عليل as חולה.

סַגִּיא • **סגיא רגלי** · **(lit., many legs); common polypody [*Polypodium vulgare* L.]:** Arab. كثير الأرجل, syn. بسبايج (cf. MIG 119) · Shem Tov ben Isaac, *Sefer ha-Shimmush*, bk. 29, list 1 (SHS 1: 368–369 (Samekh 32)): סגיא רגלי ב"ה בסבאיג וב"ל פוליפודיום (*saggi' riglei*; Arab. *basbāyij*; Lat. *polipodium*). In the sense of 'common polypody,' סגיא רגלי is a non-attested calque of Arab. كثير الأرجل. Zeraḥyah Ḥen renders the Arabic term as המרבה הרגלים (see entry [רבה]).

סְגִירוּת · **closure:** Arab. سدّ · Ibn al-Jazzār, *Zād al-musāfir wa-qūt al-ḥādir* · trans. Abraham ben Isaac, *Sefer Ṣedah la-Oreḥim*, bk. 1, ch. 22: דע כי החולי הזה הנקרא בלשון יון איפילינישיאה והוא אל צרע רטיבות מונעת[220] תסגור חדרי המוח שלראש סגירות חזקה (Know that this disease that is called in Greek 'YPYLYNYŠY'H [i.e., ἐπιληψία], i.e., [Arab.] 'L ṢR' [i.e., الصرع], [originates] from a viscous[221] fluid, which completely closes the ventricles of the brain). Hebr. סְגִירוּת only features as a modern term in EM 1214. Moses ibn Tibbon translates Arab. سدّ as סתום and Do'eg ha-Edomi translates the parallel Latin term *opilor* as סגור.

סֵדֶר · **regimen:** Lat. *ordinatio* (Arab. تدبير)[222] · Constantinus Africanus, *Viaticum* · trans. Do'eg ha-Edomi, *Sefer Ya'ir Netiv*, bk. 1, ch. 22: ואם יקרה זה לנער או לבחור לעזור להם כן כאשר הזכרנו כי לאלה יקרה יותר תמיד בסבת לחות גופם ונעשית בשני ענינים או מחבור קר ולח מושל במוח או מסדר רע (If this [i.e., epilepsy] occurs to a child or adolescent one should treat them as we have mentioned, for in two cases they are more often affected because of the moisture of their body: either a cold and moist temperament that dominates the brain or a bad regimen). Hebr. סֵדֶר does not feature in this

219 Do'eg ha-Edomi also translates the synonymous *patiens*, featuring in bk. 2, ch. 17, as סובל.

220 מונעת (= مانعة): ميّاعة a.

221 'viscous': Trans. after a.

222 See also entry גָּדוֹל.

sense in the current dictionaries. Moses ibn Tibbon translates Arab. تدبير as הנהגה and Abraham ben Isaac as נִהוּל (see entry).

סוֹבֵב (*Part.*) → סָבַב.

סוֹבֵל (*Part.*) → סָבַל.

סוֹף • סוף המוח · **the rear part of the brain**: Lat. *puppis cerebri* (Arab. مؤخّر الدماغ) · Constantinus Africanus, *Viaticum* · trans. Do'eg ha-Edomi, *Sefer Ya'ir Netiv*, bk. 1, ch. 14: וכאשר תגבר לעלות בסוף המוח אז תכבה הרוח המרגיש[223] ונקרא זה החולי ליטרגיאה (And when it [i.e, the phlegmatic superfluity] arises to the rear part of the brain and dominates it, it extinguishes the psychical[224] pneuma and this illness is called lethargy). Hebr. סוף המוח does not feature in the current dictionaries. Moses ibn Tibbon renders Arab. مؤخّر الدماغ as המאוחר מן המוח and Abraham ben Isaac as קצה מוח הראש.

[סור] • *Hof'al* **הוּסַר • קמח שהוסר המורסן ממנו** → קֶמַח.

סִיד • סיד חי · **quicklime**: Arab. جير غير مطفأ (cf. KM 1:389–391, s.v. جير, syn. نورة (cf. M 260 (200))) · Shem Tov ben Isaac, *Sefer ha-Shimmush*, bk. 29, list 1 (SHS 1:364–365 (Samekh 21)): סיד חי ב״ה ג׳יר בגיר מטפי וב״ל קאלס ויוא (*sid ḥay*; Arab. *jir bi-ghayr mutfa'*; vern. Q'LS WYW' [i.e., O.Occ. or O.Cat. *calz/cals viva*]). Hebr. סיד חי features in BCD 185 (NM 1:34) in an attestation from Hillel ben Samuel's translation of Lat. *calx viva*, featuring in the *Sefer Keritut*, i.e., his translation of Bruno Longobucco's *Cyrurgia Magna*.

• סיד מרוקח · **quicklime**: Arab. نورة (cf. KM 1:390; 2:1095–1099) · Ibn al-Jazzār, *Zād al-musāfir wa-qūt al-ḥādir* · trans. Abraham ben Isaac, *Sefer Ṣedah la-Oreḥim*, bk. 1, ch. 1: וראוי לו לשמור מאד שלא ישים שם מן הסמים שהן חמים וחדים פן יולידו שם חבורה אך ראוי להעביר תער על ראשו או הסיד המרוקח עם ארסיניצי להסיר השיער משם (He should be very careful and not use things that are hot and sharp, lest ulceration of the skin takes place. He should shave his head either with a razor or with quicklime with arsenic in order to remove the hair from that spot). Hebr. סיד המרוקח does not feature in the current dictionaries. Moses ibn Tibbon translates the parallel Arabic term نورة as טרכסיד (cf. SHS 1:241 (Ṭet 3): טרכסיד ב״ה נורה וב״ל פלדור והוא דבר מורכב מסיד וזרנך); the term תרכסיד is used as a variant reading by Do'eg ha-Edomi. See also entry אֵשׁ: אש קרה.

סַיִף • סיף העורב · **(lit., sword of the raven); cornflag** [*Gladiolus communis* L.]: Arab. صيف الغراب (cf. D 1:713; DT 4:20 (532–534); M 287 (219–220); LF 2:7) · Shem Tov ben Isaac, *Sefer ha-Shimmush*, bk. 29, list 1 (SHS 1: 367 (Samekh 29)): סיף העורב ב״ה סיף אלגראב (*sayif ha-'orev*; Arab. *ṣayf al-ghurāb*). In the sense of 'cornflag,' Hebr. סיף העורב is a non-attested calque of Arab. صيف الغراب.

---

223 המרגיש: *animatum* L النفساني a.

224 'psychical': Trans. after aL.

סֶלַע • נתק הסלע → נֶתֶק.

• *Plur.* **סלעים • הדג המתגדל בין הסלעים** → דָּג.

• **דג הסלעים** → דָּג.

סַלְעִי • הדג הסלעי → דָּג.

סַם • הסם הממרק › **the clearing medicine**: Arab. الدواء الجلّاء (cf. MMT 243) · Maimonides, *Medical Aphorisms* 23.100 · trans. Nathan ha-Me'ati (BMMN 231): הסם הרוחץ והממרק הוא אותו שעוקר הזוהמא מהשטח החיצון מן הנקבים והחורים כגון הדבש וקמח תורמוס ושעורים ופולים וכרסנה ורבים מן הזרעים (A cleansing and clearing medicine uproots sordidness from the outer layer of the pores and openings, such as honey, white lupine flour, barley, beans, bitter vetch, and a large number of seeds). Hebr. הסם הממרק features in BCD 188 (NM 4:128) in the sense of 'the detergent (cleansing, clearing) remedy' (for Arab. الدواء الجالي) in an attestation from the anonymous *Sammim Libbiyim*. Zeraḥyah Ḥen translates Arab. الدواء الجلّاء as הרפואה המטהרת (see entry רְפוּאָה).

• **הסם הרוחץ** › **the cleansing medicine**: Arab. الدواء الغسّال · Maimonides, *Medical Aphorisms* 23.100 · trans. Nathan ha-Me'ati (BMMN 231): הסם הרוחץ והממרק הוא אותו שעוקר הזוהמא מהשטח החיצון מן הנקבים והחורים כגון הדבש וקמח תורמוס ושעורים ופולים וכרסנה ורבים מן הזרעים (A cleansing and clearing medicine uproots sordidness from the outer layer of the pores and openings, such as honey, white lupine flour, barley, beans, bitter vetch and a large number of seeds). Hebr. הסם הרוחץ features in BCD 191 (NM 4:135) in the sense of 'the abluent remedy' in an attestation from the anonymous *Sammim Libbiyim*. Zeraḥyah Ḥen translates Arab. الدواء الغسّال as הרפואה המכבסת (see entry רְפוּאָה).

• *Plur.* **סמים • סמים משככים** › **repellent drugs**: Arab. الأدوية الردّاعة · Ibn al-Jazzār, *Zād al-musāfir wa-qūt al-ḥādir* · trans. Moses ibn Tibbon, *Sefer Ṣedat ha-Derakhim*,[225] bk. 2, ch. 24: ואם קרה המורסא בפה ולא יהיה בגוף מותר יטה וימשך אל המקום הכואב הנה ראוי אז שיתרפא בהתחלה במה שיתיך המורסא וישקיט הכאב ולא יביט אל הסמים המשככים[226] (If an ulcer affects the mouth but the body does not contain a superfluity that tends and streams to the painful spot, it should initially be treated with that which dissolves the ulcer and alleviates the pain; one should not consider [the use of] repellent drugs). Hebr. *Sing.* סם משכך, *Plur.* סמים משככים, is not attested for in the current dictionaries. See also entry [שכך].

סַמּוּת › **poisonous property; poisonous effect**: Arab. سمّيّة · Maimonides, *Medical Aphorisms* 13.50 · trans. Zeraḥyah Ḥen (BMMZ 150): אמר משה: זה אמת כל זמן שיהיה השלשול ברפואה בעלת סם או חזקה כמו הקולוקוינטידא והתורפד מפני סמותם או הקטפוץ מרוב כחו (Says Moses: This is correct if the purgation is done by poisonous drugs, such as pulp of colocynth or St. Thomas lidpod, because of their poisonous effect; or [by strong

225 See also entry [שכך]: שִׁכֵּךְ.

226 המשכבים: המרתיעים Ms Munich, Bayerische Staatsbibliothek, Cod. hebr. 19, fol. 50^b.

drugs, such as] bay laurel, because of its strength). Hebrew סַמּוּת, an abstract noun, coined from סַם ('poison') is not attested for in the current dictionaries. Nathan ha-Me'ati translates Arab. سمّية as ארסיות.

סִמְפּוֹן • *Plur.* סמפונים/סמפונות ‣ **pores**: Arab. مسامّ · Ibn al-Jazzār, *Zād al-musāfir wa-qūt al-ḥādir* · trans. Abraham ben Isaac, *Sefer Ṣedah la-Oreḥim*, bk. 1, ch. 2 (Ms Jerusalem, National Library of Israel, Fr. 95, fol. 84b): ואם יקרה מחמת עובי העור וסתימת[227] סימפוניו יעשה רפואות הפותחין הסימפונות ומרטיבין שרשי חורי השיער (If it [i.e., loss of hair] originates from density of the skin and obstruction of the pores, one should apply remedies that open the pores and moisten the openings of the roots of the hair). Hebr. *Sing.* סִמְפּוֹן, *Plur.* סמפונים/סמפונות, does not feature in this sense in the current dictionaries (cf. BCD 192 (NM 4:136)). Moses ibn Tibbon translates Arab. مسامّ as נקבים. The same term is used by Do'eg ha-Edomi for the parallel Latin term *poros*. Moses ibn Tibbon uses *Plur.* סמפונות for Arab. خيشوم, *Plur.* خياشيم ('[nasal] arteries;' cf. BCD ibid.); in his glossary to his translation of the *Sefer ha-Qānūn*, Nathan ha-Me'ati remarks: ורידים הם העורקים שבכבד והם הסמפונות (WRYDYM.[228] These are the veins in the liver, i.e., the SMPWNWT (large blood vessels)) (NM 2:112, 134 (Waw 1)).

סִנּוּן ‣ I. **filtration**: Arab. تصفية · Ibn al-Jazzār, *Zād al-musāfir wa-qūt al-ḥādir* · trans. Moses ibn Tibbon, *Sefer Ṣedat ha-Derakhim*, bk. 3, ch. 6: ואח"כ יסונן השמן סנון בנחת בכף ויושם בזכוכית (Then the oil should be gently filtered by hand and put into a flask). Hebr. סִנּוּן features in BM 4122 in attestations from Rashi's commentary on the Talmud, and from Tuviah ha-Kohen, *Ma'aseh Tuviah*.

‣ II. **filtrate**: Lat. *colatura* · Guillaume de Congenis, *Treatise on Surgery* · trans. Isaiah, fol. 49a: וזה מעשה המשיחה קח השומן והרתיחנו באש ויסונן ובסנון יושם האבק הנזכר וינער יפה באשפטולה ויועיל גם כנגד כל סרטן ישן לפי החכם (This is the recipe of the salve:[229] Take the fat [of an old pig], boil it on a fire, filter it, put the mentioned powder into the filtrate, and stir it well with a spatula. According to the learned [Master, i.e. Guillaume de Congenis] it is also good for an inveterate cancer). Hebr. סִנּוּן only features in the current dictionaries in the sense of 'filtration, filtering' (cf. BM 4122).

סְנוּנִית • ירק הסנונית → יֶרֶק.

סְנַפִּיר • *Plur.* סנפירים ‣ **scurf; dandruff**: Lat. *furfures* (DMLBS 1303, s.v. *furfur*: 'scurf or other scaly infection of the skin' (Arab. إبرية; cf. FL 1:3: 'furfuratio capitis')) · Constantinus Africanus, *Viaticum* · trans. Do'eg ha-Edomi, *Sefer Ya'ir Netiv*, bk. 1, ch. 5: מסנפירי הראש (On scurf [i.e., dandruff]). Subsequently, Moses ibn Tibbon uses the same Hebrew term in the *Plur.f.* סנפירות (cf. BCD 137 (NM 4:192)). Abraham ben Isaac

---

227 וסתימת סימפוניו: om a.

228 *Sing.* WRYD ('vein' and esp. 'jugular vein'): Cf. BM 1272.

229 I.e., the one mentioned under the entry יָרֹק.

renders Arab. إبرية as אלבריאה ובלשון יוון פיטרידש ([Arab.] ʾLBRYʾH [read: ʾLʾBRYʾH]; in Greek PYṬRYDŠ [i.e., πιτυρίς]).

סָפַג • *or Piʿel* **סִפֵּג** · **to rub**: Arab. مسح · Ibn al-Jazzār, *Zād al-musāfir wa-qūt al-ḥāḍir* · trans. Abraham ben Isaac, *Sefer Ṣedah la-Oreḥim*, bk. 1, ch. 1: אחר כן יספג אותו המקום בחתיכת בגד פשתן לא רכה ולא קשה אלא בינונית (After that, the spot [where the hair vanished] has to be rubbed with a linen cloth that is neither soft nor hard, but moderately so). Hebr. ספג features in the current dictionaries in the sense of 'to wipe (rub) and to dry' with attestations from Rabbinic literature (cf. JD 1011; BM 4143), medieval liturgical literature, and modern literature (EM 1260). Do'eg ha-Edomi translates the parallel Latin term *extergo* as גרד; Moses ibn Tibbon translates Arab. مسح as חפף.

סְפוֹג • אבן הספוג → אֶבֶן.

סַפִּירִי • ספירית · **crystalline moisture (i.e., lens) (in the eye)**: Lat. *cristalleidon* (Arab. جليدية) · Constantinus Africanus, *Viaticum* · trans. Do'eg ha-Edomi, *Sefer Ya'ir Netiv*, bk. 2, ch. 6: ויקרה לפעמים מהליחה הגסה המתקבצת בין הספירית והענבית (Sometimes it [i.e., nightblindness] is caused by the coarse humor that accumulates between the crystalline moisture [i.e., lens] and the grape-like moisture [i.e., lens]). In the sense of 'crystalline moisture (i.e., lens),' Hebr. ספירית features in BM 4163 in a later attestation from Me'ir Aldabi, *Shevilei Emunah*; cf. KDS 96. Moses ibn Tibbon translates Arab. جليدية as כפורית; cf. BCD 136 (NM 4:85, s.v. הלחות הכפורית).

סַפְלִיקָא · **cephalic vein**: Lat. *cephalica* (Arab. قيفال) · Constantinus Africanus, *Viaticum* · trans. Do'eg ha-Edomi, *Sefer Ya'ir Netiv*, bk. 3, ch. 1: וכאשר יכבה חדוד האדומה ויצא עם התוצאות אז יאות להקיז הספליקא עד צאת הדם הנלהב מן האדומה (When the heat of the yellow bile is extinguished and leaves [the body] through purgation, then one should bleed the cephalic vein until the blood that is heated by the yellow bile is extracted). Hebr. סַפְלִיקָא is a non-attested loan word of Lat. *cephalica*. Moses ibn Tibbon translates Arab. قيفال as הגיד העליון (cf. BCD 45 (NM 4:31)).

סֵפֶר • ספר ההשגחות → הַשְׁגָּחָה.

סְתִימָה · **obstruction**: Arab. انسداد · Ibn al-Jazzār, *Zād al-musāfir wa-qūt al-ḥāḍir* · trans. Abraham ben Isaac, *Sefer Ṣedah la-Oreḥim*, bk. 1, ch. 23: ואם יקרה החולי באבר אחד יקרה[230] על שם האבר ההוא בלבד בעבור כי הסתימה אם יהיה בשורש אחד מהגידים הדקים ויהיה שאר הגידים הקרובים סביביו בלא הזק כלום אז יהיה ההזק והרפיון באותו האבר אשר יעבור אותו הגיד הדק (If the illness [i.e., apoplexy] befalls one [specific] organ, it is named after that [specific] organ. For, if such an obstruction befalls the root of a single nerve and the other surrounding nerves remain sound, harm and looseness occur only in the organ that nerve passes through). As a medical term, Hebr. סְתִימָה features in MD 514 in the sense of 'obstruction' without any further reference, and in EM 1278 as a modern term in the sense of '[dental] filling.' Moses ibn Tibbon translates Arab.

230 יקרה: نسب a (= יקרא).

انسداد as סתום (cf. BCD 195 (NM 4:140)). Do'eg ha-Edomi translates the parallel Latin term *constipatio* as מְצוֹק (see entry).

סָתַם · **to promote cicatrization; to heal**: Arab. أدمل (Gr. ἐπουλόω; ἰάομαι; κολλάω; cf. UW 264, 303–304, 354–355) · Ibn al-Jazzār, *Zād al-musāfir wa-qūt al-ḥāḍir* · trans. Moses ibn Tibbon, *Sefer Ṣedat ha-Derakhim*, bk. 3, ch. 8: תאר עוגות ילקחו לרקיקת הדם ולסדיקת העורקים בחזה והכבד והכליות והרחם עם חלב או עם מי שעור ויסתום ויחתום והם ידועות (A recipe for well-known pastilles that are taken for spitting of blood, for a rupture of the veins in the chest, liver, intestines, and womb, [and that has to be taken] with milk, or barley gruel, and that heals [i.e., promotes cicatrization] and seals [a wound]). Hebr. סָתַם does not feature in this sense in the current dictionaries.

ע

בְּלוֹי • **בלויי עב טיט** → **עָב**.
• **כתש כתישה עבה** → **כָּתַשׁ**.

[עבד] • *Part. Hif'il* **מַעֲבִיד** · **strengthening (the stomach)** · Ms Cambridge, T-S K14.48, P7 (recto 1): הפלפל השחור לו כח מעכל המזון אם יעורב עם קצת מהקובצים האצטומכה ומעבידינה[231] (Black pepper has power to digest the food when it is mixed with ingredients that contract the stomach [muscles] and strengthen it). Hebr. *Hif'il* הֶעֱבִיד does not feature in this sense in the current dictionaries. However, in the Pi'el conjugation, the verb features in the same sense (for Arab. دبغ) in Shem Tov ben Isaac, *Sefer Almansur* (BMZ 18, 30, 56); cf. BCD 196 (NM 2:16).

עָבֶה · **frequent**: Lat. *spissus* (cf. DMLBS 3515) · Constantinus Africanus, *Viaticum* · trans. Do'eg ha-Edomi, *Sefer Ya'ir Netiv*, bk. 3, ch. 11: ואם האסטומכא יכאב או המרי הוא הושט או בועות[232] הכבד או ראש הטחול או אם הנפח והכאב יהיה תחת הקרב זהו דיאפראגמא אז הנשימה קטנה ועבה (But if the stomach, the esophagus, the convex[233] part of the liver, or the top of the spleen hurts, or there is a swelling and pain beneath the diaphragm, i.e., [Lat.] *diaphragma*, breathing will be small and frequent). In the sense of 'frequent,' Hebr. עָבֶה is a non-attested semantic borrowing from Lat. *spissus*. Moses ibn Tibbon translates the parallel Arabic term متواتر as תכוף.

עֳבִי • **בעובי** · **frequently**: Lat. *spisse* (cf. DMLBS 3515, s.v. *spissus*) · Constantinus Africanus, *Viaticum* · trans. Do'eg ha-Edomi, *Sefer Ya'ir Netiv*, bk. 3, ch. 11: ואם הוא חומד מאד האויר למשכו והחזה ימלא בעובי גדול מהנשימה אז נבין כי קוצר כלי הרוח הם (If he has a strong need to frequently inhale air and fill the chest, we know that this is because of the narrowness in [one of] the respiratory channels). In the sense of 'frequently,' Hebr. בעובי is a non-attested semantic borrowing from Lat. *spisse*. Moses ibn Tibbon translates Arab. كثرة التنفّس as להרבות הנשימה.

[עבר] • *Hif'il* **הֶעֱבִיר** · **to filter; to strain**: Lat. *colo* (Arab. صفّى) · Constantinus Africanus, *Viaticum* · trans. Do'eg ha-Edomi, *Sefer Ya'ir Netiv*, bk. 1, ch. 17: ובסוף להעבירו ולשום שם אופי כתוש די ספקו עם השמנים הנזכרים (In the end, strain [these ingredients] and add a sufficient amount of pulverized opium with the mentioned oils). Hebr. הֶעֱבִיר, which is possibly an abbreviated version for להעביר בנפה, does not feature in this sense in the current dictionaries. Moses ibn Tibbon translates Arab. صفّى as סינן and Abraham ben Isaac as הכביר בנפה יפה.

עֲגֻלָּה • *Plur.* **עגולות** · **pastilles**: Arab. أقراص · Ibn al-Jazzār, *Zād al-musāfir wa-qūt al-ḥāḍir* · trans. Abraham ben Isaac, *Sefer Ṣedah la-Oreḥim*, bk. 1, ch. 17: וזה מעשה העגולות

---

231 ומעבידינה: read ומעבידין אותה.
232 בועות (?): حدبة a.
233 'convex part': Trans. after a.

הנקראין טורשׁשכין[234] ירדימו החולה כאשר יהיה תוקף ⟨אותו⟩ נידוד שינה עם חמימות חזקה (Recipe for pastilles called ṬWRŠŠKYN [read ṬRWṢYSQY;[235] i.e., Lat. *trocisci*] that make the patient sleep when he suffers from sleeplessness and intense heat). Hebr. *Sing.* עֲגֻלָּה, *Plur.* עגולות, does not feature as a medical term in the current dictionaries. Moses ibn Tibbon translates Arab. أقراص as עוגות (cf. BCD 197 (NM 1:63–64)); the same term features in Do'eg ha-Edomi's translation of the parallel Latin term *trocisci* (see entry עוּגָה).

עֵדוּת · **prognostic sign**: Lat. *signum* (cf. DMLBS 3334 (13)) · Constantinus Africanus, *Viaticum* · trans. Do'eg ha-Edomi, *Sefer Ya'ir Netiv*, bk. 1, ch. 17: והנשימה הקטנה והמאוחרת תכבה מהר החום וזאת בהכרח כל זמן קרה ועל כן היא יותר[236] עדות מן המות (Shallow, slow breathing, which is necessarily always cold, quickly extinguishes the [innate] heat; for this reason it is a more [certain] sign of death [than other signs]). Hebr. עֵדוּת does not feature in a medical context in the current dictionaries. Moses ibn Tibbon translates the parallel Arabic term دلّ على as ראיה על.

עֲדִיפָה • **עדיפת הבשר** · **keloid (i.e., an area of irregular fibrous tissue formed at the site of a scar or injury)**: Lat. *caro superflua* · Guillaume de Congenis, *Treatise on Surgery* · trans. Isaiah, fol. 49ᵃ: לעדיפת הבשר ולפוליף: גיליטה שרופה והעצם יהיה אבק ומושמת עליה ממעט הפוליף והבשר העודף ([A remedy] for keloid and polyps: When one burns chalk[237] and the substance turns into powder and then puts the powder on the spot, it reduces the polyp and the keloid). Hebr. עדיפת הבשר does not feature in the current dictionaries. See also entry בָּשָׂר: בשר עודף.

[עדף] • *Part.* **עוֹדֵף** • **בשר עודף** · **בָּשָׂר**.

עוּגָה • *Plur.* **עוגות** · **pastilles**: Lat. *trocisci* (Arab. أقراص) · Constantinus Africanus, *Viaticum* · trans. Do'eg ha-Edomi, *Sefer Ya'ir Netiv*, bk. 1, ch. 17: גם עוגות קטנות הנקראות טרוסישקש נעשות לזה כן (Small pastilles called [in Lat.] ṬRWSYŠQŠ are also applied for [this condition, i.e., sleeplessness] as follows …). In the sense of 'pastille,' Hebr. *Sing.* עוּגָה features in BCD 197 (NM 1:63–64) in a later attestation from Moses ibn Tibbon, *Sefer Ṣedat ha-Derakhim*, bk. 7, ch. 18.4 (IJZ 156); see also ROT 26 (*trocisci*), 43 (עוגות). Moses ibn Tibbon renders Arab. أقراص as עוגות as well. Abraham ben Isaac translates Arab. as עגולות (see entry עֲגֻלָּה).

עוֹדֵף (*Part.*) → **[עדף]**.

עֲוִוּת · **colic; gripes**: Lat. *tortura* · Constantinus Africanus, *Viaticum* · trans. Do'eg ha-Edomi, *Sefer Ya'ir Netiv*, bk. 1, ch. 10: ואם כאב הראש יחול מן האסטומכ׳ ומן הליחות הנאספות

---

234 טורשׁשכין: טרוציסקי Ms Jerusalem, National Library of Israel, Fr. 95.

235 Ms Jerusalem, National Library of Israel, Fr. 95.

236 יותר: *certius* L.

237 'chalk' (גיליטה): I.e., O.Occ. **gleda* (*greda*); cf. M. McVaugh, G. Bos, and J. Shatzmiller (eds. and trans.), *The Regimen Sanitatis of "Avenzoar": Stages in the Production of a Medieval Translation* (Leiden 2019), 169, n. 7.

שם תעזור אליו כן. אם יהיה לו איסטניסות ויסבול עוות הבטן (If the headache hails from the stomach and from the humors collected there, we treat the patient as follows. If he suffers from nausea and a colic in the stomach …). In the sense of 'colic,' Hebr. עִוּוּת features in BCD 197–198 (NM 4:192) in a later attestation from Moses ibn Tibbon, *Sefer Ṣedat ha-Derakhim*.

• **עוות הפה · twisted mouth (i.e., crooked mouth; facial paresis; paralysis of the facial nerve)**: Arab. لقوة · Ibn al-Jazzār, *Zād al-musāfir wa-qūt al-ḥāḍir* · trans. Abraham ben Isaac, *Sefer Ṣedah la-Oreḥim*, bk. 1, ch. 23: וזה ריקוח הגלולות הסרוחות הנקראות בלשון ישמעאל חב אל מנתן מאת אשר ריקח סבאור המועילות מן חולי הפלג ועיוות הפה וכאב כל פרקי הגוף והפודגרא והרוחות העבות החזקות בכל הגוף ולחולי קוליקום ולליחה העבה ולכאב הגידים ולרפיון ויתיר דם הנדות וכבר ניסינוהו (Recipe of the 'stinking pill,' called in Arab. *ḥabb al-muntin*, composed by Sābūr,[238] which is beneficial for hemiplegia, facial paresis, joint pain [i.e., arthritis], gout, strong coarse winds in the whole body, colic, thick humors, neuralgia, and looseness, and which provokes menstruation. We have tested it). In the sense of 'facial paresis,' Hebr. עוות הפה features in BM 4361 in an attestation from Shabbetai Donnolo, *Sefer Ḥakmoni*. Moses ibn Tibbon translates Arab. لقوة as עקום הפה (cf. BCD 212 (NM 4:158–159)); Do'eg ha-Edomi renders Lat. *paraliticis* as פראלישין.

עוֹמֵד (*Part.*) → עָמַד.

עומק → עֹמֶק.

עוֹפֶרֶת • אבק העופרת → אָבָק.

עוֹצֵר (*Part.*) → עָצַר.

עוֹצֶר → עֹצֶר.

[עור] • *Polel* **עוֹרֵר** • **עורר העטוש · to apply a sternutatory medicine**: Lat. *sternutationem facio* (Arab. سعّط) · Constantinus Africanus, *Viaticum* · trans. Do'eg ha-Edomi, *Sefer Ya'Ir Netiv*, bk. 1, ch. 17: וטוב מאד להעביר תער על ראשו ולטבול בחלב אשה או חמורה או מבהמה אחרת ונעורר לו עטוש עשוי מחלב אשה ושמן זרע קוקורביטא (It is very beneficial if one shaves the head [of the patient], washes it with women's milk, milk of she-asses, or another animal. One should apply a sternutatory medicine prepared from women's milk and pumpkin seed oil). Hebr. עורר עטוש is not attested for in the current dictionaries. Moses ibn Tibbon translates Arab. سعّط as שם בנחיריו (cf. BCD 274 (NM 4:204)) and Abraham ben Isaac as שם באפיו (see entry [שים]).

עוֹר • *Plur.* **עורות · membranes**: Lat. *pelliculae* (Arab. غشاء) · Constantinus Africanus, *Viaticum* · trans. Do'eg ha-Edomi, *Sefer Ya'ir Netiv*, bk. 2, ch. 1: אופטלמיא הוא נפח חם הנולד על הלובן ועל עורות העינים (Ophthalmia is an inflammation that originates in the [eye] white and membranes of the eye). Hebr. *Sing.* עוֹר features in the current dic-

238 Cf. Ibn Sahl, *Dispensatorium Parvum*, ed. Kahl, no. 114 (99); and O. Kahl (ed. and trans.), *Ibn Sahl's Dispensatory*, no. 173 (186).

tionaries in the sense of 'skin, hide, leather' (cf. BDB 736; JD 1058; BM 4393–4394) and of 'folio of pergament or paper' (cf. BCD 199 (NM 3:174)). In the sense of 'membrane (of the eye),' it features in KDS 86. Moses ibn Tibbon renders Arab. غشاء as קצידה.[239]

• **מראה עור הפנים** → מַרְאֶה.

עוֹרֵב • **סיף העורב** → סַיִף.

עורף → עֹרֶף.

עוֹרֵק • **העורק אשר בין האצבע הקטן וחברו** · **(lit., the vein that is between the little finger and the next one); vena salvatella**: Arab. الأُسيلم · Ibn al-Jazzār, *Zād al-musāfir wa-qūt al-ḥādir* · trans. Abraham ben Isaac, *Sefer Ṣedah la-Oreḥim*, bk. 3, ch. 7: וממה שראוי שנתחיל בו ברפואתו שנעיין ואם היה החולי מחום והורה על זה המופת אשר אמרנו נצוה החולה להקיז הגיד התחתון או להקיז העורק אשר בין האצבע הקטן וחברו הנקרא אסילם (One of the first things one should do in order to cure [the illness] is to examine whether it arises from fever as indicated by what I mentioned [above]. [If this is the case] we should order the patient to be bled from the basilic vein or from the vena salvatella that is called [in Arabic] *usaylam*). Hebr. העורק אשר בין האצבע הקטן וחברו does not feature in the current dictionaries. A variant reading העורק אשר בין האצבע הקטן ושכנו features in BM 4748 in an attestation from Me'ir Aldabi, *Shevilei Emunah*. However, Aldabi defines this vein as מאבץ (i.e., Arab. مأبض, i.e., the inner side [of the arm]). Do'eg ha-Edomi renders the parallel Latin term *vena que inter auricularem et medicum extat* as המקור העומד בין האצבע הקטן לחבירו (see entry מָקוֹר). Nathan ha-Me'ati refers to this vein with the Hebrew loan word אסילם in the *Sefer ha-Qanun* (cf. BCD 24 (NM 4:18)).

• **העורק אשר אצל העקב** · **the saphenous vein**: Arab. الصافن · Ibn al-Jazzār, *Zād al-musāfir wa-qūt al-ḥādir* · trans. Moses ibn Tibbon, *Sefer Ṣedat ha-Derakhim*, bk. 3, ch. 8: והקזת העורק אשר אצל העקב מועיל גם כן בחולי הזה (Bleeding the saphenous vein is also useful in the case of this illness [i.e., spitting of blood]). Hebr. העורק אשר אצל העקב is not attested for in the current dictionaries. Do'eg ha-Edomi translates the parallel Latin term *vena inter auricularem et medicum* as המקור אשר בין האצבע הקטן לאחיהו (see entry מָקוֹר). Nathan ha-Me'ati renders Arab. العرق الصافن, featuring in Maimonides, *Medical Aphorisms* 12.31, as העורק הנקרא צאפן (BMMN 143) and Zeraḥyah Ḥen translates the Arabic term as גיד הצאפין (BMMZ 140).

עָזַב • **עזב מן** · **to neglect**: Arab. أغفل · Maimonides, *Medical Aphorisms* 9.45 · trans. Zeraḥyah Ḥen (BMMZ 104): מי שמזונו תפסד באסטומכא הרבה יועילנו הקיא המזון וישתה המזונות[240] המתוקים וישים מזונותיו מה שלא ימהר אליו ההפסד ויתמיד בין הזמנים לשלשל בטנו בדברים אשר ישלשלוהו ביושר ותנקה כמו הפיגרא. ואם אתה עזבת מנהוג זאת הליחה הרעה יעצור רפואתה (If someone's food often putrefies in his stomach, he benefits from emesis

239 For the term קצידה, see G. Bos, 'Two Comments on the Ben-Yehuda Dictionary' (in Hebr.), *Ha-'Ivrit* 65, nos. 3–4 (2018–2019): 106–107.

240 המזונות: الخمر a.

before eating and from drinking sweet wine.[241] He should eat those foods that are not quickly putrefied and should accustom himself to relieving the bowels from time to time with those substances that have a moderately relieving, cleansing force such as [hiera] picra. But if one neglects [to purge] the bad humor, healing is difficult). Hebr. עזב מן does not feature in the current dictionaries. Nathan ha-Me'ati translates Arab. أغفل as נעלם מן.

[עזר] • *Part. Nif'al* **נֶעֱזָר** · **to be cured:** Lat. *curor* · Constantinus Africanus, *Viaticum* · trans. Do'eg ha-Edomi, *Sefer Ya'ir Netiv*, bk. 1, ch. 5: והם נעזרים בדברים שהם הפך להם (And it [i.e., dandruff] is cured by ingredients with opposite [qualities]). Hebr. נֶעֱזָר does not feature in this sense in the current dictionaries.

עֵזֶר · **healing; treatment; cure:** Lat. *cura* (Arab. علاج) · Constantinus Africanus, *Viaticum* · trans. Do'eg ha-Edomi, *Sefer Ya'ir Netiv*, bk. 1, ch. 16: והעזר אל זה החולי הוא שלם[242] כעזר ליטירגיאה (The treatment of this illness [i.e., torpor] is the[243] same as that for lethargy). Hebr. עֵזֶר does not feature in this sense in the current dictionaries. Moses ibn Tibbon translates Arab. علاج as רפואה.

עִטּוּשׁ · **sternutatory:** Lat. *sternutatio* (Arab. سعوط) · Constantinus Africanus, *Viaticum* · trans. Do'eg ha-Edomi, *Sefer Ya'ir Netiv*, bk. 1, ch. 23: עטוש זה טוב לאפופליקשיא אפילמסיא כי יטהר המוח מהליחות הגסות (The following sternutatory is good for apoplexy [and] epilepsy because it cleanses the brain from the coarse humors). In the sense of 'sternutatory,' Hebr. עִטּוּשׁ features in BM 4121 in later attestations from Me'ir Aldabi, *Shevilei Emunah*, and Nathan ben Jo'el Falaquera, *Sefer Ṣori ha-Guf*.[244] In the *Sefer Agur*, i.e., his translation of a Latin version of Hippocrates' *Aphorisms*, Do'eg ha-Edomi uses the term דבר מעטיש in the sense of 'sternutatory' (cf. BCD 55 (NM 3: 134–135)). Moses ibn Tibbon translates Arab. سعوط as נחירה (cf. BCD 173 (NM 4:111)) and Abraham ben Isaac as רפואה להעטיש.

עֲטִישָׁה • *Plur.* **עטישות** · **sternutatories:** Arab. سعوطات · Ibn al-Jazzār, *Zād al-musāfir wa-qūt al-ḥāḍir* · trans. Abraham ben Isaac, *Sefer Ṣedah la-Oreḥim*, bk. 1, ch. 10 (Ms Jerusalem, National Library of Israel, Fr. 95, fol. 90[a]): ועל כן ראוי שיטהר הגוף קודם וישלשלנו כפי כחו וישמרנו בעת שילשולו ואם נראה שיחלש לא ישלשלנו הרבה כי אם מעט ודיו בכך ואחר כן רפא הרפש בעטישות (Therefore, his body should first be cleansed and purged according to his strength, but one should be careful during the purgation. When we see that he is weakened we should not apply many [strong] purgations but only a few [mild ones]—which should be sufficient—and then [expel] the superfluities through ster-

241 'wine': Trans. after a.

242 שלם כ-: *itidem ut* L.

243 'the same as': Trans. after L.

244 On this medical encyclopaedia, cf. G. Bos and R. Fontaine, 'Medico-philosophical Controversies in Nathan b. Jo'el Falaquera's *Sefer Ṣori ha-Guf*,' *Jewish Quarterly Review* 90, nos. 1–2 (1999): 27–60.

nutatories). Hebr. *Sing.* עֲטִישָׁה features in the current dictionaries only in the sense of 'sneezing' (cf. JD 1063; BM 4423–4424; EM 1312). Moses ibn Tibbon translates Arab. سعوطات both as משיחת הנחירים and נחירות (cf. BCD 165, 173 (NM 4:108–109, 111)).

עיוות → עִוּוּת.

עיכוב → עִכּוּב.

עַיִן • אודם אשר באחת קצוות העין → אֹדֶם.

• **צמח בלובן העין** → צֶמַח.

• *Dual* **עֵינַיִם • דם העינים** → דָּם.

• **עיני ליציא** · **boxthorn** [*Lycium* sp. L.]: Lat. *oculi lucii* (read: *lucidi*) · Constantinus Africanus, *Viaticum* · trans. Do'eg ha-Edomi, *Sefer Ya'ir Netiv*, bk. 2, ch. 19: וכאשר נרצה לעזור אל העניינים האלה נחשב גוף החולה בעבור שנטהר שפעת הליחות ואחרי העזר המחזק והמטהר נשוב לתקן השנים כן: נכתוש גטלא אין נקובה עם עיני ליציא (When we want to treat these [symptoms], we should examine the body of the patient in order to purge it from the surplus of humors. Once we have applied a strengthening and a purging drug, we should treat the teeth with the following remedy: pulverized gallnut that has no holes in it with boxthorn buds ...). Hebr. עיני ליציא is a non-attested combination of Hebr. עינים and Lat. *lucidi*. The term is a non-attested loan translation/transcription of Lat. *oculus lucidus*, Plur. *oculi lucidi*, which is a synonym of 'boxthorn.'[245]

• **חלי העינים** → חֳלִי.

• **חשיכות העינים** → חֲשֵׁיכוּת.

• **מחשך העינים** → מַחְשָׁךְ.

• **פאתי העינים** → פֵּאָה

עַכְבָּר • בצל העכבר → בָּצָל.

• **הדפק הנק' זנב העכבר • זנב העכבר** → דֹּפֶק.

עִכּוּב • עיכוב ההרגשות · **indolence**: Arab. كسل · Ibn al-Jazzār, *Zād al-musāfir wa-qūt al-ḥāḍir* · trans. Abraham ben Isaac, *Sefer Ṣedah la-Oreḥim*, bk. 1, ch. 22: ואת אשר יוולד בראש המוח מן אילו הרפשים וזה החולי יקדים לו פחד וכובד בראש ועיכוב הרגשותיו וכאילו מראית עיניו מכוסים (The illness [i.e., epilepsy] that is caused in the brain by these superfluities is preceded by anxiety, heaviness in the head, indolence, and loss of vision). Hebr. עיכוב ההרגשות does not feature in the current dictionaries. Do'eg ha-Edomi translates the parallel Latin term *pigritia* as חולשת הראש (see entry חֲלִשָׁה). Moses ibn Tibbon possibly read Arab. كسل as كسر and translated it as שברון.

עָלָה • עלה בנפח · **to swell**: Lat. *tumesco* · Constantinus Africanus, *Viaticum* · trans. Do'eg ha-Edomi, *Sefer Ya'ir Netiv*, bk. 1, ch. 17: וכאשר לא יתבשל המאכל היטב בגוף או כולו או רובו יוליד קבוצים רעים הם ג׳ימוש ועל כן פניהם ועפעפיהם יחלו לעלות בנפח (And if the entire

---

245 Cf. *Alphita*, ed. García González, 235, 465. I thank Iolanda Ventura for this reference. According to DMLBS 2359, the term signifies the 'honeysuckle' (*Lonicera periclymenum* L. or *Lonicera caprifolium* L.).

food or most of it is not well digested in the body, it produces bad chymes i.e., [Lat.]. ǦYMWŠ, and consequently their face and eyelids start to swell). Hebr. עלה בנפח does not feature in the current dictionaries. For the different meanings of נֶפַח, cf. BCD 177 (NM 3:158; 4:114). The parallel Arabic text is فيحدث من ذلك ثقل الأجفان وتهيّج الوجه (… which causes heaviness of the eyelids and facial disturbance) and is translated by Moses ibn Tibbon as ויתחדש ממנו כבדות בעפעפים וצבות בפנים (This causes heaviness of the eyelids and swelling of the face).

• *Inf.* **עֲלוֹת** · **increase (of a disease in intensity, power, severity)**: Lat. *augmentum* (Arab. منتهى; i.e., 'climax') · Constantinus Africanus, *Viaticum* · trans. Do'eg ha-Edomi, *Sefer Ya'ir Netiv*, bk. 2, ch. 1: אחר טוב בעלות האופטלמיא להסיר הכאב (Another [collyrium] that is good for ophthalmia when its becomes more severe [and] for alleviating the pain). Hebr. עָלָה, *Inf.* עֲלוֹת, does not feature in this sense in the current dictionaries. Moses ibn Tibbon translates Arab. منتهى as תכלית.

• *Inf. Hif'il* **הַעֲלוֹת • כלי מיודע להעלות זיעתו** → **כְּלִי**.

• *Part. Hif'il* **מַעֲלֶה • הרפואה המעלה הבשר** → **רְפוּאָה**.

עֲלִיָּה · **increase (of a disease in intensity, power, severity)**: Arab. صعود · Ibn al-Jazzār, *Zād al-musāfir wa-qūt al-ḥādir* · trans. Moses ibn Tibbon, *Sefer Ṣedat ha-Derakhim*, bk. 3, ch. 12: ונאמר כי ראוי שנעיין תחלה מאיזו סבה התילדה המורסא במסך ואם הורה המופת אשר זכרנו כי החולי דמי נעיין אם יעזרנו כח החולה ושניו ומזגו ומזג הפרק מן השנה וטבע האויר ההוה והמנהג נוציא הדם מהגיד התחתון מצד החולי קודם שיקח החולי בעליה (I say that first one should look for the cause of the tumor in the diaphragm; if the symptoms that I mentioned indicate that the illness comes from the blood and if the strength, age, temperament of the patient, season, current weather, and habits are helpful [i.e., favorable], one should bleed the basilic vein from the side of the illness before the illness gets worse). In the sense of 'getting worse, increase (of a disease),' Hebrew עֲלִיָּה features in BCD 202 (NM 1:176) (for Arab. تزيّد) in a later attestation from Zeraḥyah Ḥen's translation of Maimonides, *Medical Aphorisms* 9.20 (BMMZ 100). Do'eg ha-Edomi translates the parallel Latin term *augmentor* (for Arab. أخذ في الصعود) as גדל.

עֶלְיוֹן • עליון הגרון · **larynx**: Arab. حنجرة · Ibn al-Jazzār, *Zād al-musāfir wa-qūt al-ḥādir* · trans. Moses ibn Tibbon, *Sefer Ṣedat ha-Derakhim*, bk. 3, ch. 1: ונשים מה שנרפאהו בו בתחלת הכאב מה שישכך החומר הנמשך אל עליון הגרון ויחזק האבר (In the beginning of the pain, we treat [the angina] with those medications that restrain the humors [lit., matter] that descend to the larynx and that strengthen it). Hebr. עליון הגרון is not attested for in the current dictionaries. Do'eg ha-Edomi translates the parallel Latin term *guttur* as שפוי הכובע (see entry שִׁפּוּי).

• **הגיד העליון** → **גִּיד**.

• **העומק אשר בעליון אחורי הצואר** → **עֹמֶק**.

עֲלִילָה • *Plur.* **עלילות** · **causes**: Arab. سبب · Ibn al-Jazzār, *Zād al-musāfir wa-qūt al-ḥādir*, trans. Abraham ben Isaac, *Sefer Ṣedah la Orḥim*, bk. 1, ch. 23: וזה ריקוח

הגלולות שלשיטרג הוא הריקוח שתיקנתיו וניסיתיו ויועיל לחולי הפלג ולחולי העיוות ולחולי הנקרא כוזאז ולחולי שעלילותיו מן הקור (Recipe of the 'pepperwort pill' according to my own modification—I have tested it. It is beneficial for hemiplegia, facial paresis, the illness called [in Arab.] *kuzāz* [i.e., spasms], and any disease caused by coldness ...). In the sense of 'cause,' Hebr. *Sing.* עֲלִילָה features in BM 4519; however, it is not attested for in medical literature. Moses ibn Tibbon translates Arab. سبب as סבה.

עָמַד • *Inf.* עֲמֹד · **stage when a disease has ceased to develop or is fully established:** Lat. *status* (cf. DMLBS 3538) · Constantinus Africanus, *Viaticum* · trans. Do'eg ha-Edomi, *Sefer Ya'ir Netiv*, bk. 1, ch. 18: וזה יאות לעיין בתחלת החולי או בעמדו (This should be observed when the illness begins or when it is fully established). Hebr. עֲמֹד is not attested for in this sense in the current dictionaries.

• *Part.* **עוֹמֵד • המקור העומד בין האצבע הקטון לחבירו** → מָקוֹר.

עִמּוּץ · **closure:** Arab. تغميض · Ibn al-Jazzār, *Zād al-musāfir wa-qūt al-ḥādir*, trans. Abraham ben Isaac, *Sefer Ṣedah la-Oreḥim*, bk. 1, ch. 16: שער ששה עשר יזכיר חולי הנקרא בלשון ישמעאל אלסבאת ובלש' יון ליתרגוס הוא שיכה[246] האדם ויישן בעמוץ עינים וסגירתם (Chapter 16: On the illness called in Arabic *al-subāt* [i.e., lethargy, torpor] and in Greek *lethargos* [i.e., lethargy]. It is an illness in which [the patient] is[247] inclined to sleep with the eyes closed). As a synonym of סגירה in the sense of 'closure,' Hebr. עִמּוּץ only features in EM 1338 as a modern term in an attestation from Abraham Shlonsky. Moses ibn Tibbon translates Arab. تغميض as סתימה.

[עמץ] • *Hif'il* הֶעֱמִיץ · **to close:** Arab. غمّض · Ibn al-Jazzār, *Zād al-musāfir wa-qūt al-ḥādir* · trans. Abraham ben Isaac, *Sefer Ṣedah la-Oreḥim*,[248] bk. 1, ch. 16: ולזה המין לא תהיה עימו שינה כלל אם יעמיץ עיניו כדי לישן יפתחם מהרה (In the case of this second type [of torpor] one does not sleep at all; if one closes one's eyes in order to sleep, one opens them quickly). In the sense of 'to close,' Hebr. עמץ is only attested for in the current dictionaries in the Qal or Pi'el conjugation; cf. BM 4568; EM 1341. Moses ibn Tibbon translates Arab. غمّض as סתם.

עֹמֶק • העומק אשר בעליון אחורי הצואר · **the nape of the neck (fovea nuchae; Ger. *Nackengrube*):**[249] Arab. نقرة · Ibn al-Jazzār, *Zād al-musāfir wa-qūt al-ḥādir* · trans. Moses ibn Tibbon, *Sefer Ṣedat ha-Derakhim*, bk. 1, ch. 10: ואם היה חלוש ולא תהיה בו קדחת נשים לו כוסות המציצה בחיצון כל אחד משוקיו גבוה טפח מן העקב או נשים כוסות המציצה בעומק אשר בעליון אחורי הצואר ויוציא מן הדם בשיעור הכח (If [the patient] is weak and is without

246 שיכה האדם ויישן (= שיטה האדם ויישן): هو الميل إلى النوم مع a.

247 'is inclined to sleep': Trans. after a.

248 In addition to הֶעֱמִיץ, Abraham ben Isaac uses the standard term סגר for Arab. غمّض as in bk. 1, ch. 18 (Ms Florence, Biblioteca Medicina Laurenziana, Plut. 88.37, fol. 93a): ואחר כן לֹא יוסיף עוד לסוגרם.

249 Cf. FL 4:321, s.v. نقرة: 'Scrobs in occipitis inferiore parte (ubi desinit pars protuberantior occipitis);' HA 188–190.

fever we put cupping glasses on every leg, one span above the ankle or on the nape of the neck and [we] extract as much blood as he can endure). Hebr. העומק אשר בעליון אחורי הצואר is not attested for in the current dictionaries. Synonyms used by Moses ibn Tibbon are עורף and העורף אחרי הצואר (see entry עֹרֶף).

עֵנָב · **uvula (when swollen)**: Arab. عنبة (UW 634: 'geschwollenes Zäpfchen'); Gr. σταφυλή (LSG 1635: 'uvula when swollen at the end so as to resemble a grape') · Ibn al-Jazzār, *Zād al-musāfir wa-qūt al-ḥādir* · trans. Moses ibn Tibbon, *Sefer Ṣedat ha-Derakhim*, bk. 3, ch. 3: וכאשר יכלה הדבר אשר יקראו לו הענב וחזר קצת האונקלי יותר גדול ויותר עב ויותר נוטה אל הכהות וחזר מה שהוא למעלה ממנו יותר דק בעת ההוא תסמוך לחתוך האונקלי (When eventually part of the organ that is called the uvula becomes larger and thicker and more livid and its point is thinner then it is safe to cut it). Hebr. עֵנָב does not feature in this sense in the current dictionaries. Do'eg ha-Edomi renders the parallel Latin term *uvula* as להאה (= Arab. *lahāt*).

• *Plur.* **ענבים** • **רב ענבים** → רֹב.

עִנְבִּי • **הענבית** · **grape-like tunic**: Lat. *uvea* (Arab. الطبقة العنبية) · Constantinus Africanus, *Viaticum* · trans. Do'eg ha-Edomi, *Sefer Ya'ir Netiv*, bk. 2, ch. 2: זה נעשה בעינים מהנגעים או מהאבעבועות הם פושטולש וזה אין להם עזר ונעשית מן הליחות המקובצות בין הענבית והכפירית זהו אוביאה קרישטא ליאנקא והוא דק יועיל לרפואתו ויספיק מיץ פאפאבר אדום (When this [i.e., white spot on the eye (*albugo*)] affects the eye, caused by tumors or pustules, i.e., [Lat.] *pustulas*, it cannot be healed. But when it is caused by the humors coagulated between the grape-like tunic and the crystalline tunic, [Lat.] 'WBY'H QRYŠṬ' LY'NQ', and when [these humors] are thin, the juice of red poppy is sufficient to cure it). In the sense of 'grape-like tunic,' Hebr. הענבית features in BCD 204 (NM 4:148) in a later attestation from Moses ibn Tibbon, *Sefer Ṣedat ha-Derakhim*.[250] According to Masie (MD 756, s.v. 'uvea'), the term הענבית can already be found in the *Sefer Asaph ha-Rofe*. Moses ibn Tibbon renders Arab. الطبقة العنبية as הענבית, just like Do'eg ha-Edomi.

עָנִי • *Plur.* **עניים** • **חבל העניים** → חֶבֶל.

עִנְיָן • *Plur.* **עינינים** · **kinds; types**: Arab. أصناف · Ibn al-Jazzār, *Zād al-musāfir wa-qūt al-ḥādir* · trans. Abraham ben Isaac, *Sefer Ṣedah la-Oreḥim*, bk. 1, ch. 24: החולי הזה נקרא כוזאז הוא ניענוע יקרה בלא רצון בגידים המתנענעים ברצון ויבוא מחמת מילואי האיברים שיש בהם גידים דקים או מן ריקנותם והוא על שלשה ענינים (The illness called [in Arab.] *kuzāz* [i.e., spasms] consists of involuntary motions of organs that are [normally] moved voluntarily. They occur either because of repletion of the organs that have nerves, or because they are empty. There are three types of [this illness]). Hebr. *Sing.* עִנְיָן, *Plur.* ענינים, does not feature in this sense in the current dictionaries, nor in the secondary literature (cf. BM 45981–45987; KTP 3:148–150; EM 1347; EP 95–96). Moses ibn Tib-

250 For a detailed discussion of the term הענבית, cf. KDS 90–92.

bon translates Arab. أصناف as מינים. Do'eg ha-Edomi translates Lat. *est autem triplex* as והוא בשלשה ענינים.

עִסָּה · **pulp**: Arab. دماغ · Ibn al-Jazzār, *Zād al-musāfir wa-qūt al-ḥādir* · trans. Moses ibn Tibbon, *Sefer Ṣedat ha-Derakhim*, bk. 3, ch. 6 (Ms London, British Library, Add. 27542, fol. 43[a]): ומי שירצה שיהיה פעולתו לחזה יותר גדולה ויותר חזקה יקח לב זרע קשואים הנקראים קתא ולב זרע קשואים הנקראים כיאר ולב זרע אבטיח ולב זרע קרא וזרע חבושים ודרגגן לבן וזרע פפאויר מ״א י׳ דר׳ יודק עד שישוב כעיסה (If you want that its effect on the chest is greater and stronger, you should take core of the seeds of [the kind of] cucumber called *qiththā* and [core of the kind of] cucumber called *khiyār* and the core of watermelon seeds and of pumpkin seeds and quince seed and white gum tragacanth and poppy seed, ten *dirhams* of each, [and] pound these until it turns into pulp). Hebr. עִסָּה features in BM 4605–4607, a.o. in attestations from Rashi's commentary on the Talmud in the sense of 'pith' of plants, and in one attestation from Elijah de Vidas, *Reshit Hokhmah* in the sense of 'kernel' of nuts. Ms Oxford, Bodleian Library, Poc. 353, Uri Heb. 314 (cat. Neubauer 2111), the main Ms used for the edition of Ibn Tibbon's *Sefer Ṣedat ha-Derakhim*, translates Arab. دماغ as מֹחַ (see entry).

עַפְעַף • *Plur.* **עפעפים** • **עפעפים הפוכות** · **inverted eyelashes (ectropion; ectropium)**: Lat. *palpebra inversa* · Guillaume de Congenis, *Treatise on Surgery* · trans. Isaiah, fol. 47[b]: לעפעפים ההפוכות או הגסות לפעמים לזקנים ביותר תעשה משיחה בזאת: קח אלואין סיטרין צירושא ב׳ דרכבמו׳ מ״א שומן[251] חזיר חדש בלי מלח אוקי׳ ירקח ביחד בכלי זך וחזק ואחר שחוק במדוכה וישאר לעת הצורך בכלי זכוכית (For eyelashes that are inverted or rough and that sometimes [affect] especially old people, one should prepare the following salve: Take two *dirhams* each of aloe, citron, ceruse, one ounce of the unsalted fat of a young pig, mix [these ingredients] in a strong clean vessel, pound [the mixture] in a mortar and [put it] in a glass and leave it there until you need it). Hebr. עפעפים הפוכות does not feature in the current dictionaries. Masie (MD 244, s.v. 'ectropium') refers to three different kinds of ectropion: הפיכת העפעף שמשתוק (e. *paralyticum*), הפיכת העפעף של הקנים (e. *senile*), and הפיכת העפעף שמעוית (e. *spasticum*).

עֵץ • **תותי העץ** → **תּוּת**.

עֵצָה • **לקח עצה** → **לָקַח**.

עִצּוּם · **substance**: Lat. *substantia* (Arab. جرم) · Constantinus Africanus, *Viaticum* · trans. Do'eg ha-Edomi, *Sefer Ya'ir Netiv*, bk. 1, ch. 25: ותרדמת האברים מחוברת בין התולדת והחולי והסבה היא קרירות שיקבוץ עצום הגידים ויקרר ויעצור שלא יוכל הכח המרגיש לנקוב שם (Numbness [occurs because of] a combination of nature and a disease. Its cause is coldness, which coagulates the substance of the nerves. It cools them down and blocks [them], so that the power of sensory perception cannot pass through them anymore). Moses ibn Tibbon translates Arab. جرم as גרם, Abraham ben Isaac as גוף.

---

251 שומן: Ms[1].

In the sense of 'substance,' Hebr. עִצּוּם features in the current dictionaries with attestations from Rabbinic and medieval philosophical literature only (cf. JD 1073–1074, s.v. עיצום: 'strengh; essence, self;' BM 5640; KTP 3:153).

• **בעצומו** • *Plur.* **בעצומן** • **(lit., in their substance); substantially; basically**: Lat. *substantialiter* (Arab. في جوهره) · Constantinus Africanus, *Viaticum* · trans. Do'eg ha-Edomi, *Sefer Ya'ir Netiv*, bk. 1, ch. 15: מאשר אמר גיאלינוס דעתנו הוא כי נכון לעזור אל החולי הזה בטהרת שתי הליחות המונחות זו כנגד זו בעצומן (For this reason, Galen maintained that the main purpose of the therapy of this disease has to be the cleansing of the brain of those two humors that are substantially opposed to each other). Moses ibn Tibbon translates Arab. في جوهرهما as בעצמיהם.

עָצוּר (*Part. Pass.*) → עָצַר.

עִצּוּר • **בעצור** • **(through) contraction**: Lat. *constringendum* (Arab. إذا انقبض) · Constantinus Africanus, *Viaticum* · trans. Do'eg ha-Edomi, *Sefer Ya'ir Netiv*, bk. 3, ch. 11: ועל כן היו לו שתי תנועות הפוכות אשר בהרחבה ימשוך האויר ובעצור יגרש החום (For this reason, [the heart] has two opposite movements, through its expansion [i.e., diastole] it attracts the air, and through its contraction [i.e., systole] it expels the heat). Hebrew עִצּוּר features in BCD 207 in the sense of 'constipation' (cf. NM 2:179), 'cramps' (cf. NM 1:64), and 'pressure' (cf. NM 1:64). The term features in the sense of 'extract' in Moses ibn Tibbon's Hebrew translation of Maimonides, *On Hemorrhoids* 5.4 (BMH 42) in the combined term עצור העופרת ('lead extract') for Arab. عصارة الرصاص. Moses ibn Tibbon (*Sefer Ṣedat ha-Derakhim*) translates Arab. إذا انقبض as כשיתקבץ.

עַצְלוּת • **inability**: Arab. عجز · Ibn al-Jazzār, *Zād al-musāfir wa-qūt al-ḥādir*, trans. Abraham ben Isaac, *Sefer Ṣedah la-Oreḥim*, cf. bk. 1, ch. 16: ודע כשעניין השיני שתהיה שנתו קלה שאמרנו לא שינה ממש אך היא עצלות מלהקיץ (Know that the second [kind of torpor], i.e., the one in which—as we said—one's sleep is light, is not a real sleep but an inability to wake up). Hebr. עַצְלוּת does not feature in this sense in the current dictionaries. Moses ibn Tibbon translates Arab. عجز as חולשה ועצלה.

עֶצֶם • *Plur.* **עצמות** • **kernels; stones (of fruits)**: Lat. *ossa* (Arab. نوى) · Constantinus Africanus, *Viaticum* · trans. Do'eg ha-Edomi, *Sefer Ya'ir Netiv*, bk. 1, ch. 2 (fol. 9ᵇ): ועוד תקח לאדנום אישנץ[252] עצמות תמרים ותשרפם לאבק ותכרוך הכל בבגד רחב ותשים לשרות בשמן ז' ימים ותתמיד למשוח בו (Another remedy: Take labdanum, absinth wormwood, date palm kernels, burn them into a powder, bind everything in a wide cloth, macerate it in oil for seven days, and rub it regularly [on the affected spot]). In the sense of 'kernels, stones,' Hebr. עצמות is a semantic borrowing from Lat. *os*, Plur. *ossa* (cf. DMLBS 2417). Moses ibn Tibbon renders Arab. نوى as גרעינים. Ben-Yehuda (BM 4652) cites the term in the sense of 'substance (of a radish)' in a quotation from Shem Tov Falaquera, *Sefer ha-Mevakkesh*.

---

252 אישנץ: *absinthium* L.

עָצַר • *Part.* **עוֹצֵר** · **astringent; stiptic:** Lat. *stipticus* (Arab. قابض) · Constantinus Africanus, *Viaticum* · trans. Do'eg ha-Edomi, *Sefer Ya'ir Netiv*, bk. 2, ch. 20: ואם החולה מלא מאלה הליחות יאות לטהרו ואחרי כן לשוב לעזור אל השינים בדברים עוצרים ומיבשים (If the patient [suffering from toothache] is full with these [putrid] humors, he should be purged, and then his teeth should be treated with astringent, drying remedies). In the sense of 'astringent,' Hebr. עוֹצֵר features in BCD 211 (NM 3:181–182) in later attestations, a.o. from Hillel ben Samuel's translation of Hippocrates' *Aphorisms* 7.37. Moses ibn Tibbon translates Arab. قابض as קובץ.

• *Part. Pass.* **עָצוּר** · **suffering from constipation:** Lat. *patior constipationem* · Constantinus Africanus, *Viaticum* · trans. Do'eg ha-Edomi, *Sefer Ya'ir Netiv*, bk. 3, ch. 7: ואם הוא עצור תשיבנו במזג לחות עם אישרוף ותשומת כלי מלחלח (If the patient suffers from constipation, one should change his constitution into a moist one with a moistening syrup or clyster). In the sense of 'suffering from constipation,' Hebr. עָצוּר features in BM 4641, a.o. in an attestation from Rashbam (Samuel Ben Meir) (c. 1085–c. 1158). Moses ibn Tibbon translates the parallel Arabic term for Lat. *patior constipationem*, i.e., حصر في الطبيعة, as עוצר הטבע (see entry עֹצֶר).

עֹצֶר • **עוצר הטבע** · **constipation:** Arab. حصر في الطبيعة · Ibn al-Jazzār, *Zād al-musāfir wa-qūt al-ḥādir* · trans. Moses ibn Tibbon, *Sefer Ṣedat ha-Derakhim*, bk. 3, ch. 7: ואם יקרה לחולה עוצר הטבע ראוי שישולשל טבעו לא בדברים חזקים אבל בכמו המשקים והקלוחים הרכים (If the patient suffers from constipation, one should not give him a strong purgative [but a mild one], such as a mild potion or clyster). Hebr. עוצר הטבע does not feature in the current dictionaries. The Arabic synonym حبس البطن is translated by Shem Tov ben Isaac as עצור המעים in the *Sefer ha-Shimmush*, bk. 27 (cf. BCD 207 (NM 4:152)). Do'eg ha-Edomi translates the parallel Latin term *patior constipationem* as עצור (see entry עָצַר).

עָקֵב • **העורק אשר אצל העקב** → עוֹרֵק.

עִקּוּם • **עקום בפנים** · **twisting of the face:** Arab. اعوجاج في الوجه · Ibn al-Jazzār, *Zād al-musāfir wa-qūt al-ḥādir* · trans. Moses ibn Tibbon, *Sefer Ṣedat ha-Derakhim*, bk. 1, ch. 23: ואם יהיה בפנים עקום ורפיון עם שאר הגוף או בקצת האיברים נדע אז כי שרש החולי מפני שרש החוש והתנועה ר״ל המוח (If twisting or looseness occurs in the face—just like in the rest of the body, respectively, one of its organs—, we know that the root of the disease hails from the origin of sensory perception and motion, i.e., the brain). Hebr. עקום בפנים does not feature in the current dictionaries. The term עִקּוּם features in Rabbinic literature in the sense of 'curve;' cf. JD 1074; BM 4672. For the identification of the root עקם as اعوجاج, see SMK 432, s.v. עקם. Abraham ben Isaac translates the Arabic term as עיוות בפנים (cf. BCD 198 (NM 4:142–143)); Do'eg ha-Edomi translates the parallel Latin term *faciei tortura* as עקימת הפנים (see entry עֲקִימָה).

עֲקִימָה • **עקימת הפנים** · **twisting of the face:** Lat. *faciei tortura* (Arab. اعوجاج في الوجه) · Constantinus Africanus, *Viaticum* · trans. Do'eg ha-Edomi, *Sefer Ya'ir Netiv*, bk. 1, ch. 23: אם עקימת הפנים או הרכות יהיה בכל הגוף או בחלק אחד הכרח הוא להבין שהמוח

סתום (If twisting or looseness [occurs] in the face, or the whole body, or one [of the organs], one should necessarily conclude that the brain is affected by an obstruction). Hebr. עֲקִימָה is not attested for in medieval medical literature. The term features in Rabbinic literature in the sense of 'curvature, crookedness;' cf. JD 1106; BM 4674 (also with an attestation from Rashi: עקימת השפתים). Moses ibn Tibbon translates Arab. اعوجاج في الوجه as עקום בפנים (see entry עִקּוּם) and Abraham ben Isaac as עיוות בפנים (cf. BCD 198 (NM 4:142–143)).

עֲקִיצָה · **fracture**: Lat. *ruptura* · Constantinus Africanus, *Viaticum* · trans. Do'eg ha-Edomi, *Sefer Ya'ir Netiv*, bk. 2, ch. 18 (Ms Oxford, Bodleian Library, Can. Or. 26, fol. 268[a]): והחולי משתנה והחלק השנוי נגלה[253] בתולדתו כמו הדברים הבלוים והבואשה והעקיצה והנקיבה והתנועה ושאר דברים דומים לאלה (There are different clearly visible [symptoms in the case of toothache] such as putrefaction, bad smell, fractures, cavities, movement, and other similar things). Hebr. עֲקִיצָה only features in the current dictionaries in the sense of 'sting, cutting fruit by the stalk' (JD 1106) or 'biting or stinging (by an animal or insect)' (BM 4674). Shem Tov ben Isaac also uses the term in the sense of 'burning, biting [pain]' in the *Sefer ha-Shimmush*, bk. 27 (cf. BCD 212 (NM 4:151)).

עֶרֶב • **בשתי וערב** → שְׁתִי.

עִרְבֵּב • **ערבב ונענע** · **to stir**: Arab. ضرب · Ibn al-Jazzār, *Zād al-musāfir wa-qūt al-ḥādir*, trans. Abraham ben Isaac, *Sefer Ṣedah la-Oreḥim*, bk. 1, ch. 17 (Ms Florence, Biblioteca Medicina Laurenziana, Plut. 88.37, fol. 93[b]):[254] ושים עמהן שמן זנבק ויניחהו בשמן י׳ ימים ויבללהו וינענעהו בכל יום בכלי זכוכית ואחר כן תצלילהו וקח מן אופיאו כפי הצורך וכותשנו ושימנו באותו שמן ועוד יערבבהו וינענעהו עשרה ימים ואחר כן תחזיר הכל אל השמרים ויוסיף על הכל עוד אופייו וינענעהו בכל יום (Add saffron oil to [the mentioned ingredients], leave it in the oil for ten days, stir it every day in a glass flacon and purify it. Take opium as much as you need, pound it and add it to the oil. Stir it for [another] ten days, then return everything to the lees [from which it was purified before], and add again opium. Stir this every day …). Hebr. ערבב ונענע is not attested for in the current dictionaries. Moses ibn Tibbon translates Arab. ضرب as הכה.

עֵרוּב · **composition**: Arab. أخلاط · Ibn al-Jazzār, *Zād al-musāfir wa-qūt al-ḥādir* · trans. Moses ibn Tibbon, *Sefer Ṣedat ha-Derakhim*, bk. 3, ch. 5: ומזה תואר רפואה חברה בן מאסויה לנחור הקול אשר יקרה בגרון ושפלות הקול והפסק הקול ערובו (Recipe of a remedy composed by Ibn Māsawayh for roughness of the voice, hoarseness, and loss of voice occurring in the throat, its composition …). Hebr. עֵרוּב is not attested for in medieval medical literature in the current dictionaries. It features in Rabbinic literature in the sense of 'interweaving, mixture, conjunction,' and 'erub' in Rabbinical literature (cf. JD 1075–1076).

---

253 נגלה בתולדתו: *palam est visui* L.

254 Ms Jerusalem, National Library of Israel, Fr. 95, fol. 96[b], has a variant reading בלבל ונענע. See also entry בָּלַל: בלל ונענע.

עֶרְוָה • גיד הערוה → גִּיד.

עֵרוּת · **insomnia**: Arab. سهر · Ibn al-Jazzār, *Zād al-musāfir wa-qūt al-ḥādir*, trans. Abraham ben Isaac, *Sefer Ṣedah la-Oreḥim*, bk. 1, ch. 17: ואם הערות מיובש מרה שחורה אז נריק לו על ראשו מים מרותחין עם כמומילון ואכליל אל מלך הוא עשב סוריצילה וקליפת כשכאש ואניטו וזרע מלווא ודומ׳ ויגלח ראשו וימשחנו מחלב נשים או חלב אתון או חלב צאן וישים באפיו חלב אשה (If insomnia originates from dryness of the black bile, we pour water on [the head of the patient], in which camomile, melilot, i.e., the plant SWRYṢYLH, poppy calyces, dill, common marshmallow seeds, and the like have been cooked. After the head has been shaved, one should rub on it women's milk, milk of a she-ass, or milk of a goat. One should apply a sternutatory of women's milk). Hebr. עֵרוּת only features in the sense of 'vigilance' in BM 4720 in an attestation from Shabbetai Donnolo, *Sefer Ḥakmoni*. Do'eg ha-Edomi translates the parallel Latin term *uigilie* as תעורה. Moses ibn Tibbon uses the same term for Arab. سهر.

[ערם] • *Hifʿil* הֶעֱרִים · **to employ artful means; to use one's skill; to contrive; to make an effort**: Arab. احتال · Ibn al-Jazzār, *Zād al-musāfir wa-qūt al-ḥādir* · trans. Moses ibn Tibbon, *Sefer Ṣedat ha-Derakhim*, bk. 3, ch. 2: הנה ראוי לנו כשראינו מופתי הבשול במורסא המתהוה תוך הגרון וידענו כי כבר קבצה המוגלא שנערים אז ונדקדק לפתחה ולא נעשה לה רפואות חזקות אבל נכון בו בקלות כמו שיגרגר בחלב עז חלוב (Once we see signs that the tumor in the throat has concocted [i.e., ripened] and know that the pus has accumulated, we should use our skill and expertise to open it. However, we should not apply strong medications but light ones, such as a gargle of fresh goat's milk). Hebr. הֶעֱרִים is not attested for in medieval medical literature.

עֹרֶף · **the nape of the neck (fovea nuchae; Ger. *Nackengrube*)**: Arab. نقرة (cf. HA 188–190, FL 4:321, s.v. نُقْرَة: 'Scrobs in occipitis inferiore parte (ubi desinit pars protuberantior occipitis')) · Ibn al-Jazzār, *Zād al-musāfir wa-qūt al-ḥādir* · trans. Moses ibn Tibbon, *Sefer Ṣedat ha-Derakhim* bk. 2, ch. 22 (fol. 65b): ואם ימנע מן ההקזה מונע כמו חולשת הכח ומה שדומה לזה נצוהו לשים כלי המציצה בעורף (If it is impossible to bleed [the patient] because his strength is weak or for similar reasons, we order him to put a cupping glass on the nape of his neck). Hebr. עֹרֶף features in the current dictionaries in the sense of 'neck, back of neck' (cf. JD 1059; BM 4741–4742). Lowinger (Low LXVIII) mentions it as featuring in Rabbinic literature in the sense of 'neck, nape, nucha.' In addition to עֹרֶף, Moses ibn Tibbon renders Arab. نقرة as העורף אחרי הצואר (see next entry) and as העומק אשר בעליון אחורי הצואר (see entry עֹמֶק). Do'eg ha-Edomi translates the parallel Latin term *collum* as צואר.

• **העורף אחרי הצואר** · **the nape of the neck (fovea nuchae; Ger. *Nackengrube*)**: Arab. نقرة · Ibn al-Jazzār, *Zād al-musāfir wa-qūt al-ḥādir* · trans. Moses ibn Tibbon, *Sefer Ṣedat ha-Derakhim* bk. 2, ch. 20: ואם היה הלחות ההוא חד נצוה להקיז הגיד העליון או לשים כלי המציצה בעורף אחרי הצואר (If that moisture is sharp we order to bleed the cephalic vein or to put a cupping glass on the nape of the neck). Hebr. העורף אחרי הצואר is not attested for in the current dictionaries. In addition to העורף אחרי הצואר, Moses ibn Tibbon renders Arab. نقرة as העומק אשר בעליון אחורי הצואר (see entry עֹמֶק) and as עֹרֶף (see previous entry). Do'eg ha-Edomi translates the parallel Latin term *cervix* as צואר.

עֵשֶׂב • עשב יוחנן · bearded or perforate St. John's wort [*Hypericum barbatum* Jacq. or *Hypericum perforatum* L.] · *Shinnui ha-Shemot ha-Niqra'im Synonimi*, Ms Florence, Bibliotheca Laurenziana, Or. 17, fol. 69[a]: אפירקון הוא אנפודלי ס״א או היופאריקון הנק׳ עשב יוחנן ('PYRQWN [read 'WP'RYQWN; i.e., Arab. *ūfārīqūn*]; i.e. 'NPWDLY(?); another version: HYWP'RYQWN [i.e., Arab. *hayūfārīqūn*], which is called [in Hebr.] *'esev yoḥanan*). In the sense of bearded or perforate St. John's wort, Hebr. עשב יוחנן is a non-attested loan translation of Ital. *erba san giovanni* (cf. LF 4:407).[255] See also *Shemot ha-Asavim*, Ms Leiden, Universiteitsbibliotheek, Or. 4732/1 (SCAL 15), fol. 2[a] (entry 48): איפיריקון ב״א יהנש קרוט חם ב״ב ('YPYRYQWN [i.e., Lat. *hypericum*]; Ger. YHNŠ QRWṬ [i.e., *iohanis krut* = 'Johanniskraut']; hot in the second degree).[256]

• עשב השוטה · common purslane [*Portulaca oleracea* L.]: Arab. بقلة حمقا (cf. DT 2:106 (270–271)) · [*Synonima*], Ms Vatican, Biblioteca Apostolica, ebr. 550, fol. 126[a] (127[a]): פרפך הוא עשב השוטה בערב בקלה חמקא ונקר׳ בורטוליגא ([Arab.] *farfaḥ* (cf. DT 2:106 (271, n. 5)); i.e., [Hebr.] *'esev ha-shoṭeh*; Arab. *baqla ḥamqā*; called BWRṬWLYG' [O.Occ. *bortolaiga* (cf. SHS 1:218 (Ḥet 16))]). In the sense of 'common purslane,' Hebr. עשב השוטה is a non-attested calque from Arab. *baqla ḥamqā*.

עָשָׂה • עשה גרשׂא · to apply scarification: Lat. *scarifico* (Arab. حجامة ('cupping')) · Constantinus Africanus, *Viaticum* · trans. Do'eg ha-Edomi, *Sefer Ya'ir Netiv*, bk. 2, ch. 22: ואם הוא מנפח חם יאות לעשות לו גרשא (If it [i.e., the softness (weakness) of the gums] is caused by a hot tumor, one should apply scarification). Aram. גרשׂא is not attested for in the current dictionaries. Moses ibn Tibbon translates Arab. حجامة as לעשות ונטושא (cf. וינטוסי for Lat. *ventose* ('cupping glasses') in Hillel ben Samuel's *Sefer Keritut* (BCD 79 (NM 1:43))). See also entry עשה וינטושא below.

• עשה גרשׂה · to apply scarification: Lat. *scarifico* · Constantinus Africanus, *Viaticum* · trans. Do'eg ha-Edomi, *Sefer Ya'ir Netiv*, bk. 2, ch. 22 (Ms Oxford, Bodleian Library, Can. Or. 26, fol. 272[b]): לעזור לרכות יאות לחסר דם הספליקא אם אין דבר אחר מונע ואם ימנע אותנו דבר נעשה לו גרשה בצואר (To treat the softness [i.e., weakness (of the gums)], one should bleed from the cephalic vein, if there is no hindrance, but if there is a hindrance one should apply scarification on the neck [of the patient]). Hebr. גרשׂה is not attested for in the current dictionaries. The term has possibly been coined from the verb גרשׂ 'to bray, pound, grind coarse' (BDB 176).

• עשה וינטושא · to apply cupping glasses: Arab. احتجم · Ibn al-Jazzār, *Zād al-musāfir wa-qūt al-ḥādir* · trans. Moses ibn Tibbon, *Sefer Ṣedat ha-Derakhim*, bk. 3, ch. 6: ואם

---

255 Cf. O. Penzig, *Flora Popolare Italiana* (Genova 1924), 1:237.

256 Cf. G. Bos and Kl.-D. Fischer (eds.), *A Glimpse into Medical Practice among Jews around 1500: Latin-German Pharmaceutical Glossaries in Hebrew Characters Extant in Ms Leiden, Universiteitsbibliotheek, Cod. Or. 4732/1* (SCAL 15), *fols. 1a–17b* (Leiden 2021), 11, 67.

ימנע מן ההקזה מונע או ענין זולתו נמצא מחולשת הכח או זולת זה נצוהו שיעשה וינטושא אלכהאל ואלכרעין (If bleeding is impossible because of weak [bodily] strength or for another reason, we order to put cupping glasses on the sacrum or legs of the patient). Hebr. וינטושא is a non-attested loan word from O.Occ. *ventosa/ventoza* or O.Cat. *ventosa*, 'cupping glass' (FEW 14:254a; DCVB 10:717b–718a). Constantine the African translates Arab. احتجم as *scarifico* ('to scarify'); the latter term is translated by Do'eg ha-Edomi as עשה גרשׂא (cf. entry above).

• **עשה קיא** · **to foment**: Lat. *facio fomentationem* · Guillaume de Congenis, *Treatise on Surgery* · trans. Isaiah, fol. 46b: לנתק: קח ליטרגיר שרוף וסיד חי מ״א ב׳ דרכמו׳ דע והבן שבתחלה יעשה קיא מן דקונקציאון האיישינץ (Against scurfy or scabby disease of the scalp: Take two *dirhams* each of burnt litharge and quicklime, but know and understand that first one has to foment [the head] with a decoction of absinth wormwood ...). Hebr. עשה קיא does not feature in this sense in the current dictionaries.

• *Part. Pass.* **עָשׂוּי • ההנחות העשויות למטה** → הֲנָחָה.

עָשׂוּי (*Part. Pass.*) → עָשָׂה.

עָשָׁן · **vapor**: Lat. *fumus* (Arab. بخارات) · Constantinus Africanus, *Viaticum* · trans. Do'eg ha-Edomi, *Sefer Ya'ir Netiv*, bk. 1, ch. 21: העיטוש נולד מליחות משתנות כי לפעמים התולדת פועל בחזקתו לדחות הליחות המקובצות או עשן המוח אותם שהם סבת חולי או סבת ההשחתה העתידה לבא (Sneezing may originate from various fluids, for sometimes nature becomes active to repel with all its force the humors or vapors that are aggregated in the brain and that are the cause of the [current] illness or of the bodily defects that will occur later on). In the sense of 'vapor,' Hebr. עָשָׁן features in BM 4753–4754 in later attestations from medical literature, a.o. from Joseph ben Meir ibn Zabara, *Sefer Sha'ashu'im*. Moses ibn Tibbon translates Arab. بخارات as אידים and Abraham ben Isaac as עשנים.

עֲשָׁנִיּוּת · **gaseous [substance]**: Arab. دخانية · Maimonides, *Medical Aphorisms* 10.67 · trans. Nathan ha-Me'ati (BMMN 133): הקבסא שמשתנה בה המאכל אל חמיצות לא יתחדש ממנה קדחת. ואמנם אפשר שתתחדש קדחת מן הקבסא שמשתנה בה המאכל אל העשניות (No fever develops from an indigestion in which the food turns sour. But fever can occur from an indigestion in which the food turns into a gaseous substance). Hebr. עֲשָׁנִיּוּת features in BM 4756 in an attestation from the *Sefer ha-Qanun*. Zeraḥyah Ḥen translates Arab. دخانية as אדיית (see entry אֲדִיּוּת).

עֶשֶׂר • עשרה מאמרות · **'Ten Treatises'**: Arab. العشر المقالات[257] · Ibn al-Jazzār, *Zād al-musāfir wa-qūt al-ḥādir* · trans. Moses ibn Tibbon, *Sefer Ṣedat ha-Derakhim*, bk. 1, ch. 10: תאר גירא פיגרא לגאלינוס והיא כתובה בספר העשרה מאמרות תנקה האצטומכא והראש והגוף ממותרות האדומה והליחה הלבנה (Recipe of the hiera picra by Galen from the 'Ten

257 With the term العشر المقالات, Ibn al-Jazzār apparently meant the ten books of Galen's *De compositione medicamentorum secundum locos*, normally referred to by Arabic authors as *K. al-Mayāmir*.

Treatises,' which cleanses the stomach, the head, and the body from yellow bile and phlegm). The Hebrew title עשרה מאמרות, a loan translation of Arab. العشر المقالات, is not attested for in the dictionaries or secondary literature. Abraham ben Isaac translates Arab. العشر المقالات as עשרה מאמרות as well. Do'eg ha-Edomi translates Constantine the African's parallel Latin term *decalogus* as עשרת הפקודים (see next entry).

• **עשרת הפקודים** · **'Ten Treatises'**: Lat. *decalogus* (Arab. العشر المقالات)[258] · Constantinus Africanus, *Viaticum* · trans. Do'eg ha-Edomi, *Sefer Ya'ir Netiv*, bk. 1, ch. 10: גירא מגילי הכתובה בספר עשרת הפקודים לטהר האסטומכא והראש וכל הגוף מן האדומה והלבנה (A hiera by Galen from the 'Ten Treatises,' which cleanses the stomach, the head, and the whole body from yellow bile and phlegm). The Hebrew title עשרת הפקודים, a loan translation of Lat. *decalogus*, is not attested for in the dictionaries or secondary literature. Moses ibn Tibbon and Abraham ben Isaac both translate Arab. العشر المقالات as עשרה מאמרות (see previous entry).

עֵת · **age**: Lat. *etas* (Arab. سنّ) · Constantinus Africanus, *Viaticum* · trans. Do'eg ha-Edomi, *Sefer Ya'ir Netiv*, bk. 1, ch. 22 (Ms Oxford, Bodleian Library, Can. Or. 26, fol. 246[a]): ואם יחל מיום הולדו הנה הוא מגדול רע או מסבה אחרת רעה וזרה ונעזור לו כפי אשר יסבול כחו ועתו (If [epilepsy] develops from the moment of a child's birth, it is caused by a bad regimen or by something else that is bad and external and we treat him according to his strength and age). Hebr. עֵת does not feature in this sense in the current dictionaries. Moses ibn Tibbon translates Arab. سنّ as שנות.

---

258 See previous note.

פ

פֵּאָה • *Plur.* **פאתים** • **פאתי העינים** · **canthi of the eyes**: Lat. *anguli oculorum* (Arab. مأقان) · Constantinus Africanus, *Viaticum* · trans. Do'eg ha-Edomi, *Sefer Ya'ir Netiv*, bk. 2, ch. 6: ויקרה לפעמים מהליחה הגסה המתקבצת בין הספירית והענבית ועל הענין הזה יאות לחתוך המקור הספליקא ולחסר מהדם כפי כחו וראוי לתת לו הגירש הגדולות לטהר המוח ולהקיז דם המקורות אשר בפאתי העינים ולהניח העלוקות ברקות (If the disease [i.e., dimsightedness] is caused by a coarse fluid that aggregates between the lens and the uvea, one should cut the cephalic vein and extract blood according to his strength. He should be administered one of the great hieras that cleanse the brain. Blood should be extracted from the veins in the canthi of the eyes and leeches should be placed on the temples). Hebr. *Sing.* פאת העין, *Plur.* פאתי העינים, does not feature in the current dictionaries. Moses ibn Tibbon translates Arab. مأقان as קצה העין. The latter term also features as *Plur.* קצוות העין in Nathan ha-Me'ati's *Sefer ha-Qanun* (cf. BCD 248 (NM 4:188)).

פַּגּוּת · **the state of not being ripe or cooked**: Arab. فجاجة (Lane 2340; D 2:242) · Shem Tov ben Isaac, *Sefer ha-Shimmush*, bk. 29, list 1 (SHS 1:418 (Pe 30)): פגות ב"ה פג'אג'ה (*pagut*; Arab. *fajāja*). Hebrew פַּגּוּת only features in BM 4811 in the sense of 'congelation.'

פֶּה • **נענע בפיו** → **נִעְנַע**.
• **נשימת האויר על הנחירים והפה** → **נְשִׁימָה**.
• **עוות הפה** → **עִוּוּת**

פּוּךְ · **collyrium**: Lat. *collyrium* (Arab. شياف) · Constantinus Africanus, *Viaticum* · trans. Do'eg ha-Edomi, *Sefer Ya'ir Netiv*, bk. 2, ch. 1 (fol. 27ᵃ): ונשים הפוך הלבן בעינים הוא קוללירי (And we apply a white collyrium, i.e., QWLLYRY,[259] to the eyes). Hebr. פּוּךְ features in the current dictionaries in the sense of 'antimony, stibium, eye dye, eye-paint' (BDB 806; JD 1141; BM 4847). Ben-Yehuda (ibid.) brings an attestation from medieval medical literature but without further explanation. Moses ibn Tibbon translates Arab. شياف as עגול (cf. BCD 196 (NM 1:63)).

פּוֹל • *Plur.* **פולים** · **pills**: Arab. حبّ · Ibn al-Jazzār, *Zād al-musāfir wa-qūt al-ḥāḍir* · trans. Abraham ben Isaac, *Sefer Ṣedah la-Oreḥim*, bk. 1, ch. 4 (Ms Jerusalem, National Library of Israel, Fr. 95, fol. 85ᵇ): פולים של משטיכי (mastic pills). In the sense of 'pills,' Hebr. פולים features in BM 4849 in an attestation from *Sefer Refu'ot*, Ms Florence. Moses ibn Tibbon translates Arab. حبّ as גרגרים.

פִּיל • **ביצי הפיל** → **בֵּיצָה**.

פיסי · **1. natural condition**: Arab. الحالة الطبيعية (Gr. dat. φύσει, nom. φύσις) · Ibn al-Jazzār, *Zād al-musāfir wa-qūt al-ḥāḍir* · trans. Abraham ben Isaac, *Sefer Ṣedah la-Oreḥim*,

259 'QWLLYRY': Cf. the Rabbinic term קילור, קילורית, from Gr. κολλύριον, Lat. *collyrium* (cf. HM 203–204).

bk. 1, ch. 18: וכאשר יתגדל החולי ויגיע לתוקפו יקרה לחולה מקראות רעות כגון צמא גדולה ויובש הפה ועובי הלשון ושחרותו ... ושינוי מראות פניו מפיסי שלו (When the illness increases and becomes more severe, the patient suffers from bad symptoms such as severe thirst, dryness of the mouth, thickness and blackness of the tongue ... His face loses its natural color). Hebr. פיסי is a non-attested loan word from Gr. dat. φύσει, pronounced as φίσι by medieval speakers,[260] from nom. φύσις, 'nature.' Moses ibn Tibbon translates Arab. الحالة الطبيعية as הענין הטבעי.

‣ II. **nature:** Arab. طبيعة · Ibn al-Jazzār, *Zād al-musāfir wa-qūt al-ḥāḍir* · trans. Abraham ben Isaac, *Sefer Ṣedah la-Oreḥim*, bk. 1, ch. 21 (Ms Jerusalem, National Library of Israel, Fr. 95, fol. 100[b]): העיטוש יבוא מחמת כמה עניינים פעמים שיבוא תדיר מחמת הפיסי שלגופות בעלי חיים כאשר תתנענע להוציא ולדחות רפשי הגוף או עשנים המתקבצים במוח (Sneezing may occur for various reasons. Sometimes its constant occurrence is caused by the nature of the body of a living being. It becomes agitated and [tries to] repel bodily humors or vapors aggregated in the brain). Moses ibn Tibbon translates Arab. طبيعة as טבע. Do'eg ha-Edomi translates the parallel Latin term *natura* as תּוֹלֶדֶת/תּוֹלָדָה (see entry).

פישוט → פְּשׁוּט.

[פלג] • *Part. Pass.* **מְפְלוּג** ‣ **suffering from hemiplegia:** Arab. مفلوج · Ibn al-Jazzār, *Zād al-musāfir wa-qūt al-ḥāḍir* · trans. Abraham ben Isaac, *Sefer Ṣedah la-Oreḥim*, bk. 1, ch. 23: ואם הסתימה באחד צד מחוט השדרה או ימין או שמאל אז יהיה למטה מן הצואר מן הצד הנלקה הסתום מפלוג (If the obstruction occurs in one of the two sides of the spinal cord—either the left or the right side—, he will suffer from hemiplegia in that which lies beneath the neck on the affected, obstructed side). In the sense of 'suffering from hemiplegia,' Hebr. מְפְלוּג is a non-attested semantic borrowing from Arab. مفلوج. Moses ibn Tibbon translates Arab. كان ما دون العنق من ذلك الشقّ المنسدّ مفلوجًا as יהיה הפלג במה שלמטה מן הצואר מן הפלח ההוא האטום.

• *Part. Nif'al* **נִפְלָג** ‣ **suffering from hemiplegia:** Arab. مفلوج · Ibn al-Jazzār, *Zād al-musāfir wa-qūt al-ḥāḍir* · trans. Abraham ben Isaac, *Sefer Ṣedah la-Oreḥim*, bk. 1, ch. 23: ויבשלום באש רפה קלה עד שיאכל המים וישאר השמן ויורידוהו וישימוהו בזכוכית נקיה וימשח בו הנפלגים (Boil [these ingredients] on a low fire, until the water evaporates and only the oil remains. Remove it [from the fire] and put it in a clean flask and anoint persons suffering from hemiplegia). Hebr. נִפְלָג does not feature in this sense in the current dictionaries. Moses ibn Tibbon translates Arab. المفلوج as מי שבו הפלג.

• *Part. Hif'il* **מַפְלִיג** • **הדברים המפליגים** → דָּבָר.

פלגמון ‣ **swelling; tumor:** Arab. ورم · Ibn al-Jazzār, *Zād al-musāfir wa-qūt al-ḥāḍir* · trans. Abraham ben Isaac, *Sefer Ṣedah la-Oreḥim*, bk. 1, ch. 10 (Ms Jerusalem, National Library of Israel, Fr. 95, fol. 89[b]): ויש שיכאב מחמת פלגמון שיהיה בראש ונקר'

260 I thank Petros Boutros Gallianatos for this explanation.

בלשון ישמעאל אוראם (The head may also hurt because of a tumor in it that is called in Arab. [*waram*, Plur.] *awrām*). Hebr. פלגמון is possibly a non-attested loan word from Lat. *phlegmon* (cf. DMLBS 2622: 'extavasation of blood, inflammation, abscess, or similar resulting from extavasation') or from Gr. φλεγμονή (in this case פלגמון should be read as פלגמוני (see next entry)). The same term פלגמון features in the anonymous adaptation in Ms Berlin, Staatsbibliothek Preußischer Kulturbesitz, Or. fol. 1058, as פלגמון הוא צבות (see entry צְבוּת). Moses ibn Tibbon translates Arab. ورم as מורסא.

פלגמוני · **swelling; tumor**: Arab. ورم (Gr. φλεγμονή) · Ibn al-Jazzār, *Zād al-musāfir wa-qūt al-ḥādir* · trans. Abraham ben Isaac, *Sefer Ṣedah la-Oreḥim*, bk. 1, ch. 10 (Ms Jerusalem, National Library of Israel, Fr. 95, fol. 90[b]): ועשה תחבושת על הפלגמוני (And put a plaster on a tumor). Hebr. פלגמוני is a non-attested variant of the term פלגמון. It is possibly a loan word from the Arabic, i.e., فلغموني or from Gr. φλεγμονή; cf. previous entry. Moses ibn Tibbon translates Arab. ورم as מורסא.

פלומיצול · **feather-pad; pledget; compress**: Rom. *plumaceol* · Guillaume de Congenis, *Treatise on Surgery* · trans. Isaiah, fol. 44[a]: כאשר שבירת העצם גדולה ונכרת באותות אז יאות לקחת אבק לבונה ולשים על האם קשה ואחר יושם עליו בגד טבול בלובן ביצה בין העצם והאם הקשה ואחר לפי כמות העצם יתכן לשום פלומצול מאישטופאש רחוצות במים לבדה (When the fracture of the bone [in the head] is large and can be diagnosed [i.e., recognized] from the symptoms, one should take incense powder and put this on the dura mater. Then, one should put a cloth dipped in egg white between the bone and the dura mater and then one can—according to the size of the bone—put a pledget on it that is made from [fibres of] tow and has been washed with water only). Hebr. פלומצול is a non-attested loan word from Rom. *plumaceol* (and var.).

פַּלָּצוּת • **פלצות הלב** · **palpitation (i.e., cardialgia)**: Lat. *tremor cordis* (Arab. خفقان القلب) · Constantinus Africanus, Viaticum · trans. Do'eg ha-Edomi, *Sefer Ya'ir Netiv*, bk, 3, ch. 13: פלצות הלב הוא מהליחות המקובץ בדפים הסובבים הלב (Palpitation is caused by moisture that collects in the pericardium). Hebr. פלצות הלב features in BM 4966 in an attestation from Moshe Narboni (ca. 1300–1362 CE),[261] *Sefer Oraḥ Ḥayyim*: דפיקת הלב נקרא קרדיאקה ר״ל פלצות במי שיצא חוץ מגדרו תנועה רעידית תקרה ללב בסבה מה שיזיק ללב. The term דפיקת הלב already features in Moses ibn Tibbon's translation of Arab. خفقان القلب (cf. BCD 58 (NM 4:39)).

פָּנִים • **מראה עור הפנים** → מַרְאֶה.

• **עקום בפנים** → עִקּוּם.

• **עקימת הפנים** → עֲקִימָה.

• **רעימת פנים** → רעימה.

261 On the author and the *Sefer Oraḥ Ḥayyim*, see G. Bos, 'R. Moshe Narboni, Philosopher and Physician: A Critical Analysis of *Sefer Oraḥ Ḥayyim*,' *Medieval Encounters* 2, no. 1 (1995): 219–251.

פניס · **sugar candy; a sweetmeat:** Lat. *panis* (Arab. فانيذ) · Constantinus Africanus, *Viaticum* · trans. Do'eg ha-Edomi, *Sefer Ya'ir Netiv*, bk. 3, ch. 1: ונתן לו לאכול במדה מועטת מאיזה מרק או מזרע מילונש וכן אמידום דרגגן עם שמן שקדים מכל אלה יעשה מרק שינתן לו בצום או אמידום עם חלב ועם פניס ושמן שקדים (We let him eat a little bit of broth from common melon seed. Similarly from starch, gum tragacanth with almond oil. The broth prepared from all these ingredients should be given to the patient on an empty stomach. One can also make it from starch with milk, sugar candy, and almond oil). Hebr. פניס, a loan word from Lat. *panis* features in BCD 222 (NM 4:166) in later attestations, a.o. from Shem Tov ben Isaac's *Sefer ha-Shimmush*, bk. 27. Moses ibn Tibbon uses the same term to translate Arab. فانيذ.

[פסד] • *Part. Hif'il* **מַפְסִיד** • **מפסיד הראות בנטית השמש** · **night blindness (nyctalopia):** Lat. *amittens visum ab occasu solis* (Arab. عشا / Gr. νυκταλωπίασις)[262] · Constantinus Africanus, *Viaticum* · trans. Do'eg ha-Edomi, *Sefer Ya'ir Netiv*, bk. 2, ch. 5 (Ms Oxford, Bodleian Library, Can. Or. 26, fol. 257[b]): ממפסידי הראות בנטית השמש (On night blindness). Hebr. מפסיד הראות בנטית השמש does not feature in the current dictionaries. Moses ibn Tibbon translates Arab. عشا as לילית (cf. BCD 137 (NM 4:91)).

פִּסְקוֹן · **disappearance** · Ibn al-Jazzār, *Zād al-musāfir wa-qūt al-ḥāḍir* · trans. Abraham ben Isaac, *Sefer Ṣedah la-Oreḥim*, bk. 1, ch. 2 (fol. 89[b]): אמ׳ כי זה החולי מין אחר מנפילת השיער אך אינו גדול כאותו האמור למעלה אך הוא קטן ובזה לא יפול לרוב אך יפול מעט מעט והוא מהחלאים הבאים מחמת חסרון דבר אחד מעניני הגוף ומן פסקון כולו (He said that this illness is another type of hair loss but not so severe as the one mentioned before [i.e., alopecia]. It does not occur in a drastic way, but slowly slowly. It is an illness that occurs because of a decrease or a complete disappearance of one of the things that concern the body [i.e., that the body needs; i.e., nourishment]). Hebr. פִּסְקוֹן does not feature in this sense in the current dictionaries.

פִּקּוּד • **עשרת הפקודים** → עֶשֶׂר.

פַּרְגּוֹד · **diaphragm:** Arab. حجاب (cf. DKT 30, 350; FAL 69:1549) · Shem Tov ben Isaac, *Sefer ha-Shimmush*, bk. 29, list 1 (SHS 1:422 (Pe 38)): פרגוד ב״ה חג׳אב והיא הטרפשה (*pargod*; Arab. *ḥijāb*; [Hebr.] *ṭarpashah*). In the sense of 'diaphragm,' Hebr. פַּרְגּוֹד is a non-attested semantic borrowing from Arab. حجاب. The latter term features a.o. in Maimonides, *Medical Aphorisms* 6.53, and is translated by Nathan ha-Me'ati as טרפשא (BMMN 73) and by Zeraḥyah Ḥen as מסך (BMMZ 67). The term טרפשה is a Hebraization of Aram. טרפשא, which features in SDA 519 in the sense of 'membrane.'

פָּרוּר · **metal pot; cauldron:** Lat. *cacabus* (var. *caccabus* < κάκκαβος) (DMLBS 306) · Guillaume de Congenis, *Treatise on Surgery* · trans. Isaiah, fol. 59[a]: כנגד ארטיטיקה ופרלשי קח עצמות החמור הנמצאות בשדה ודע כי יש להם קשי גדול על כן הנה טובות ויתרחצו יפה ויתיבשו לשמש ואחר יבושלו בפרור במים וירתחו יפה והשומן הצף על פני המים ההם תקח

262 Cf. MMT 253; LSG 1183; UW 438–439.

ותצניעהו לעת הצורך (To [treat] arthritis and paralysis: Take donkey bones that can be found in the fields—you should know that they are very hard and for this reason they are useful—wash them thoroughly, dry them in the sun, then cook them well with water in a metal pot. Take the fat that floats on the water and store it for when you need it). Hebr. פָּרוּר features in BM 5149 in the sense of 'pot' with attestations from the Bible (cf. KB 965: 'cooking-pot'), Rabbinic literature (cf. JD 1222: 'a [round] pot'), and Ben Sira.

פרוּגָה* • *Plur.* **פרוגות** · **young chickens**: Arab. فراريج · Isḥāq ibn ʿImrān, *Treatise on Melancholy* · trans. Anonymous, fol. 51[a] (52[a]): בשר הפרוגות הנקבות (The meat of young chickens). Hebr. *Plur.* פרוגות is possibly coined after Arab. فرّوج, 'young chicken,' by adding the *f. Plur.* ending *-ot*. The regular corresponding Hebrew term is פרגית, *Plur.* פרגיות (cf. BM 5132 (esp. n. 3); JD 1214; KA 9:335; KG 2:477; SD 443–444).

פֶּרַח • **פרח המלח** · **efflorescence of salt; scum of salt**: Arab. زهرة الملح (KM 2:684–686) · Ibn al-Jazzār, *Zād al-musāfir wa-qūt al-ḥādir* · trans. Moses ibn Tibbon, *Sefer Ṣedat ha-Derakhim*, bk. 1, ch. 25: וירחץ במים שנתבשלו בהם סמים חמים וימשח במה שזכרנו מן השמנים אחר שיצא ממים חמים שהושלך בהם פרח המלח ([The spots affected by twitching] should be washed with water in which hot ingredients have been cooked. The oils mentioned should be applied after bathing in hot water to which salt scum has been added). Hebr. פרח המלח is a non-attested calque from Arab. زهرة الملح. Abraham ben Isaac translates the latter term as קצף המלח (see entry קֶצֶף).

• **פרח הנחושת** · **copper oxide [*CuO*]**: Arab. زهرة النحاس (cf. KM 2: 686–691) · *Shinnui ha-Shemot ha-Niqra'im Synonimis*, Ms Munich, Bayerische Staatsbibliothek, Cod. hebr. 8, fol. 197[b]: זהרה אלנחס הוא פרח הנחושת ([Arab.] *zahra al-nuḥās* is [Hebr.] *peraḥ ha-neḥoshet*). In the sense of 'copper oxide,' Hebr. פרח הנחושת is a non-attested calque from Arab. زهرة النحاس.

• *Plur.* **פרחים** • **הזלת הפרחים** → הַזָּלָה.

פריפליומוניא • **פריפליומוניא ⟨בעל⟩** · **pneumonia [patient]**: Lat. *peripleumonicus* (Arab. صاحب قرحة الرئة) · Constantinus Africanus, *Viaticum* · trans. Do'eg ha-Edomi, *Sefer Ya'ir Netiv*, bk. 3, ch. 7: והרופאים נחלקו בנגעי[263] הריאה כי האחרים אומרים שאין להם עזר והעיר גיאלינוס ואמר: אם איזה רופא יעזור אל ⟨בעל⟩ פריפליומוניא קודם שהנפח יתעכב שם ויבלה יתרפא הנפח (The physicians disagree [in the matter of] pneumonia. Some of them say that it cannot be cured. Galen remarks and says that if a physician treats a pneumonia [patient] before a tumor settles in and putrefies, he can be cured). In the sense of 'pneumonia patient,' Hebr. בעל פריפליומוניא is a non-attested partial loan word from Lat. *peripleumonicus*. For פריפליומוניא, see also entry נֶגַע: נגעי הריאה. Moses ibn Tibbon translates Arab. صاحب قرحة الرئة as בעל נגע הריאה.

פִּרְנוּס • **חסרון הפרנוס** → חֶסְרוֹן.

263 בנגעי הריאה: פריפליומוניא Ms Oxford, Bodleian Library, Can. Or. 26, fol. 289[b].

פַּרְנָסָה · **food; nourishment**: Arab. غذاء · Ibn al-Jazzār, *Zād al-musāfir wa-qūt al-ḥādir* · trans. Abraham ben Isaac, *Sefer Ṣedah la-Oreḥim* bk. 1, ch. 2: וכאשר נראה אם נפילת השיער מחמת חסרון הפרנסה אז נצוה אותו שיכנס למרחץ תדיר ויתפרנס מאכילות קלות המיישרין והמתקנין עובי הד׳ יסודי הגוף (If the hair loss originates from a lack of nourishment, we order frequent visits to the bathhouse and a diet consisting of light foods that balance and correct the coarseness of the four humors of the body). Hebr. פַּרְנָסָה only features in the current dictionaries in the sense of 'provision, maintenance, outfit' (JD 1231), or 'subsistence, livelihood' (BM 5195–5196). Subsequent to Abraham ben Isaac, the term פַּרְנָסָה features in the sense of 'food, nourishment' in Zeraḥyah Ḥen's translation of Maimonides, *Medical Aphorisms* 9.124 (BMMZ 117; cf. BCD 223 (NM 1:180)). Moses ibn Tibbon translates Arab. غذاء as מזון.

פַּרְפֶּרֶת • *Plur.* פַּרְפְּרָאוֹת · **dessert**: Arab. نُقْل · Ibn al-Jazzār, *Zād al-musāfir wa-qūt al-ḥādir* · trans. trans. Abraham ben Isaac, *Sefer Ṣedah la-Oreḥim* bk. 1, ch. 19: ותהיה הפרנסה שלו תרנוגלים קטנים גם דראג׳ מבושלים עם מי ענבי הבוסר ועם מי שריגי הפרפחינים הרעננים ומי ענבי הבוסר עם חומץ אתרוגים ויאכל מן הפרפראות הרימונים החמוצים ומן הזערור והתפוחים (The [patient's] food should consist of young chickens, francolins cooked in juice of unripe grapes, juice made from fresh common purslane stalks, and from unripe grapes and citron pulp. As dessert, he should take sourish pomegranates, common medlars, and apples). Hebr. פַּרְפְּרָאוֹת is not attested for in medieval medical literature. Abraham ben Isaac translates Arab. نُقْل as אֲפִיקוֹמָן (see entry).

פְּשׁוּט · **dilatation of the palpebral membrane**: Arab. انتشار (D 2:671) · Maimonides, *Medical Aphorisms* 23.69 · trans. Zeraḥyah Ḥen (BMMZ 226): המים אשר יתקבץ בעין והוא אשר יקראוהו הרופאים פישוט בערבי אנתשאר יתקבץ במה שבין הלחות הכפורי והקרום הקרניי. בעשירי מהתועלת (The cataract that occurs in the eye and that the physicians call 'extension' [i.e., dilatation], Arab. *intishār*, lies between the crystalline humor and the horn-like tunic. *De usu partium* 10[264]). Hebr. פְּשׁוּט does not feature in this sense in the current dictionaries; cf. BM 5265. In addition to פְּשׁוּט, Zeraḥyah Ḥen (ibid. 22.40) renders the same Arabic term as פשוט הראות (BMMZ 212; see next entry). Nathan ha-Me'ati (a.l.) translates Arab. انتشار as הִתְפַּשְּׁטוּת (BMMN 227; see entry).

• **פשוט הראות** · **dilatation of the palpebral membrane**: Arab. انتشار (D 2:671) · Maimonides, *Medical Aphorisms* 22.40 · trans. Zeraḥyah Ḥen (BMMZ 212): מי שיכחל עינו באשרוב שלהוורדים החדשים[265] ימנע מן הרמד ויחזק הראות ואם יתמיד זה ירפא מהחולי הנקרא פשוט הראות. התאמת זה בניסיון ולא סרתי מעשותו בחזוק הראות (The anointment of the

---

264 Galen, *De usu partium* 10.1, ed. Helmreich, 2:55. Cf. MIG 55: الانتشار في العين هو اتّساع الحدقة من الأدوية في ذكر النبات الذي يقال له سطوبي (*Al-intishār* (synchysis, lit., "widening") of the eye is a dilation (*ittisā'*) of the pupil (*ḥadaqa*)—from the entry on the plant called στοιβή in (sc. Galen's) "Drugs" (*al-Adwiya*)).

265 החדשים (a السكري): הסוכרי marginal note in Ms Vatican, Biblioteca Apostolica, Urb. ebr. 38.

eyelids with rose syrup made[266] with sugar prevents ophthalmia and strengthens vision.[267] Its permanent use cures dilatation of the palpebral membrane. This has been verified by experience; I have not ceased to use it for strengthening vision). Hebr. פשוט הראות is not attested for in the current dictionaries. Nathan ha-Me'ati (a.l.) translates Arab. انتشار as הִתְרַחֲבוּת (see entry).

[פשט] • *Part. Hof'al* **מֻפְשָׁט** • **מופשט מן** · **free from**: Arab. معرّى من · Maimonides, *Medical Aphorisms* 3.4 · trans. Zeraḥyah Ḥen (BMMZ 32): גוף האדם כולו מתנפש ניפוש טוב והוא נקי מופשט מן המותרות ומן הלחיצה (The whole body of a man breathes well when it is clean and free from superfluities and pressure). Hebr. מֻפְשָׁט features in medieval philosophical literature as 'abstract' (i.e., devoid of all attributes) (cf. KT 2:250; BM 5274; EP 70). In addition to מופשט מן, Zeraḥyah translates Arab. معرّى من as ערום מן. Nathan ha-Me'ati translates Arab. معرّى من as נמנע מן (BMMN 40; see entry [מנע]).

פָּתַח · **to burst; to break forth**: Arab. انفجر · Ibn al-Jazzār, *Zād al-musāfir wa-qūt al-ḥādir* · trans. Moses ibn Tibbon, *Sefer Ṣedat ha-Derakhim*, bk. 1, ch. 25 (Ms London, British Library, Ar. Or. 26, fol. 99[a]): רקיקת מוגלא בלויה תהיה מסבות רבות פעמים תהיה ממורסא תתחדש בכלי הנשימה ותפתח המורסא וימשך מה שיצא ממנה (Spitting of pus can occur because of many things, sometimes because of an abscess that is formed in the respiratory organs and that bursts, and [the pus] that oozes out [of the abscess] streams [to the lungs]). In the sense of 'to burst,' Hebr. פָּתַח features in BCD 225 (NM 3:190–191) in a later attestation from Zeraḥyah Ḥen's translation of Maimonides, *Medical Aphorisms* 5.15 (BMMZ 58).

---

266 'made with sugar': Trans. after a and Ms Vatican, Biblioteca Apostolica, Urb. ebr. 38.

267 The fourteenth century French surgeon Guy de Chauliac (Guigonis de Caulhiaco) possibly refers to this remedy (in the Latin translation) for strengthening vision in his *Inventarium sive Chirurgia Magna*. Cf. ed. McVaugh (Leiden 1997), 1:230, ll. 1–2; 2:188.

צ

צָבוּעַ · **corrupt**: Lat. *infectus* (Arab. فاسد) · Constantinus Africanus, *Viaticum* · trans. Do'eg ha-Edomi, *Sefer Ya'ir Netiv*, bk. 1, ch. 6: מן פושטוליש הוא מן גרב נולד בראש בשפעת ליחות חמות או מן פליקמא צבועה (On PWŠṬWLYŠ, i.e., a kind of ulcer that originates on the head because of a surplus of hot humors or of corrupt phlegm). In the sense of 'corrupt,' Hebr. צָבוּעַ is a non-attested semantic borrowing from Lat. *infectus*, which can mean both 'dyed, colored' and 'spoiled, corrupted, infected;' cf. LS 945, s.v. *inficio*.

צְבוּת · **inflammation**: Lat. *phlegmon* (inflammation; h.l., tumor)[268] (Arab. ورم) · Ibn al-Jazzār, *Zād al-musāfir wa-qūt al-ḥādir* · trans. Abraham ben Isaac, *Sefer Ṣedah la-Oreḥim*, Adaptation, bk. 1, ch. 10 (Ms Berlin, Staatsbibliothek Preußischer Kulturbesitz, Or. fol. 1058, fol. 92[b]): ויש שיכאב מחמת פליגמון הוא צבות הנולדת בראש (One may also suffer from a [headache] because of a PLYGMWN [i.e., Lat. *phlegmon*, 'inflammation'], i.e., tumor, occurring in the head). In the sense of 'tumescence, tumor,' Hebr. צְבוּת features in BM 5357 in an attestation from Samuel Jaffe's midrashic commentary *Yefeh To'ar* and from Y. Tovim, *Ha-Diphteriah*. Do'eg ha-Edomi renders Lat. *apostema*, as it features in the *Viaticum*, as נפח, Abraham ben Isaac renders Arab. ורם as פלגמון (see entry), and Moses ibn Tibbon translates it as מורסא.

צַוָּאר • **העוּמק אשר בעליון אחורי הצואר** → עֹמֶק.

• **העורף אחרי הצואר** → עֹרֶף.

[צום] • *Part.* **צָם** • **בהיותו צם** · **on an empty stomach**: Arab. على الريق (Lat. *ienuno*) · Ibn al-Jazzār, *Zād al-musāfir wa-qūt al-ḥādir* · trans. Moses ibn Tibbon, *Sefer Ṣedat ha-Derakhim*, bk. 3, ch. 6: ואמ' גאלי' כי אצטרקה ליקידא כשילחך ממנה בהיותו צם מי שהיה בו שעול או ירידה או רבמאס יקבל תועלת בו (Galen said that if someone who is suffering from cough, catarrh, or rheum licks liquid styrax, he will benefit from it). Hebr. בהיותו צם does not feature in the current dictionaries. Do'eg ha-Edomi translates Lat. *ienuno* as קודם אכילה (see entry קֹדֶם).

צוֹר • *Plur.* **צורים** • **דג הצורים** → דָּג.

צָלַל · **to clarify; to clear; to purify; to filter**: Arab. صفّى · Ibn al-Jazzār, *Zād al-musāfir wa-qūt al-ḥādir* · trans. Abraham ben Isaac, *Sefer Ṣedah la-Oreḥim*, bk. 1, ch. 14 (Ms Jerusalem, National Library of Israel, Fr. 95, fol. 94[a]): ויחבוש עליו חובש זה כי יועיל לשכחה ויצלול הדעת (And apply the following plaster, which is beneficial for forgetfulness and which purifies the intellect [i.e., brain]). Hebr. צָלַל is attested for in Rabbinic literature (JD 1284; LW 4:192; BM 5494–5495) a.o. in the sense of 'to settle; to sink; to clarify; to be clear.' It is also attested for in medieval literature in Maimonides' *Commentary on the Mishnah*: צוללין היין בסודר. Moses ibn Tibbon translates Arab. صفّى as זיכך.

268 Note that the *Viaticum* has *apostema* and not *phlegmon* featuring in the adaptation.

• *Part. Pu'al* מְצֻלָּל • **filtered**: Arab. مصفّى · Ibn al-Jazzār, *Zād al-musāfir wa-qūt al-ḥāḍir* · trans. Abraham ben Isaac, *Sefer Ṣedah la-Oreḥim*, bk. 1, ch. 10 (Ms Jerusalem, National Library of Israel, Fr. 95, fol. 90^b^): ג׳ אונק׳ ממי ענבי שועל מרותח ומצולל (Three ounces of decocted and filtered nightshade juice). Hebr. מְצֻלָּל does not feature in this sense in the current dictionaries. Moses ibn Tibbon translates Arab. مصفّى as מזוכך.

• *Hif'il* הִצְלִיל • **to clarify; to clear; to purify; to filter**: Arab. صفّى · Ibn al-Jazzār, *Zād al-musāfir wa-qūt al-ḥāḍir* · trans. Abraham ben Isaac, *Sefer Ṣedah la-Oreḥim*, bk. 1, ch. 14 (Ms Jerusalem, National Library of Israel, Fr. 95, fol. 94^a^): וישתה כל דבר המתיר והמכנע חדות מרה אדומה כגון שיקח תרנג׳בין ובנפסג׳ מרבא מכל א׳ ה׳ שקלים ולב כיאר שנבר מטוהר ב׳ שקל׳ וחצי ותמעכם במי הדלעת הצלויה בתוך המים ויצליל אותם (Drink anything that dissolves and subdues the sharpness of the yellow bile, such as five *shekels* each of manna and preserve of violets; two and a half *shekels* of purified pulp of purging cassia; macerate this in the juice of roasted pumpkins and purify it). Hebr. הִצְלִיל features in BM 5496 in the sense of 'to sink' or 'to purify,' but is not attested for in medieval medical literature.

צֶלַע • *Plur.* **צלעות** • **צמח בין הצלעות** → **צֶמַח**.

צִלְצוּל • **(האזנים) צלצול** • **צלצול** • **tinnitus**: Lat. *tinnitus aurium* (Arab. دويّ) · Constantinus Africanus, *Viaticum* · trans. Do'eg ha-Edomi, *Sefer Ya'ir Netiv*, bk. 2, ch. 8 (Ms Oxford, Bodleian Library, Can. Or. 26, fols. 259^b^–260^a^): מצלצול האזנים. אם האזנים אינם סובלות נפח גם שאר הדברים הכתובים למעלה וראוים לקבל הקול אז יש להבין כי הצלצול הוא מרוח גס או מליחות דביקות או מאפיסת השמע או מאיזה דבר יקרה (On tinnitus. If the ears do not suffer from a tumor nor from the other things mentioned above but seem to retain the sound, one should understand that the tinnitus hails from a coarse wind, or viscous superfluities, or from a loss of hearing, or from something else). In the sense of 'tinnitus,' Hebr. (האזנים) צלצול features in MD 722, s.v. 'tinnitus': צלילה/צלצול/צלילת האזנים.[269] Moses ibn Tibbon renders Arab. دويّ as צלילה (see BCD 229 (NM 4:172)).

צָם (*Part.*) → **[צום]**.

צֶמַח • **צמח אדמדם** • **inflamed tumor;**[270] **inflammation**: Arab. فلغموني (Gr. φλεγμονή; cf. UW 736; SN 98) · Shem Tov ben Isaac, *Sefer ha-Shimmush*, bk. 29, list 1 (SHS 1:440 (Ṣade 24)): צמח אדמדם ב״ה פלגמוני (*ṣemaḥ adamdam*; Arab. *falghamūnī*). Hebr. צמח אדמדם, lit., 'a reddish, inflamed tumor,' is not attested for in the current dictionaries.

• **צמח בטרפשה** • **(lit., an inflammation of the diaphragm); pleurisy**: Arab. شوصة (cf. UWS 2:130, s.v. πλευριτικός)[271] · Shem Tov ben Isaac, *Sefer ha-Shimmush*, bk. 29,

---

269 Cf. the anonymous *Sefer ha-Yosher* (Ms Oxford, Bodleian Library, Opp. 180 (cat. Neubauer 2134), fol. 17b): שער בצלצול האוזן (On tinnitus).

270 For the different meanings of צמח, cf. BCD 231.

271 M. Ullmann (ed. and trans.), *Rufus von Ephesos: Krankenjournale* (Wiesbaden 1978), 125, remarks: '*šawṣa* designates a disease that has not been defined accurately. According to

list 1 (SHS 1:438–439 (Ṣade 21)): צמח בטרפשה ב״ה שוצה וב״ל פלבירשין וירא (*ṣemaḥ ba-ṭarpashah*; Arab. *shawṣa*; vern. PLBYRŠYN WYR' [i.e., O.Occ. (compound term) **plevesin/pleu(re)sin vera* ('real pleurisy')]). Hebr. צמח בטרפשה is not attested for in the current dictionaries (see also entry צמח בין הצלעות).

• **צמח בלובן העין** · **(lit., an inflammation of the whites of the eye (sclera)); cataract**: Arab. زرقة (UW 181, s.v. γλαύκωσις) · Shem Tov ben Isaac, *Sefer ha-Shimmush*, bk. 29, list 1 (SHS 1:439–440 (Ṣade 23)): צמח בלובן העין ב״ה ודקה (*ṣemaḥ be-loven ha-ʿayin*; Arab. WDQH [read: ZRQH; i.e. *zurqa*; cf. MMT 248ff.]). Hebr. צמח בלובן העין is not attested for in the current dictionaries.

• **צמח מתחת הלשון** · **(lit., an inflammation beneah the tongue); ranula**: Arab. ضفدع (SN 106; cf. al-Zahrāwī, *Kitāb at-taṣrīf*, bk. 30, pt. 2, ch. 35 (SpLA 298f.): قد يحدث تحت اللسان ورم يشبه الضفضع الصغير يمنع اللسان عن فعله الطبيعي (Sometimes there occurs under the tongue a swelling resembling a small frog that hinders the natural movements of the tongue); cf. Hebrew translation, MS Paris, BN, héb. 1163, fol. 214[a]: לפעמים ימצא תחת הלשון צבות ידמה הצפרדע הקטון ימנע הלשון מפעולתו הטבעית) · Shem Tov ben Isaac, *Sefer ha-Shimmush*, bk. 29, list 1 (SHS 1:441 (Ṣade 27)): צמח מתחת הלשון ב״ה צפרדע (*ṣemaḥ mi-taḥat ha-lashon*; Arab. ṢPRDʿ [i.e., *ṣefardeʿa*; read: ṢPDʿ, i.e., *ḍifḍiʿ*]). Hebr. צמח מתחת הלשון features in BM 5607 in an attestation from Nathan ben Jo'el Falaquera, *Sefer Ṣori ha-Guf*.[272]

• **צמח המוח** · **(lit. inflammation of the brain); phrenitis**: Arab. شرسام / سرسام (cf. MIG 1002) · Shem Tov ben Isaac, *Sefer ha-Shimmush*, bk. 29, list 1 (SHS 1:439 (Ṣade 22)): צמח המוח ב״ה שרסאם (*ṣemaḥ ha-moaḥ*; Arab. *shirsām/sirsām*). Hebr. צמח המוח is not attested for in the current dictionaries.

• **צמח בין הצלעות** · **(lit., an inflammation between the ribs); (costal) pleurisy**: Arab. ذات الجنب (cf. UW 535, s.v. πλευρίτις) · Shem Tov ben Isaac, *Sefer ha-Shimmush*, bk. 29, list 1 (SHS 1:438 (Ṣade 20)): צמח בין הצלעות ב״ה דאת אלג׳נב (*ṣemaḥ beyn ha-ṣelaʿot*; Arab. *dhāt al-janb*). Hebr. צמח בין הצלעות is not attested for in the current dictionaries (see also entry צמח בטרפשה).

• **צמח בציפורן האצבע** · **(lit., an inflammation in the fingernail); paronychia; whitlow**: Arab. داحس (Gr. παρωνυχία; cf. MIG 587) · Shem Tov ben Isaac, *Sefer ha-Shimmush*,

Ibn Wāfid in Dozy suppl. I 803a, it is a growth in the thoracic diaphragm. The pain caused by this disease can radiate as far as the collarbones. According to Ibn Sīnā (*Qānūn* I 400,35), *šawṣa* is a growth in the membranes, diaphragms, and muscles of the thorax. He names them in conjunction with *birsām* and *ḏāt al-ǧanb*. Ibn Manẓūr (Lis. 7,50b 4ff.) speaks of a wind that is trapped between the ribs and is experienced as a shooting pain. On the whole, 'pleurisy' can be considered as the right translation;' M.W. Dols, *Medieval Islamic Medicine* (Berkeley 1984), 123, distinguishes between *shauṣa* and *dhāt al-janb* as: 'pleurisy' and 'true pleurisy.'

272 For the author and the *Sefer Ṣori ha-Guf*, cf. Bos and Fontaine, 'Medico-philosophical Controversies,' 27–60.

bk. 29, list 1 (SHS 1:441 (Ṣade 26)): צמח בצפורן האצבע ב״ה דאחס ב״ל גלאיי (*ṣemaḥ be-ṣipporen ha-eṣba'*: Arab. *dāḥis*; vern. GL'YY [unclear; perhaps a corruption or a dialectal variant belonging to Provençal *unglàdo* (Haute Loire, FEW 14:40a, var. *oyàda*), 'engourdissement douloureux du bout des doigts, causée par un grand froid' (painful numbness of the fingertips); 'apostume aux racines des ongles, panaris' (abscess at the roots of the fingernails, whitlow); cf. M.Fr. and Mod. Fr. *onglée*]). Hebr. צמח בצפורן האצבע is not attested for in the current dictionaries.

צָמִיד • *Plur.* **צמידים** • **צמידי הראש** · **collar bones (clavicles)**: Lat. *furculae* (cf. DMLBS 1303) (Arab. ترقوة) · Constantinus Africanus, *Viaticum* · trans. Do'eg ha-Edomi, *Sefer Ya'ir Netiv*, bk. 3, ch. 12: העזר בראותינו נפח הקרב שהוא מהדם אם העת ושנותיו והנהגתו וכחו נחסר דמו מהמקור הבסליקא מהצד ההוא באשר יסבול בטרם יגדל הנפח ויותר אם הכאב יעלה עד צמידי הראש הם פורקולי של הצואר (If we notice that the swelling of the diaphragm hails from blood and the time [of the year], age, habits, and strength [of the patient are favorable], we bleed him from the basilic vein at the side of the illness before the tumor grows, especially when the pain reaches the collar bones, i.e., the *furculae*). Hebr. *Sing.* צמיד הראש, *Plur.* צמידי הראש, is not attested for in the current dictionaries. Moses ibn Tibbon translates Arab. ترقوة as אורגנא.

צִנּוֹר • *Plur.* **צנורות** • **צנורות הנחירים** · **nostrils**: Lat. *canales narium* (Arab. قصبة الأنف) · Constantinus Africanus, *Viaticum* · trans. Do'eg ha-Edomi, *Sefer Ya'ir Netiv*, bk. 1, ch. 21: ולפעמים נעשה העטוש בדברים אחרים שאינם חולי כי צנורות נחירי האדם הם קצרות ועל כן הדברים אשר יזיקו באים מן החוץ מהרה אל המוח כמו האבק וקרירות האויר וזריחת השמש ודומיהם (Sometimes sneezing is caused by other things than illness. Since the human nostrils are short, harmful things—such as dust, cold air, smoke, sunrays, and the like—can easily pass from without to the brain). Hebr. צנורות הנחירים is an unattested loan translation of Lat. *canales narium*. Moses ibn Tibbon translates Arab. قصبة الأنف as קנה החוטם (see entry קָנֶה) and Abraham ben Isaac as קנה האף (see also entry קָנֶה).

• **צנורות הריאה** · **trachea**: Lat. *canalis pulmonis* (Arab. قصبة الرئة) · Constantinus Africanus, *Viaticum* · trans. Do'eg ha-Edomi, *Sefer Ya'ir Netiv*, bk. 3, ch. 6: והשעול שאינו רע כזה הוא יוצא מהחבור הרע מכלי הרוח או מניחור הגרון או מצנורות הריאה (Cough that is not that bad originates from a bad temperament of the respiratory organs or roughness of the throat or trachea). Hebr. *Sing.* צנור הריאה, *Plur.* צנורות הריאה, is not attested for in the current dictionaries. Moses ibn Tibbon translates Arab. قصبة الرئة as קנה הריאה.

[צנע] • *Hof'al* **הוּצְנַע** · **to be put aside; be conserved; to be kept**: Arab. رُفِعَ · Ibn al-Jazzār, *Zād al-musāfir wa-qūt al-ḥāḍir* · trans. Moses ibn Tibbon, *Sefer Ṣedat ha-Derakhim*, bk. 3, ch. 6: יודקו הסמים וינופו ויולשו במשקה ויאולד או ברב ענבים ויוצנע בכלי זכוכית ויקח ממנו שני שקלים בעת הצורך בקר וערב כי הוא מועיל ומנוסה (Pound these ingredients, sieve them and knead them with violet juice or with a rob prepared from grapes; keep this in a glass vessel and take, when necessary, two *shekels* in the morning and evening, because it is beneficial and tested). Hebr. הוּצְנַע does not feature in this sense in the current dictionaries. However, in the *Hifʿil* conjugation it features as 'to put aside; to keep' in BM 5556–5557 with attestations from Rabbinic literature.

[צער] • *Part. Hitpaʿel* **מִצְטַעֵר** · **disturbed**: Arab. مضطرب (Gr. θορυβώδης) · Maimonides, *Medical Aphorisms* 6.37 · trans. Zeraḥyah Ḥen (BMMZ 64): סימני קראניטס י״ו עלאמה והם התעורה או השינה המצטערת ובלבול הדעת ויתחיל מעט אחר מעט והקדחת החדה אשר לא תרפה בזמן מן הזמנים והשכחה לדברים ההוים ומיעוט הצמא (The signs of phrenitis are sixteen: sleeplessness or disturbed sleep, delirium manifesting itself gradually, acute fever that never subsides, short-term memory loss, lack of thirst ...). Hebr. מִצְטַעֵר does not feature in this sense in the current dictionaries. Nathan ha-Me'ati translates Arab. مضطرب as מִתְנוֹעֵעַ (see entry [נוע]).

צף • **צף הים** · **sea froth**: Lat. *escuma maris* (Arab. زبد البحر) (Gr. ἁλκυόνιον, which refers to a variety of marine substances, such as cuttlebones or spongy corals; cf. MIG 325) · Constantinus Africanus, *Viaticum* · trans. Do'eg ha-Edomi, *Sefer Ya'ir Netiv*, bk. 1, ch. 1: ואם הוא מליחה קרה נעביר תער על ראשו ונכרות עליו כריתות קטנות עד צאת הדם ועם שומים כתושים היטב נמשח עליו ונרחץ אותו ונטיח עליו אבפורבי מזוג עם שמן לברין וכן שורש קנים או נשטורש שחוק לאבק ומעורב עם שמן ועם צף הים (If this disease [i.e., alopecia] originates from a cold humor, we shave his head with a razor and make small incisions in the [bald] spot until blood comes forth. Then we rub finely pounded garlic on it and wash it and anoint it with resin spurge mixed with laurel oil. Reed roots, or garden cress pounded into a powder and mixed with olive oil and with sea froth [may also be rubbed on it]). Hebr. צף[273] הים does not feature in the current dictionaries. In addition to צף הים, Do'eg ha-Edomi renders the Latin synonym *spuma marina* as צף מרינא (see next entry). Shem Tov ben Isaac renders the Arabic equivalent زبد البحر as חלאת הים (cf. SHS 1:228 (Ḥet 33)). Moses ibn Tibbon renders it as Rom. אשקומא דמר.

• **צף מרינא** · **sea froth**: Lat. *spuma marina* (Arab. زبد البحر) · Constantinus Africanus, *Viaticum* · trans. Do'eg ha-Edomi, *Sefer Ya'ir Netiv*, bk. 2, ch. 1: אחר: סירקא קולא ה׳ דרכמ׳ אמידום ד׳ דרכמ׳ צף מרינא ג׳ סוקרי ב׳ ותשחוק לאבק (Ms London, British Library, Add. 18969, fol. 24[a]): אחר: סירקא קולא ה׳ דרכמ׳ אמידום ד׳ דרכמ׳ קצף מרינא ג׳ סוקרי ב׳ ותשחוק לאבק (Another [remedy for ophthalmia]: [Take] five *dirhams* of sarcocol, four *dirhams* of starch, three [*dirhams*] of sea froth, two [*dirhams*] of sugar, and grind them into a powder). The term צף מרינא, a combination of Hebr. צף and Lat. *marina* is not attested for in the current dictionaries. In addition to צף מרינא, Do'eg renders the Latin synonym *escuma maris* as צף הים (see previous entry). Moses ibn Tibbon renders Arab. زبد البحر as Rom. אשקומא דמאר. Additionally, Ibn Tibbon renders Arab. زبد البحر as קצף הים (see entry קֶצֶף).

צִפּוֹר • **אצבע צפור** → **אֶצְבַּע**.

• **לשון הצפור** → **לָשׁוֹן**.

273 Hebr. צף is possibly *Part.* from צוף, meaning 'floating'.

צפורן → צִפֹּרֶן.

צִפֹּרֶן • **צמח בצפורן האצבע** → צֶמַח.

• *Dual* צִפָּרְנַיִם ‣ **hoofs**: Lat. *ungulae* (Arab. ظلف) · Constantinus Africanus, *Viaticum* · trans. Do'eg ha-Edomi, *Sefer Ya'ir Netiv*, bk. 1, ch. 1:[274] ונפזר אבק קליפת לוזים קלויים על הדם או אבק צואת תישים וצפרניה (Then, we have to sprinkle pulverized shells of roasted hazelnuts [on the spot with] the blood or pulverized goat dung or goat hoof). As a body part, Hebr. *Sing.* צִפֹּרֶן, *Dual* צִפָּרְנַיִם, only features in the current dictionaries in the sense of 'nail, talon (of a bird)' (cf. JD 1296; BM 5607–5609). For the meaning of 'pterygium,' cf. BCD 233 (NM 1:111–112). Moses ibn Tibbon translates Arab. ظلف as צפרנים as well. Abraham ben Isaac translates it as *Sing.* צפרן.

צָרוּת • **צרות הנשימה** ‣ **breathlessness; shortness of breath (orthopnea)**: Arab. بهر · Ibn al-Jazzār, *Zād al-musāfir wa-qūt al-ḥāḍir* · trans. Moses ibn Tibbon, *Sefer Ṣedat ha-Derakhim*, bk. 3, ch. 6: תואר משקה אישופי נעשה בשרשים חברתיו לשעול המתהוה מאדים כרכומיים ולכאב הצדדים ולצרות הנפש ולצרות הנשימה (Recipe of a hyssop potion that is prepared with roots and that I have composed [and that is good] for cough caused by choleric vapors, for pleurisy, for anxiety, and for breathlessness). Hebr. צרות הנשימה features in BCD 233–234 (NM 4:176) in an attestation from Shem Tov ben Isaac, *Sefer ha-Shimmush*, bk. 27, as a translation of Arab. ضيق النفس ('orthopnea'). The latter term is translated by Moses ibn Tibbon as קצר הנשימה (see entry קֹצֶר). For Arab. بهر, cf. the definition given by Nathan ha-Me'ati in his glossary to the *Sefer ha-Qanun*: בהאר הוא שם לקוצר הנשימה החזק (BH'R. This is the term for severe shortness of breath) (cf. NM 2:110, 128 (Bet 10)).

צְרִי • **צרי הגדול** ‣ **the great theriac**: Lat. *tiriaca maior* · Constantinus Africanus, *Viaticum* · trans. Do'eg ha-Edomi, *Sefer Ya'ir Netiv*, bk. 2, ch. 18 (Ms Oxford, Bodleian Library, Can. Or. 26, fol. 269^b): ואם הכאב לא ינוח נשים על השנים פלוני[275] או שוקרי[276] גינא או צרי הגדול הוא טריאקא מנגנא (If the [toothache] does not alleviate, we should put philonium[277] or sucriginem[278] or the great theriac, i.e., *theriaca magna*, on the teeth). Hebr. צרי הגדול is not attested for in the current dictionaries. The term צֳרִי on its own features in the sense of 'antidote, theriac' in the anonymous *Sefer ha-Refu'ot ha-Libbiyot* (cf. BCD 234 (NM 4:176)).

---

274 Do'eg ha-Edomi consistently uses צִפֹּרֶן in the sense of 'hoof,' as in bk. 1, ch. 22 (וכן צפרניו שרופות), and in bk. 2, ch. 21 (צפרני התיש).

275 פלוני: *philonium* L.

276 שוקרי גינא: *sucriginem* L.

277 'philonium': I.e., Arab. *fīlūniyā* (Gr. Φιλώνια or (correctly) Φιλώνειος), a remedy invented by Philo of Tarsos, a poet-physician and pharmacist of the late Hellenistic period, which comes in a 'Greek' and a 'Persian' variety (cf. KR 180, n. 66); for Arabic prototypes, see O. Kahl (ed. and trans.), *Ibn Sahl's Dispensatory*, nos. 7 and 8; see also KR 180, n. 66.

278 'sucriginem': I.e., Arab. شخزنايا, a compound remedy; for its composition, cf. IJZ 85, n. 62.

ק

קִבּוּץ • **coagulation:** Lat. *coagulatio* (Arab. انعقاد) · Constantinus Africanus, *Viaticum* · trans. Do'eg ha-Edomi, *Sefer Ya'ir Netiv*, bk. 3, ch. 14: לפעמים יקרה צמח או נפח בדדים וזה בענינים משתנים או מהדם הנשחת והבלוי או מליחה אחרת או מקבוץ החלב ומבלויו (Sometimes an abscess or tumor occurs in the breasts from different causes; either from blood that is spoiled and putrefied or from another humor or from coagulated and putrefied milk). Hebr. קִבּוּץ does not feature in this sense in the current dictionaries. For other meanings in a medical context, see BCD 235 (NM 1:66, 182; 2:78, 168; 4:177). Moses ibn Tibbon translates Arab. انعقاد as קפיאה.

• **קבוץ הגידין** • **spasms; tetanus:** Arab. تشنّج · Isḥāq ibn ʿImrān, *Treatise on Melancholy* · trans. Anonymous, fol. 49b (50b): ועוד תוסיף על אלה מכה והיא גדולה יותר מדאי[279] והיא[280] תוליד החולי טאט⟨נ⟩יס והוא אלתשנג' והוא קבוץ הגדין (To the afflictions [mentioned before], one should add one that is even more severe, namely the illness [called] *Ṭ'Ṭ[N]YS* [i.e., tetanus], i.e., [Arab.] *al-tashannuj*, i.e., [Hebr.] *qibbuṣ ha-gidin*). In the sense of 'spasm' (for Lat. *spasmus*), Hebr. קבוץ הגידים features in BCD 235 (NM 3:197) in an attestation from Do'eg ha-Edomi's *Sefer Agur*, i.e., his translation of a Latin version of Hippocrates' *Aphorisms*. For the definition of تشنّج as meaning both 'spasms' and 'tetanus,' see Ibn al-Jazzār, *Zād al-musāfir wa-qūt al-ḥāḍir* · trans. Abraham ben Isaac, *Sefer Ṣedah la-Oreḥim*, bk. 1, ch. 24: ועל זה אמר איפוקרט בספר המאמרות שלו: כל מי שיבוא לו חולי זה הנקר' תשנג' או תמדד הנקר' בלשון יון טיטנוש ולאחר כן יבוא לו קדחת אז תמיס הקדחת לאותו חולי (Accordingly, Hippocrates said in his *Book of Aphorisms*: If someone is afflicted by this illness [i.e., spasms] that is called *tashannuj* [lit., cramps] or *tamaddud* [lit., stretching] and that is called in Greek *tetanos* [i.e., tetanus], and if fever occurs after this, the latter will dissolve his disease). See entry מַאֲמָר above.

• *Plur.* **קבוצים** • **chymes; superfluities:** Lat. *chimus*, Plur. acc. *chimos* ('chymes') (Arab. فضول) · Constantinus Africanus, *Viaticum* · trans. Do'eg ha-Edomi, *Sefer Ya'ir Netiv*, bk. 1, ch. 17 (Ms London, British Library, Add. 18969, fol. 12b): וכאשר לא יתבשל המאכל היטב בגוף או כולו או רובו יוליד קבוצים רעים הם ג'ימוש ועל כן פניהם ועפעפיהם יחלו לעלות (And if the food is not well digested in the body, all of it or most of it, it produces bad chymes, i.e., [Lat.]. ǦYMWŠ, and their face and eyelids start to swell). Hebr. *Sing.* קִבּוּץ, *Plur.* קבוצים, does not feature in this sense in the current dictionaries. Moses ibn Tibbon translates Arab. فضول as מותרות; Abraham ben Isaac uses the term כמוס (cf. Gr. χυμός).

[קבל] • *Pi'el* **קִבֵּל** • **to take:** Lat. *accipio* (Arab. أخذ) · Constantinus Africanus, *Viaticum* · trans. Do'eg ha-Edomi, *Sefer Ya'ir Netiv*, bk. 3, ch. 1: ועוד נקבל צואת הכלב הלבן ונשחקנה

279 מדאי: من ذلك a.

280 והיא: emendation editor והוא Ms. והיא תוליד: وهو حدوث a.

לאבק ונמזוג אותה עם מרת הפר וניבש אותה ונשיבנה לאבק ונגרש אותו לפנים בתוך הפה (Then we should take from the excrements of a white dog, pulverize it, mix it with the gall of a bull, dry it, turn it into a powder, and blow the powder into the mouth). In the sense of 'to take,' Hebr. קִבֵּל is a non-attested semantic borrowing from Lat. *accipio*. Moses ibn Tibbon translates Arab. أخذ as לקח.

קָבַץ · **to coagulate**: Lat. *coagulo* (Arab. جمع) · Constantinus Africanus, *Viaticum* · trans. Do'eg ha-Edomi, *Sefer Ya'ir Netiv*, bk. 1, ch. 25: ותרדמת האברים מחוברת בין התולדת והחולי והסבה היא קרירות שיקבוץ עצום הגידים ויקרר ויעצור שלא יוכל הכח המרגיש לנקוב שם (Numbness [occurs because of] a combination of nature and a disease. Its cause is coldness, which coagulates the substance of the nerves. It cools them down and blocks them, so that the power of sensory perception cannot pass through it anymore). Hebr. קָבַץ does not feature in this sense in the current dictionaries. For its occurrence in the sense of 'to be astringent,' see BCD 136 (NM 2:79). Moses ibn Tibbon translates Arab. جمع as קָבַץ (*Qal*) or קִבֵּץ (*Pi'el*) and Abraham ben Isaac as התקבץ.

קֶדֶם • **קודם אכילה** · **on an empty stomach**: Lat. *ienuno* (Arab. على الريق) · Constantinus Africanus, *Viaticum* · trans. Do'eg ha-Edomi, *Sefer Ya'ir Netiv*, bk. 3, ch. 6: וגיאלינוס אמר כי אשטורקש גם שיגיא[281] רקיקה נתון לחולה בבקר קודם אכילה יועיל לשעול הקר גם אלכורישא (Galen said that if someone who is suffering from cough caused by cold or from catarrh takes liquid styrax in the morning on an empty stomach, he will benefit from it). Hebr. קודם אכילה does not feature in the current dictionaries. Moses ibn Tibbon translates Arab. على الريق as בהיותו צם (see entry [צום]).

[קדש] • *Pi'el* קִדֵּשׁ · **to invite**: Lat. *invito* (Arab. أحضر) · Constantinus Africanus, *Viaticum* · trans. Do'eg ha-Edomi, *Sefer Ya'ir Netiv*, bk. 1, ch. 20: ואמרו כי אורפיוש אמר: המלכים מקדשים אותי לשולחנם בעבור שיתענגו בי ואני בהיותי מתענג בם אוכל להכריע לבם למה שארצה כמו מכעס להנחה (They said that Orpheus said: Kings invite me to their banquets so that they get delighted by me. I equally get delighted by them; I am able to bend their heart to what I want, like from anger to mildness). Hebr. קִדֵּשׁ does not feature in this sense in the current dictionaries. Moses ibn Tibbon translates Arab. أحضر as הביא.

קַו • *Plur.* קווים • חכמת הקווים → חָכְמָה.

קודם → קֶדֶם.

קוֹל • חסרון הקול → חֶסְרוֹן.

• נחור הקול → נְחוֹר.

[קוץ] • *Part. Hof'al* מֻקָץ · **(lit., being awake); h.l., coma vigil:**[282] Arab. المنتبه · Ibn al-Jazzār, *Zād al-musāfir wa-qūt al-ḥāḍir* · trans. Moses ibn Tibbon, *Sefer Ṣedat ha-Derakhim*, bk. 1, ch. 15: השער הט"ו בחולי הנקרא המוקץ: כשיתחדש במאוחר מן המוח ליחה

---

281 שיגיא: *sigia* L.

282 Cf. entry חֲרָדָה: חרדת הישן.

לבנה עם מרה אדומה וימזגו יחד יקרה מזה שיהיה החולה מושלך על ערפו כמת ועיניו פתוחות (Bk. 15: On the illness called 'being awake' (coma vigil): If the rear part of the brain suffers from phlegm and yellow bile and if they intermingle, there follows that the patient lies on his back like a dead man, with his eyes open). Hebr. מֵקֶץ is not attested for in the current dictionaries. Do'eg ha-Edomi translates Lat. *expergefactio a somno* as חרדת הישן (see entry חֲרָדָה).

קוֹץ • *Plur.* **קוצים** · **tooth-stick (miswak):**[283] Arab. مسواك, *Plur.* مساويك (*miswāk*) · Ibn al-Jazzār, *Zād al-musāfir wa-qūt al-ḥāḍir* · trans. Moses ibn Tibbon, *Sefer Ṣedat ha-Derakhim*, bk. 2, ch. 23: ויתמיד לנקות שניו בקוצים ובראש החד מעלי הדקל (And he should clean his teeth regularly with a tooth-stick (miswak) or the sharp ends [i.e., tips] of palm leaves). Hebr. *Sing.* קוֹץ, *Plur.* קוצים, does not feature in this sense in the current dictionaries.

קוצר → קֹצֶר.

קטון → קָטֹן.

קָטָן • **המקור העומד בין האצבע הקטן לאחיהו** → מָקוֹר.
• **העורק אשר בין האצבע הקטן וחברו** → עוֹרֵק.

קָטֹן • **המקור העומד בין האצבע הקטון לחבירו** → מָקוֹר.

[קטר] • *Hif'il* **הִקְטִיר** · **to fumigate:** Lat. *fumigo* (Arab. استنشق دخانا) · Constantinus Africanus, *Viaticum* · trans. Do'eg ha-Edomi, *Sefer Ya'ir Netiv*, bk. 2, ch. 14: וכן יאות להקטירו עם סובין ועם קמח שעורין טבול בחומץ (One should also fumigate him with bran and barley meal soaked in vinegar). In the sense of 'to fumigate,' Hebr. הִקְטִיר features in BM 5896 in a later attestation from Me'ir Aldabi, *Shevilei Emunah*. Moses ibn Tibbon translates Arab. استنشق دخانا as הריח.

קִיא • **עשה קיא** → עָשָׂה.

קִיטוֹר • *Plur.* **קיטורים** · **vapors:** Arab. بخار · Isḥāq ibn 'Imrān, *Treatise on Melancholy* · trans. Anonymous, fol. 41ᵃ (42ᵃ): וסבתו הוא שקיטורי השחורה כשיגיעו למוח וידבקו במקום השכל יחשיכו אורו ויבלבלוהו ויפסישוהו ([Melancholy occurs] when melancholic vapors rise to the brain and reach the location of reason, darken its light, disturb and corrupt it). In the sense of 'vapor,' Hebr. קִיטוֹר features in BCD 242 (NM 4:181) for Arab. بخار and Lat. *vapor*, in attestations from Shem Tov ben Isaac, *Sefer ha-Shimmush*, bk. 27, and the *Sefer ha-Refu'ot ha-Libbiyot*. Constantine the African translates Arab. بخار as *fumus*.

קַל • **קל בשכל** · **light-headed:** Arab. متهوّر · Isḥāq ibn 'Imrān, *Treatise on Melancholy* · trans. Anonymous, fol. 45ᵃ (46ᵃ): משל למה הדבר דומה לאיש אחד שידענוהו בטבעו נעצב[284] או משוגע או קל בשכלו דברן בעל אף (One can compare this to a man who was known as

283 For the miswak, made from toothbrush tree leaves [*Salvadora persica* L.]; cf. G. Bos, 'The *miswāk*, an Aspect of Dental Care in Islam,' *Medical History* 37 (1993): 68–79.

284 נעצב: خرفا a.

childish,[285] foolish, light-headed, talkative, irascible by nature). Hebr. קל בשכל is not attested for in the current dictionaries.

קַלּוּת · **courage**: Arab. شجاعة · Isḥāq ibn ʿImrān, *Treatise on Melancholy* · trans. Anonymous, fol. 45ª (46ª): וכמו כן אלו היה מאחר לענות דומם חלש[286] ואחר כך ראינוהו ממהר לענות ומרבה לדבר והראה קלות וגבורה הורנו מעשיו אלו שהגיע זה החולי אליו (Likewise, if someone is slow to answer [a question], silent, lacking[287] courage [i.e., anxious] and then we see that he is quick to answer [a question], talkative, and that he shows courage and bravery, we learn from this that he is affected by this disease [i.e., melancholy]). Hebr. קַלּוּת does not feature in this sense in the current dictionaries. Constantine the African translates the Arabic synonym شجاعة وإقدام as *audax*.

קליפה → קְלִפָּה.

[קלף] • *Hif'il* הִקְלִיף · **to peel off**: Arab. تقشّر · Ibn al-Jazzār, *Zād al-musāfir wa-qūt al-ḥādir* · trans. Abraham ben Isaac, *Sefer Ṣedah la-Oreḥim*, bk. 1, ch. 5 (Ms Jerusalem, National Library of Israel, Fr. 95, fol. 87ª): או קח שקדים מרים ושים במים פושרים עד שיקליפו (Or take bitter almonds, put them in lukewarm water until [their skins] peel off). In the sense of 'to peel off,' (intrans.) Hebr. הִקְלִיף features in EM 1608 in an attestation from modern literature only.

קְלִפָּה · **hyposphagma (i.e., bloodshot eyes)**: Lat. *crustula* (Arab. طرفة) · Constantinus Africanus, *Viaticum* · trans. Do'eg ha-Edomi, *Sefer Ya'ir Netiv*, bk. 2, ch. 3: הקליפה היא דם היורד אל הכתונת החוברת זהו קונגוקטיבא ואל[288] הארטיריאש שלה בהבקעם (Hyposphagma is blood that streams to the conjunctiva, i.e., [Lat.] QWNGWQṬYB', [from][289] blood vessels torn in it). In the sense of 'hyposphagma,' Hebr. קְלִפָּה is a non-attested semantic borrowing from Lat. *crustula*, which in addition to its regular meaning of 'a little crust, crumb' can als mean 'speck of matter (in the eye);' cf. DMLBS 694–695. In addition to קְלִפָּה, Do'eg ha-Edomi renders the Latin synonym *sanguis in oculis* as דם העינים (see entry דָּם). Moses ibn Tibbon renders Arab. طرفة as דם and as אודם אשר באחת קצוות העין (see entry אֹדֶם).

קֶמַח · **powder**: Arab. سفوف · Ibn al-Jazzār, *Zād al-musāfir wa-qūt al-ḥādir* · trans. Abraham ben Isaac, *Sefer Ṣedah la-Oreḥim*, cf. bk. 1, ch. 23: וזה מעשה קמח מאשר עשה יצחק יועיל לפלג ולרפיון ולכאב הפרקים ולחולי הנקר׳ ארתעאש[290] ולכל רפש עב (Recipe of a powder composed by Isaac, beneficial for hemiplegia, looseness, joint pain, tremor, and any coarse superfluity). Hebr. קֶמַח is only attested for in the current dictionaries in the sense of 'meal, flour, mould;' cf. JD 1384, BM 5983–5984. Do'eg ha-Edomi

285 'childish': Trans. after a.
286 חלש: جبانا a.
287 'lacking courage': Trans. after a.
288 ואל הארטיריאש: *a suis arteriis* L.
289 '[from]': Trans. according to Lat. *a*.
290 ארתעאש: الارتعاش a = ארתעאש.

translates the parallel Latin term *pulvis* as אָבָק (see entry). The same term is used by Moses ibn Tibbon for Arab. سفوف (cf. BCD 15 (NM 4:11)).

• **קמח שהוסר המורסן ממנו** · **fine bran-free wheat flour**: Arab. حوّارى (cf. NA 561) · Ibn al-Jazzār, *Zād al-musāfir wa-qūt al-ḥādir* · Moses ibn Tibbon, *Sefer Ṣedat ha-Derakhim*, bk. 2, ch. 25 (fol. 70[b]): תאר עוגות מועילות לכלף ויטהר מראה העור וייפה הפנים יקח מקמח פולים וקמח שהוסר המורסן ממנו הנקרא חוארי (A recipe of pastilles that are good for freckles that cleanse the complexion and embellish the face: Take bean flour and fine bran-free wheat flour that is called [in Arab.] *ḥuwwārā* ...). Hebr. קמח שהוסר המורסן ממנו does not feature in the current dictionaries.

קנבי · **hemp**: Rom. *canve* · Guillaume de Congenis, *Treatise on Surgery* · trans. Isaiah, fol. 43[b]: הראש בהדקר בחרב אך בזאת יאות להתחיל העזר מהמ׳ב׳ה (מהמקום ברוך הוא) ביום הראשון צריך לשום שם נעורת של קנבי רחוצות במים קרים מעורב או בלובן ביצה וסחוטות היטב (When the head is stabbed by a sword, one should—with God's help—begin its treatment on the first day by putting chaff of hemp on the spot. The chaff should be washed in cold water and mixed with egg white and wrung out thoroughly). Hebr. קנבי is a non-attested loan word from Rom. *canve* (and var.).

קָנֶה · **throat**: Lat. *guttur* · Guillaume de Congenis, *Treatise on Surgery* · trans. Isaiah, fol. 53[b]: מן האשקינניציאה: האשקינניציאה היא אפושטימא נולדת בגרון יועיל מאד הקזה מן הזרוע מן אותו הצד או מן מקור אשר תחת הלשון או וונטושא עם אשקריפקציון מונחת על הקנה (On quinsy: Quinsy is an abscess that originates in the throat. A very useful [treatment] is to apply venesection from the arm at the same side or to bleed a vein beneath the tongue or to put cupping glasses on the throat and apply scarification). Hebr. קָנֶה does not feature in this sense in the current dictionaries. In Rabbinic literature it features as 'windpipe' (JD 1338–1339; BM 6019). For its different meanings as an anatomical term, cf. BCD 245 (NM 4:184–185).

• **קנה האף** · **nostrils**: Arab. قصبة الأنف · Ibn al-Jazzar, *Zad al-musafir wa-qūt al-ḥādir* · trans. Abraham ben Isaac, *Sefer Ṣedah la-Oreḥim*, bk. 1, ch. 21: ויש[291] שיבוא מרוב נחיצות הפיסי מלא חולי בעבור שהקנה שלאפו שלאדם היא קצרה ולזה ימהרו להיכנס משם אל המוח הדברים המזיקים מבחוץ כגון האבק והקור החזק והעשן ואלשעאע[292] והדומה להם (Sometimes [sneezing] is caused by nature without an illness. Since the human nostrils are short, harmful things—such as dust, intense coldness, smoke, sunrays, and the like—can easily pass from without to the brain). Hebr. קנה האף is an unattested calque from Arab. قصبة الأنف. Moses ibn Tibbon translates the Arabic term as קנה החוטם (see next entry). Do'eg ha-Edomi translates the parallel Latin term *canales narium* as צנורות הנחירים (see entry צִנּוֹר).

• **קנה החוטם** · **nostrils**: Arab. قصبة الأنف · Ibn al-Jazzār, *Zād al-musāfir wa-qūt al-ḥādir* · trans. Moses ibn Tibbon, *Sefer Ṣedat ha-Derakhim*, bk. 1, ch. 21: ופעמים יבא פתאום

---

291 ויש שיבוא מרוב נחיצות הפיסי מלא חולי: وربّما كان من حفز من غير مرض a.
292 ואלשעאע: والشعاع a.

בלתי חולי וזה כי קנה חוטם האדם קצר ויגיעו בעבור זה דברים מזיקים מחוץ למוח כמו אבק וקור חזק והעשן וזריחת השמש ומה שדומה להם (Sometimes [sneezing] comes suddenly without an illness. Since the human nostrils are short, harmful things—such as dust, intense coldness, smoke, sunrays, and the like—can [easily] pass from without to the brain). Hebr. קנה החוטם is an unattested calque from Arab. قصبة الأنف. Abraham ben Isaac translates the Arabic term as קנה האף (see previous entry). Do'eg ha-Edomi translates the parallel Latin term *canales narium* as צנורות הנחירים (see entry צִנּוֹר).

קָצָה • *Plur.* **קצוות העין** • **אודם אשר באחת קצוות העין** → אֹדֶם.

קצידה · **inflammation or watering of the eyes**: Lat. *lippitudo* (DMLBS 1972) · Guillaume de Congenis, *Treatise on Surgery* · trans. Isaiah, fol. 48ª: לקצידה יושם שם חלב אשה פושר או יתרחצו ביין לבן ודבש מבושלים יחד או במים ודבש מבושלים יחד ([To treat] an inflammation or watering of the eyes: Put lukewarm breast milk on them or wash them with white wine that has been cooked together with honey or with water that has been cooked together with honey). Hebr. קצידה features in BCD 248 (NM 3:206) in an attestation from Moses ibn Tibbon's translation of Maimonides' *Commentary on Hippocrates'* Aphorisms 3.21 (127) (BMHA 1:354), where it stands for Arab. رمد ('ophthalmia').[293]

קָצַף • *Part. Puʿal* **מְקֻצָּף** • **דבש מקוצף** → דְּבַשׁ.

קֶצֶף · **mucilage**: Arab. رغوة · Ibn al-Jazzār, *Zād al-musāfir wa-qūt al-ḥādir* · trans. Moses ibn Tibbon, *Sefer Ṣedat ha-Derakhim*, bk. 3, ch. 6: או יוציא קצף שיליום וקצף זרע חבושים וקצף זרע מלוישקלי וילחוך אותו עם מעט סוכר ודרגגן או עם פניס וגומא אראביקא (Or extract mucilage from fleawort or quince seed or common marshmallow seed and lick this with some sugar and gum tragacanth, or with sugar candy and gum Arabic). Hebr. קֶצֶף features in BM 6105–6106 in the sense of 'froth' only.

• **קצף הים** · **sea froth**:[294] Arab. زبد البحر (Gr. ἀλκυόνιον, which refers to a variety of marine substances, such as cuttlebones or spongy corals, cf. MIG 325) · Ibn al-Jazzār, *Zād al-musāfir wa-qūt al-ḥādir* · trans. Moses ibn Tibbon, *Sefer Ṣedat ha-Derakhim*, bk. 2, ch. 21: וממה שיועיל לזה שיקח חרס ולימסא וישחוק אותה יחד אחר שישרפם וישנן בהם השנים או יקח חרס התנור קצף הים וישחקם יחד ויערב עמהם מעט מלח וישנן בהם שניו (Good for this [affliction] is to take potsherds and snails, to burn them and pound them together, and to apply this as a dentifrice to the teeth. Or take potsherds from the oven [and] sea froth, pound them together, mix it with some salt, and apply this as a dentifrice to the teeth). Hebr. קצף הים features in BM 6106 in the sense of Ger. *Meerschaum* in an attestation from the *Sefer ha-Qanun*. See also BCD 248 (NM 1:72), where it has been

---

293 See also Bos, 'Two Comments,' 106–108.

294 Ibn Tibbon also renders Arab. زبد البحر as Rom. אשקומא דמאר (see entry צף מרינא: צף).

wrongly translated as 'sepiolite.' In addition to קצף הים, Ibn Tibbon renders Arab. زبد البحر as Rom. אשקומא דמאר (see entry צף מרינא :צף).

• **קצף המלח** · **efflorescence of salt; scum of salt; flower of salt**: Arab. زهرة الملح (KM 2:684–686) · Ibn al-Jazzār, *Zād al-musāfir wa-qūt al-ḥādir*, trans. Abraham ben Isaac, *Sefer Ṣedah la-Oreḥim*, bk. 1, ch. 25: וירחוץ במים מבושלים עם בשמים חמים וימשח בכל מה שאמרנו מן אילו המשיחות אחרי שירחוץ במים חמין המרותחין עם קצף המלח הטוב ([The spots affected by twitching] should be washed with water in which hot ingredients have been cooked. The oils mentioned should be applied after bathing in hot water to which salt scum has been added). Hebr. קצף המלח is not attested for in the current dictionaries. Moses ibn Tibbon translates Arab. زهرة الملح as פרח המלח (see entry פֶּרַח).

[קצר] • *Nif'al* **נִקְצַר** · **to be blocked**: Lat. *constipor* (cf. DMLBS 605 (3)) · Constantinus Africanus, *Viaticum* · trans. Do'eg ha-Edomi, *Sefer Ya'ir Netiv*, bk. 2, ch. 17: הלשון תפסיד לפעמים התנועה ועל כן תרגיש הפסד הדבור והסיבה היא מאפיסת הכח הנע הבא מן המוח או מן הגיד באשר הכח יעבור והוא נקצר בסבת הנפח או בסבה אחרת (Sometimes the tongue looses [the ability] to move and consequently someone [suffering from this] experiences a loss of speech. It is caused by the collapse of the power that moves [the tongue] that comes from the brain or because the nerve through which that power moves is blocked through a tumor. There may also be another cause). Hebr. נִקְצַר does not feature in this sense in the current dictionaries. Moses ibn Tibbon renders the parallel Arabic term سدد ('blockage, obstruction') as אוטם.

קֹצֶר · **narrowness; blockage**: Lat. *constipatio* · Constantinus Africanus, *Viaticum* · trans. Do'eg ha-Edomi, *Sefer Ya'ir Netiv*, bk. 3, ch. 11: ואם הוא חומד מאד האויר למשכו והחזה ימלא בעובי גדול מהנשימה אז נבין כי קוצר כלי הרוח הם (If he has a strong need to [frequently] inhale air but the lungs are only filled with great exertion, we know that this is because of the narrowness in [one of] the respiratory channels). Hebr. קֹצֶר features in BM 7118 in the sense of 'shortness, insufficiency' only. Moses ibn Tibbon translates the parallel Arabic term ضيق as צרות.

• **קוצר הנשימה** · **breathlessness; shortness of breath (orthopnea)**: Lat. *strictura in flatu* (Arab. ضيق نفس) · Constantinus Africanus, *Viaticum* · trans. Do'eg ha-Edomi, *Sefer Ya'ir Netiv*, bk. 3, ch. 7: ואם הליחות האלה תהיינה חמות ומחודדות יסבול החולה אודם בלחיים וקוצר הנשימה וצמאון והקדחת תמוח במשיכת האויר הקר (If these humors are hot and sharp, the patient will suffer from redness of the cheeks, breathlessness (orthopnea), thirst, and fever that will abate through inhaling cold air). Hebr. קוצר הנשימה features in the sense of 'asthma' in BM 6119 in an attestation from Jacob Emden, *Megillat Sefer*. Moses ibn Tibbon translates Arab. ضيق نفس as קוצר הנשימה as well. The Arabic synonym بهر is translated by Moses ibn Tibbon as צרות הנשימה (see entry צָרוּת).

קַר • **אש קרה** → **אֵשׁ**.

• **טפה קרה** → **טִפָּה**.

קראסיס[295] · **temperament**: Arab. مزاج (Gr. κρᾶσις) · Ibn al-Jazzār, *Zād al-musāfir wa-qūt al-ḥādir* · trans. Abraham ben Isaac, *Sefer Ṣedah la-Oreḥim*, bk. 1, ch. 3 (Ms Jerusalem, National Library of Israel, Fr. 95, fols. 84ᵇ–85ᵃ): וישקנו ממשקה המקרר הקראסיס שלו הוא אל מזאג׳ ויפרנסהו בדלעת ופרפחינים (Give him a potion that cools the temperament, i.e., [Arab.] *al-mizāj*, and feed him with pumpkin and common purslane). Hebr. קראסיס is a non-attested loan word from Gr. κρᾶσις. In addition to קראסיס, Abraham ben Isaac once uses the term מִדָּה (see entry). Moses ibn Tibbon translates the parallel Arabic term مزاج as מזג.

קֶרֶב · **stomach**: Arab. معدة · Ibn al-Jazzār, *Zād al-musāfir wa-qūt al-ḥādir* · trans. Abraham ben Isaac, *Sefer Ṣedah la-Oreḥim*, bk. 1; ch. 4 (Ms Jerusalem, National Library of Israel, Fr. 95, fol. 85ᵇ): והשיבה המתילדת בלא עתה מחמת ריבוי הליחה הנולדה בקרב ובראש (Premature greying of the hair results from a surplus of phlegm originating in the stomach and the head). Hebr. קֶרֶב features in the current dictionaries in the general sense of 'inward part (of human body), entrails, intestines,' cf. BDB 899; JD 1411; BM 6149–6150; Low LXXVIII.

קָרוֹב · **specific; special**: Lat. *proprius* (Arab. أخصّ) · Constantinus Africanus, *Viaticum* · trans. Do'eg ha-Edomi, *Sefer Ya'ir Netiv*, bk. 1, ch. 14 (Ms Oxford, Bodleian Library, Can. Or. 26, fol. 234ᵃ): והעזר הקרוב אל החולי הזה (A medicine specific for this illness). Hebr. קָרוֹב does not feature in this sense in the current dictionaries. Moses ibn Tibbon renders the parallel Arabic term أخصّ as היותר מיוחד.

• **כח קרוב אליו** → כֹּחַ.

קָרַע · **to cut; to dissect**: Arab. شقّ (Gr. ἐντέμνω; UWS 1:360–361) · Maimonides, *Medical Aphorisms* 15.31 · trans. Zeraḥyah Ḥen (BMMZ 157): כשתהיה קורע הקרום הקרני יהיה תחלת מה שיפגושך הלחות הדק הרקיק ויהיה ניגר וזב והוא הלחות אשר הרבה פעמים אנו רואים שיגר ויצא מן הנקב אשר ינקב בעין אשר ימחט המים (If you dissect the horn-like tunic, the first thing you find is a fine and thin liquid streaming and pouring out. It is the moisture that you often see flowing out from the opening made in the eye that is being operated [on] for a cataract). In the sense of 'to cut, to dissect,' Hebr. קָרַע is a non-attested semantic borrowing from Arab. شقّ. Nathan ha-Me'ati translates Arab. شقّ as שָׁסַע (see entry [שסע]).

קַרְקָעִית · **bottom**: Arab. قعر · Isḥāq ibn 'Imrān, *Treatise on Melancholy* · trans. Anonymous, fol. 47ᵃ (48ᵃ): עד שמא אלו הרוחות שבהם המעיטו[296] המזון והדפוהו והוא כך מתחת האסטומ׳ לצד מעלה עד שלא תוכל לרדת ותדבק בקרקעיתה (Sometimes those winds [that

295 See also bk. 1, ch. 18 (Ms Jerusalem, National Library of Israel, Fr. 95 fol. 97ᵇ; Ms Florence, Biblioteca Medicina Laurenziana, Plut. 88.37, fol. 94ᵇ): על קרסי מוח הראש, where the term קרסי reflects Gr. dat. κράσει, pronounced as κράσι in the Middle Ages. In the anonymous adaptation (Ms Berlin, Staatsbibliothek Preußischer Kulturbesitz, Or. fol. 1058, fol. 90ᵃ) we find the same term as קראסיש.

296 המעיטו: قلبت a.

are in the intestines] return[297] the food that is in the bottom of the stomach by pushing it upward so that it cannot go down anymore and adhere to its bottom [i.e., of the stomach]). Hebr. קַרְקָעִית does not feature as a medical term in the current dictionaries. In their translations of Maimonides, *On the Regimen of Health* 1.8, Moses ibn Tibbon and Anonymous render Arab. قعر المعدة as תחתית האסטומכא/ההאצטומכא (BMR 156, 196).

קָשֶׁה • אֵם → אם קשה.

קֶשֶׁר • *Plur.* קשרים • **ligaments:** Lat. *ligamenta* (Arab. رباطات) · Constantinus Africanus, *Viaticum* · trans. Do'eg ha-Edomi, *Sefer Ya'ir Netiv*, bk. 2, ch. 19: השנים לפעמים נקובות או שבורות או צבעם מתחלף למכורכם או ירוק או שחור. וכל זה נולד מליחה רעה מהדבר הבלוי אשר ירוץ דרך הגידים אל קשרי השינים ברוע המאכלים הבאים באסטומכא (Teeth may be affected by cavities or fractures, their color may change to yellow, green, or black. All this originates from a bad superfluity of putrefied matter that streams through the nerves to the ligaments of the teeth. It is caused by the bad food that reaches the stomach). In the sense of 'ligaments,' Hebr. קשרים features in BCD 253 (NM 1:186) in a later attestation from Zeraḥyah Ḥen's translation of Maimonides, *Medical Aphorisms* 1.7 (BMMZ 16). Moses ibn Tibbon translates Arab. رباطات as מיתרים (cf. BCD 149 (NM 4:99)).

---

297 'return': Trans. after a.

ר

רֵאָה • נגעי הריאה → נֶגַע.

• צנורות הריאה → צִנּוֹר.

רְאוּת • כהות הראות → כֵּהוּת.

• מחשך הראות → מַחְשָׁךְ.

• מפסיד הראות בנטית השמש → [פסד].

ראֹשׁ • ראש המוח • the front part of the brain: Lat. *prora cerebri* (Arab. مقدّم الدماغ) · Constantinus Africanus, *Viaticum* · trans. Do'eg ha-Edomi, *Sefer Ya'ir Netiv*, bk. 1, ch. 22: והיא משלשת סבות: או מלחות לבנות או משחורות נולדות בראש המוח או מרוח קר (And it [i.e., epilepsy] is caused by [one of] three things, either because of phlegmatic superfluities or because of melancholic superfluities that originate in the front part of the brain or because of a cold wind). Hebr. ראש המוח does not feature in this sense in the current dictionaries. Moses ibn Tibbon translates Arab. مقدّم الدماغ as הקודם מהמוח.

• חולשת הראש → חֻלְשָׁה.

• עמידי הראש → עָמִיד.

• *Plur.* **ראשים • pods**: Arab. غلف · Isḥāq ibn ʿImrān, *Treatise on Melancholy* · trans. Anonymous, fol. 50[a] (51[a]): ראשי כשכאש (poppy pods). Hebr. *Sing.* ראֹשׁ, *Plur.* ראשים, does not feature in this sense in the current dictionaries. Constantine the African translates Arab. غلف as *cortices*.

רֹב • rob (i.e., fruit juice boiled down to syrup): Arab. ربّ · Ibn al-Jazzār, *Zād al-musāfir wa-qūt al-ḥādir* · trans. Moses ibn Tibbon, *Sefer Ṣedat ha-Derakhim*, bk. 3, ch. 1: וכאשר שככנו המותר הנוטה אל האבר במה שזכרנו נשתדל אז להתיך המותר ולהמס המורסא כמו שעשינו למעלה וזה כשיצוה החולה שיגרגר רב אגוז עם פליטרי או רב ענבים נקרא שפא ובער׳ מי בגתאג (Once we have repelled the superfluity that streams towards the organ with [the ingredients] I mentioned, we should try to dissolve the superfluity and tumor as we [mentioned] before, namely, by ordering the patient to gargle with a rob prepared from walnuts with pellitory or a rob of grapes [i.e., syrup] called ŠP' [read: ŚP'] and in Arabic MY BGT'G). In the sense of 'rob,' Hebr. רֹב, a loan word from Arab. ربّ, features in BM 6352 in attestations from Moshe Narboni (ca. 1300–1362 CE), *Sefer Oraḥ Ḥayyim*.[298] A regular Hebrew term used by Moses ibn Tibbon for Arab. ربّ is בשול יין (see entry בִּשּׁוּל).

• רב ענבים • (lit., rob of grapes); syrup: Arab. ميبختج (from Pers. مى پخته; cf. VL 2:1246: 'syrupus, et sec. al. vinum cum aliis medicamentis bullitum et defaecatum' (syrup, according to others wine boiled and purified with other medications) · Ibn al-Jazzār, *Zād al-musāfir wa-qūt al-ḥādir* · trans. Moses ibn Tibbon, bk. 3, ch. 1: וכאשר שככנו המותר היורד אל האבר במה שזכרנו נשתדל אז להתיך המותר ולהמס המורסא כמו שעשינו למעלה

298 On the author and the *Sefer Oraḥ Ḥayyim*, see Bos, 'R. Moshe Narboni,' 219–251.

וזה כשיצוה החולה שיגרגר רב אגוז עם פליטרי או רב ענבים נקרא שפא ובער׳ מי בגתאג (Once we have repelled the superfluity that streams towards the organ with [the ingredients] I mentioned, we should try to dissolve the superfluity and tumor as we [mentioned] before, namely, by ordering the patient to gargle with a rob prepared from walnuts with pellitory or a rob of grapes [i.e., syrup] called ŠP' [read: ŚP'][299] and in Arabic MY BGT'G). The term רב ענבים does not feature in the current dictionaries. In his glossary to the *Sefer ha-Qanun*, Nathan remarks: טלא הוא יין מבושל שלא נתערב וכשנתעבה נקרא מיבכתג׳ כלומר שפא או קרינו בלשון (ṬL'. This is unmixed boiled wine; when it is thickened it is called MYBKTǦ; i.e., ŠP' [read: ŚP'] or QRYNW in [Romance]); cf. NM 2:114, 140 (Ṭet 6)). In addition to רב ענבים, Moses ibn Tibbon translates Arab. ميبختج as יין מבושל (see entry יַיִן).

[רבה] • *Part. Pu'al* **מְרֻבֶּה** • **המרובה הרגלים** · **polypus**: Arab. الكثير الأرجل · Maimonides, *Medical Aphorisms* 23.74 · trans. Zeraḥyah Ḥen (BMMZ 227): המורסא אשר תתחדש בתוך האף וכאילו היא בשר נוסף הוא אשר נקרא נאסור ונקרא המרובה הרגלים. בשלישי מהמיאמיר (The tumor that forms inside the nose as if it were a fleshy excrescence is called *nāṣūr*[300] and also polypus. *Mayāmir* 3). Hebr. המרובה הרגלים is not attested for in the current dictionaries. Nathan ha-Me'ati translates Arab. الكثير الأرجل with the variant reading מַרְבֶּה רגלים. This reading features in BM 3305 in an attestation from Nathan ha-Me'ati's translation of this particular aphorism and in an earlier one from Solomon ibn Ayyub's Hebrew translation of Ibn Rushd's commentary on Ibn Sīnā's *'Urjūza*, which he completed in the year 1261. See also MD 589; EM 1672.

רַבָּה · **gum tragacanth (i.e., gum resin from some kinds of milkvetch [*Astragalus* sp. L.], e.g., gum tragacanth milkvetch [*Astragalus gummifer* Labill.], Cooper's milkvetch [*Astragalus neglectus* (Torr. & A. Gray) E. Sheld.])**: Arab. كثيرا (M 191; DT 3:21; LF 2:419 ff.) · a) Shem Tov ben Isaac, *Sefer ha-Shimmush*, bk. 29, list 1 (SHS 1:479 (Resh 1)): רבה ב״ה כתירא וב״ל דרגגנת ([Hebr.] *rabbah*; Arab. *kathıra*; vern. DRGGNT [i.e., O. Occ./O. Cat. *dragagan(t)*]). In the sense of 'tragacanth,' Hebr. רַבָּה is possibly an unattested calque from Arab. كثيرا.

b) *Shinnui ha-Shemot ha-Niqra'im Synonimis*, Ms Munich, Bayerische Staatsbibliothek, Cod. hebr. 8, fol. 199ª: כתירה הוא דראגגן ובלשונינו רבה ([Arab.] *kathīrā*; i.e., [Rom.] *dragagan*; [Hebr.] *rabbah*).

[רגל] *Hif'il* **הִרְגִּיל** · **to apply**: Lat. *uti* · Constantinus Africanus, *Viaticum* · trans. Do'eg ha-Edomi, *Sefer Ya'ir Netiv*, bk. 2, ch. 14: ולא ירגיל לישן מאד כי השינה פותחת הארובות (And he [i.e., someone suffering from a cold (coryza)] should not sleep [lit., apply sleeping] much because sleep opens the catarrhs [i.e., makes them flow]). In the sense

---

299 ŚP': I.e. Lat. *sapa*; cf. DMLBS 3283: 'new wine boiled down to a fraction of its original volume; b) (other beverage); c) moisture, sap.' See also entry שפא.

300 *nāṣūr* normally means 'fistula.'

of 'to apply,' Hebr. הִרְגִּיל features in BCD 257 (NM 1:114–115; 2:18–19) in later attestations only, a.o. from Hillel ben Samuel, *Sefer Keritut* and Shem Tov ben Isaac, *Sefer ha-Shimmush*, bk. 30. Moses ibn Tibbon translates the original Arabic term ويتباعد عن النوم الكثير as וירחיק רבוי השינה.

רֶגֶל • *Plur.* **רגלים** • **המרובה הרגלים** → [**רבה**].

רוּחַ • **הרוח החמוץ היוצא מן הגרון** ׳ **eructation:** Arab. جشاء · Ms Cambridge, T-S K14.48, P7 (verso): כראת ... מפסיק הרוח החמוץ היוצא מן הגרון (Leek stops eructation). Hebrew הרוח החמוץ היוצא מן הגרון does not feature in the current dictionaries

• **הרוח הנדחה** ׳ **eructation:** Lat. *ructatio* (Arab. جشاء) · Constantinus Africanus, *Viaticum* · trans. Do'eg ha-Edomi, *Sefer Ya'ir Netiv*, bk. 2, ch. 18 (Ms Oxford, Bodleian Library, Can. Or. 26, fol. 268b): גם כאב האסטומכ׳ והרוח הנדחה חמוץ אלה יורו כי החולי בו מליחות קרות (Stomach pain and sour eructation indicate that the illness [i.e., toothache] is caused by cold humors). Hebr. הרוח הנדחה does not feature in the current dictionaries. In addition to this term, Do'eg ha-Edomi translates the Latin variant *eructatio* as הרוח הנדחה מהגרון (see next entry). Moses ibn Tibbon translates Arab. جشاء as קבסא (cf. BCD 236 (NM 3:198)) and Shem Tov ben Isaac as געש in the *Sefer ha-Shimmush*, bk. 27 (cf. BCD 48 (NM 4:33–34)).

• **הרוח הנדחה מהגרון** ׳ **eructation:** Lat. *eructatio* (Arab. جشاء) · Constantinus Africanus, *Viaticum* · trans. Do'eg ha-Edomi, *Sefer Ya'ir Netiv*, bk. 3, ch. 14: אם הוא עשוי בכל הגוף נראה בכל האברים עיפות וכובד ואם הוא מהאסטומ׳ יתראו תמיד כל היום תמונות לנגד עיניו והרוח הנדחה מהגרון והאיסטניסות והכאב במצח אם הוא מהמעים יהיה כובד ונפח לבעלי השחורה והחורפה לבעלי האדומה (If the whole body [is full with superfluous matter], we observe that all the limbs of [someone suffering from fainting] are tired and heavy; if [only] the stomach [is full], he will see images in front of his eyes the whole day long and he will [suffer] from eructation, vomiting, and headache. If the intestines [are full of] melancholic matter, the patient will suffer from heaviness and swellings; if they [are full of] bilious matter, he will suffer from gripes). Hebr. הרוח הנדחה מהגרון does not feature in the current dictionaries. In addition to this term, Do'eg ha-Edomi translates the Latin variant *ructatio* as הרוח הנדחה (see previous entry). Moses ibn Tibbon translates Arab. جشاء as קבסא (cf. BCD 236 (NM 3:198)).

• **רוח הנפש** ׳ **the spiritual pneuma:** Arab. الروح النفسانية · Ibn al-Jazzār, *Zād al-musāfir wa-qūt al-ḥāḍir* · trans. Abraham ben Isaac, *Sefer Ṣedah la-Oreḥim*, bk. 1, ch. 22 (Ms Florence, Biblioteca Medicina Laurenziana, Plut. 88.37, fol. 96b): על כי יוולד מאחד מאילו האיברים הכימוס הרע ומהרתחתו הבל ועשן עב שיעלה בגידים הדקים אל המוח ומרוב עוביו יסתום שבילי רוח הנפש (When in one of these organs a bad chyme originates and boils, a thick vapor ascends via the nerves to the brain. Through its thickness it obstructs the channels of the spiritual pneuma). Hebr. רוח הנפש is not attested for in the current dictionaries. Moses ibn Tibbon translates Arab. الروح النفسانية as הרוח הנפשיי. The latter is the current term for 'spiritual pneuma' in medieval philosophical literature (cf. KTP 4:26; BM 6493; KDS 106). Do'eg ha-Edomi translates the parallel Latin term *spiritus animans* as רוח האדם.

• זרות הרוח → **זָרוּת**.

• כלי הרוח → **כְּלִי**.

רוּחָנִי • האברים הרוחניים → **אֵבֶר**.

רוֹחֵץ (*Part.*) → **רָחַץ**.

רוטא • שרף רוטא מדברית → **שְׂרָף**.

רוך → **רֹךְ**.

רוֹעֶה • מזמר הרועה → **מזמר**.

[רוץ] • רָץ · to flow; to stream: Lat. *discurro* (Arab. جرى) · Constantinus Africanus, *Viaticum* · trans. Do'eg ha-Edomi, *Sefer Ya'ir Netiv*, bk. 1, ch. 22: והאיפלמסיא שכינה אל האפופלקשיא כי המקום ההוא עצמו והטבע מאשר נולדת הוא קר וגס אבל האיפופלקשיא תגזול כל הכח הרץ באברים (Epilepsy is closely related to apoplexy because [both originate from] that same place and the matter [i.e., bodily fluid] from which they originate is cold and coarse. The only [difference] is, that apoplexy takes away all the power that flows to the nerves). In the sense of 'to flow,' Hebr. רָץ is a non-attested semantic borrowing from Lat. *discurro*, which, in the same sense, is a non-attested borrowing from Arab. جرى. Moses ibn Tibbon translates the Arabic term as הלך and Abraham ben Isaac as נע והתנודד.

רושה • טפה רושה → **טִפָּה**.

[רחב] • *Inf. Hif'il* **הַרְחִיב • הרחיב הטבע · to soften the stools; to purge the bowels**: Arab. إحدار الطبيعة · Ibn al-Jazzār, *Zād al-musāfir wa-qūt al-ḥādir* · trans. Moses ibn Tibbon, *Sefer Ṣedat ha-Derakhim*, bk. 3, ch. 12: וישמר מהרחיב הטבע בכמו החולי הזה אלא בעת הצורך כי הוא פעמים יבוא מעצמו ושיקשה מעצמו (One should take care not to soften the stools in this kind of illness [i.e., pleurisy] unless when it is necessary, because sometimes they become soft by themselves and sometimes hard). Hebr. הרחיב הטבע is not attested for in the current dictionaries. Do'eg ha-Edomi translates Lat. *mollicies naturae* as הרחבת התולדת (see entry הַרְחָבָה).

• *Part. Hif'il* **מַרְחִיב · laxative**: Lat. *laxativus* (Arab. مسهّل) · Constantinus Africanus, *Viaticum* · trans. Do'eg ha-Edomi, *Sefer Ya'ir Netiv*, bk. 3, ch. 14: וכאשר יהיה אפיסת הלב כענין זה יאות לראות אם יהיה המלוי בכל הגוף ונתן לו קטרטיק וכל דבר שיסיר מעליו השפע ההוא כמו אוקשימל מליקרט אוקשימל מרחיב (When the fainting is as I have said, one should look whether the whole body is congested and [if that is the case] one should give the patient a cathartic medicine and any other medicine that removes the superfluous matter, such as oxymel, honey water, laxative oxymel …). Hebr. מַרְחִיב is not attested for in this sense in the current dictionaries. Moses ibn Tibbon translates Arab. مسهّل as משלשל.

רִחוּץ · cleansing; rinsing: Arab. جلاء · Maimonides, *Medical Aphorisms* 13.6 · trans. Zeraḥyah Ḥen (BMMZ 143): אמר משה: ראוי שתהיה הרחיצה הזאת אחר כלות פעולת הרפואה קודם התפרנסו במרק התרנגול כדי שלא יתערב עם המזון אותו שנשאר מהרפואה המשלשלת

אשר נשאר מהרפואה ויחריב[301] האסטומכא. וראוי שתהיה הרחיצה בדברים שיהיה בהם דבקות בלטין וויסקוזיטטי וריחוץ ולחלוח (Says Moses: This rinsing should be done after the effect of the purgative has worn off but before the intake of soup of young chickens, so that the food does not mix with the residue of the purgative in the lining[302] of the stomach. The rinsing should be done with a viscous substance, Lat. *viscositate*, that has a cleansing and moistening effect). Hebrew רִחוּץ features in BM 6527 in the sense of 'ablution' in an attestation from Rabbinic literature only; see also EM 1703. Nathan ha-Me'ati translates Arab. جلاء as מרוק.

רָחַץ · **to clean**: Arab. غسل (Gr. πλύνω; cf. UW 539–540; UWS 2:141) · Ibn al-Jazzār, *Zād al-musāfir wa-qūt al-ḥādir* · trans. Moses ibn Tibbon, *Sefer Ṣedat ha-Derakhim*, bk. 3, ch. 7: תואר לחיכה תקנה אסחק בן סלימן למי שיש בו שעול מבעלי הסל וכש"כ כשיהיה בשעול שלהם ירידות ירדו אל חזיהם ויולידו בהם ליחות עבות דבקות צריכות אל מה שינקה אותם וירחצם וכבר נסיתיה ושבחתיה (Recipe of a linctus that was prepared by Isḥāq ibn Sulaymān [al-Isrā'īlī] for someone who suffers from phtisis and cough, especially when the cough comes with catarrhs that descend to the chest and produce thick, viscous humors that need [a remedy] that purifies and cleans them. I have tried it and found it to be good). In the sense of 'to clean,' Hebr. רָחַץ features in BM 6547 in a later attestation from the *Qibbuṣei Galenus*, the Hebrew translation of Galenic summaries by Shimshon ben Shlomo, written in 1322.

• *Part.* **רוֹחֵץ • הסם הרוחץ → סַם.**

[רחק] • *Hif'il* **הִרְחִיק מן • הרחיק מן** · **to abstain from**: Lat. *abstineo* (Arab. احتمى عن) · Constantinus Africanus, *Viaticum* · trans. Do'eg ha-Edomi, *Sefer Ya'ir Netiv*, bk. 2, ch. 23: וירחיק מכל מיני דגים גם מכל בשר (And he [i.e., someone suffering from bad breath] should abstain from all kinds of fish and meat). Hebr. הרחיק מן features in BM 6553 as synonymous with התרחק מן in the sense of 'to remove oneself from, to keep away from' with attestations from Rabbinic literature. Moses ibn Tibbon translates Arab. احتمى عن as נשמר מן.

ריאה → רֵאָה.

ריחוץ → רִחוּץ.

ריקוח → רִקּוּחַ.

רֵיקָנוּת · **emptiness**: Arab. استفراغ · Ibn al-Jazzār, *Zād al-musāfir wa-qūt al-ḥādir* · trans. Abraham ben Isaac, *Sefer Ṣedah la-Oreḥim*, bk. 1, ch. 24: החולי הזה נקרא כוזאז הוא ניענוע יקרה בלא רצון בגידים המתנענעים ברצון ויבוא מחמת מילואי האיברים שיש בהם גידים דקים או מן ריקנותם והוא על שלשה עניינים (The illness called [in Arab.] *kuzāz* [i.e., spasms] consists of involuntary motions of organs that are [normally] moved voluntarily. They occur either because of repletion of the organs that have nerves or because they

301 ויחריב: في خمل a.
302 'lining': Trans. after a.

are empty. There are three types of [this illness]). Hebr. רֵיקָנוּת features in the current dictionaries with attestations from Rabbinic literature, from Tuviah ha-Kohen, *Maʿaseh Tuviah*, and from modern Hebrew literature (cf. JD 1477; BM 6584; EM 1713). Moses ibn Tibbon translates Arab. استفراغ as הרקה. The same Hebrew term is used by Do'eg ha-Edomi for Lat. *inanitio*.

רִיר · **mucilage**: Lat. *viscum* (Arab. رغوة) · Constantinus Africanus, *Viaticum* · trans. Do'eg ha-Edomi, *Sefer Ya'ir Netiv*, bk. 3, ch. 2 וכאשר יבקע הנפח יאות לתת לו אודם ביצה אין מבושל עם אמידום דרגאגן ושמן ויאולד ריר זרע חבושים וארנולוגשא (When the tumor bursts, one should give [the patient] fresh egg yolk with starch, gum tragacanth, violet oil, mucilage of quince seed, and plantain). In the sense of 'mucilage,' Hebr. רִיר features in BCD 262 (NM 1:68) in a later attestation from Moses ibn Tibbon's *Sefer Ṣedat ha-Derakhim*.

רֹךְ · **softness**: Lat. *mollities* (Arab. شدّة استرخائه) · Constantinus Africanus, *Viaticum* · trans. Do'eg ha-Edomi, *Sefer Ya'ir Netiv*, bk. 2, ch. 17: ואל קרירות ולחות מהצמח אשר יורה הלובן והרוך ניתן לו ג׳ירא פורטישימא[303] טריאקה מנגנא (If the tumor is cold and moist—which is indicated by whiteness and softness of the tongue—we administer [the patient] a very strong hiera, [i.e.,] the great theriac). Hebr. רֹךְ is not attested for in medieval medical literature; cf. BM 6587. Moses ibn Tibbon translates Arab. شدّة استرخائه as חוזק רפיון.

[רכך] • *Piʿel* **רִכֵּךְ** · **to rub; to anoint**: Arab. مرخ · Ibn al-Jazzār, *Zād al-musāfir wa-qūt al-ḥādir* · trans. Abraham ben Isaac, *Sefer Ṣedah la-Oreḥim*, bk. 1, ch. 23: גם יועיל לחולי אל כוזאז ולריפיון הגידין הדקין ולחולי הפלג אם ישחוק פילטרו בשמן וירככו בו המקום (Also beneficial for the illness [called in Arab.] *al-kuzāz* [i.e., spasms], looseness of the nerves, and hemiplegia, is pulverized pellitory [mixed] with oil and applied as an ointment to the affected spot). Hebr. רִכֵּךְ features in the current dictionaries in the sense of 'to soften, mollify' with attestations from medieval literature (cf. EM 1717). Moses ibn Tibbon translates Arab. مرخ as משח.

[רעד] • *Part Nifʿal* **נִרְעָד** · **frightening; terrible**: Lat. *terribilis* (Arab. مهوّل) · Constantinus Africanus, *Viaticum* · trans. Do'eg ha-Edomi, *Sefer Ya'ir Netiv*, bk. 1, ch. 18: ובעלות החולי עד מעלתו העליונה יסבול החולה מקרים נרעדים כמו צמאון רב ויבשות גם שחרות הפה נחור הלשון (When the disease reaches its climax, the patient suffers from frightening symptoms, such as severe thirst, dryness, blackness of the mouth, roughness of the tongue ...). Hebr. נִרְעָד is not attested for in this sense in the current dictionaries. Moses ibn Tibbon renders the parallel Arabic term مهوّل as מפחיד and Abraham ben Isaac as רע.

• **הדפק הנרעד** → **דֹּפֶק**.

• *Part Hitpaʿel* • **מִתְרַעֵד** • **הדפק המתרעד** → **דֹּפֶק**.

303 פורטישימא: *fortissima* L.

רַעַד · **shaking**: Arab. ارتعاد · Maimonides, *Medical Aphorisms* 23.92 · trans. Zeraḥyah Ḥen (BMMZ 229): כשיהיו המותרות המזיקות לטבע לחות ידחם הכח הדוחה בזה הרעד החזק אשר יהיה בדפק[304] או בשעול וישובו אל כל המקומות אשר מטבעם שתקבלם (If the superfluities that are harmful for nature are moist, the expulsive faculty eliminates them by the severe and violent shaking, which happens during a rigor[305] or cough, and then they go to all the sites that have the property to receive them). Hebr. רַעַד features in the current dictionaries with attestations from the Bible (KB 1259), Rabbinic literature (BM 6641), and modern literature (EM 1727) in the sense of 'quivering, quaking, trembling' only. In the sense of 'twitching of muscles and their tendons' (for Arab. اختلاج), the term features in BCD 263 (NM 4:196) in an attestation from Moses ibn Tibbon, *Sefer Ṣedat ha-Derakhim*, bk. 1, ch. 24. Nathan ha-Me'ati translates Arab. ارتعاد as התנועעות (BMMN 230).

רַעְיָא (*Aram.*) • **אבובא דרעיא** → **אֲבוּבָא**.

רַעְיוֹן · **reflection; rational thought; reason**: Arab. فكر · Isḥāq ibn 'Imrān, *Treatise on Melancholy* · trans. Anonymous, fol. 41[b] (42[b]):[306] וזה החולי שמא יהיה בכל הגוף או שמא יהיה במזג המוח עצמו כשיהיה בטבעו יבש ויהיו כוחותיו המנהיגים אותו והם כח הדמיון וכח הרעיון וכח הזכרון חלשים (This illness [i.e., melancholy] can either be in the whole body or in the temperament of the brain itself when its nature is dry. Then the faculties that rule over it, i.e., the imaginative faculty, the reflective faculty, and the memorative faculty, are weakened). Hebr. רַעְיוֹן features in medieval philosophical literature in the sense of 'imagination' (as opposite to strict rational thinking) (cf. KD 4:46–47; EP 110). Constantine the African translates Arab. فكر as *ratio*.

רעימה • **רעימת פנים** · **contraction, contortion of the face**: Arab. قطوب الوجه (cf. Lane 2541: 'frowning or contracting the face, and looking sternly, austerely, or morosely') · Shem Tov ben Isaac, *Sefer ha-Shimmush*, bk. 29, list 1 (SHS 1:486 (Resh 14)): רעימת פנים ב"ה קטוב אלוג'ה (*re'imat panim*; Arab. *quṭūb al-wajh*). Hebrew רעימת פנים, derived from Biblical Hebrew and not attested for in secondary literature, was possibly coined by Shem Tov ben Isaac on the basis of the expression in Ez 27:35: רעמו פנים (Their faces contorted) (cf. KB 1267: 'to be troubled').

[רעם] • *Part. Hitpa'el* **מִתְרַעֵם** • **מתרעם מן הכבד** · **suffering from a liver disease**: Arab. مكبود · Ibn al-Jazzār, *Zād al-musāfir wa-qūt al-ḥādir* · trans. Moses ibn Tibbon, *Sefer Ṣedat ha-Derakhim*, bk. 3, ch. 6: תואר בשול מועיל למי שהיה בו שעול או כמישות והיה עם זה מתרעם מן הכבד (Recipe of a decoction that is good for someone suffering from cough

---

304 בדפק (في النبض): في النافض a.

305 'rigor': Trans. after a.

306 The same term features on fol. 46[a] (47[a]): הכחות השכליות והם שלש כח הדמיון וכח הרעיון וכח הזכרון (The three rational faculties: imagination, reflection [i.e., reason], and memory), and on fol. 48[a] (49[a]) it features as כח הרעיון והמחשבה.

or emaciation while he also suffers from a liver disease). Hebr. *Hitpaʿel* הִתְרַעֵם only features in the current dictionaries in the sense of 'to complain about' (cf. BM 6657–6658).

[רפא] • *Part. Nifʿal* **נִרְפָּא** • **הנרפאין מחליים** · **convalescents**: Arab. الناقهون من الأمراض · Isḥāq ibn ʿImrān, *Treatise on Melancholy* · trans. Anonymous, fol. 51ᵇ (52ᵇ): כמו שיצטרכו לזה גופי החולי היבש וכל חי[307] הגוף והנרפאין מחליים (As this is needed by those suffering from phthisis, by those whose body is emaciated,[308] and by convalescents). Hebr. *Sing.* הנרפא מחליי, *Plur.* הנרפאין מחליים, does not feature in the current dictionaries. The synonym הנמלט מחליי features in Nathan ha-Me'ati's translation of Maimonides, *Medical Aphorisms* 3.71 (BMMN 50; cf. BCD 151 (NM 2:67)).

רְפוּאָה • **רפואה לבבית** · **a remedy that is good for the heart**: Arab. دواء قلبي · Maimonides, *Medical Aphorisms* 13.6 · trans. Zeraḥyah Ḥen (BMMZ 144): והיא רפואה לבבית כמו כן ובצאת זה מהאסטומכא יקח המרק ואם מצא צמא ישים במקום זרע ההדס זרע השיליאו (Moreover, it [i.e., the compond mentioned before] is a remedy that is good for the heart. Once this [compound medicine] leaves the stomach, eat the soup; and if the myrtle seed causes thirst, take fleawort seed instead). Hebr. רפואה לבבית does not feature in the current dictionaries. In a medical sense, the term לבבי features in MD 184, s.v. 'cordial.' Ben-Yehuda (BM 2602; cf. EM 790) mentions the term לבבי in an attestation from the *Sefer Nofet Zufim*, composed by Judah Messer Leon. Nathan ha-Me'ati translates Arab. دواء قلبي as רפואה ליבית.

• **הרפואה המדביקה** · **the remedy that closes a wound with flesh**: Arab. الدواء الملحم (cf. MMT 245, s.v. الدواء الملحّم: 'remedy making flesh grow, promoting cicatrization') · Maimonides, *Medical Aphorisms* 15.56 · trans. Nathan ha-Me'ati (BMMN 163): הרפואה המדביקה ראוי שתהיה יותר חזקת הנגוב מהמצמיחה הבשר ושלא יהיה בה מרוק ונקוי כמו שיצטרך לזה המצמיחה הבשר אבל יהיה המדביקה קובצת (A remedy that closes a wound with flesh should be more drying than a remedy that makes the flesh grow and does not need the same cleansing and purifying action as a remedy that makes the flesh grow. Rather, a remedy that makes the flesh grow should be astringent). Hebr. הרפואה המדביקה does not feature in the current dictionaries. A variant reading הסם המדבק features in BCD 188 (NM 4:125) in the sense of 'the agglutinant remedy' (for Lat. *inviscativa medicina*) in an attestation from the anonymous *Sefer ha-Refuʾot ha-Libbiyot*. The *Hifʿil* הִדְבִּיק (for Arab. ألحم) features in BCD 53 (NM 2:36) in an attestation from Nathan ha-Me'ati's translation of *Medical Aphorisms* 15.17 (BMMN 156) in the sense of 'to cause to heal up;' for הִדְבִּיק in the sense of 'to apply' (for Arab. ألزق) or 'to make something thick, viscous, adhesive' (for Arab. لزّج) see entry [דבק]. Zeraḥyah Ḥen translates Arab. الدواء الملحم as הרפואה המעלה הבשר (see entry below).

---

307 חי הגוף: المهازيل a.
308 'emaciated': Trans. after a.

• **הרפואה המחליקה** · **the softening remedy**: Arab. الدواء الملين (cf. MMT 245) · Maimonides, *Medical Aphorisms* 21.64 · trans. Zeraḥyah Ḥen (BMMZ 201): הרופאים יקראו הרפואה המחליקה על כל מה שיחליק הגוף הקשה אשר נתקשה בעבור הקרירות וכל שכן בהיות באותם הגופות לחות כלוא ועצור כמו שהוא במורסות הקשות (The physicians apply the name 'softening remedy' to all that which softens hard bodies, whose hardness was caused by cold, especially if moisture is retained in these bodies, as in the case of a hard tumor). Hebr. הרפואה המחליקה does not feature in the current dictionaries. A variant reading הסם המחליק features in BCD 188 (NM 4:125) in the sense of 'the mollifacient remedy' (for Lat. *lenificativa*) in an attestation from the anonymous *Sefer ha-Refu'ot ha-Libbiyot*. Nathan ha-Me'ati translates Arab. الدواء الملين as הרפואה המרככת.

• **הרפואה המטהרת** · **the clearing medicine**: Arab. الدواء الجلاء · Maimonides, *Medical Aphorisms* 23.100 · trans. Zeraḥyah Ḥen (BMMZ 230): הרפואה המכבסת והמטהרת היא אשר יסיר הלכלוך משטח הנקבים והפורי כמו הדבש וקמח הלופיני והשעורים והפולין והכרסנה והרבה מהזרעים (A cleansing and clearing medicine uproots sordidness from the outer layer of the openings and pores, such as honey, white lupine flour, barley, beans, bitter vetch, and a large number of seeds). Hebr. הרפואה המטהרת does not feature in the current dictionaries. The *Pi'el* טִהֵר features in BM 1849 in an attestation from Ibn Ezra's commentary on Ec 12:3 in the sense of 'to clean the body from internal superfluities.' Nathan ha-Me'ati translates Arab. الدواء الجلاء as הסם הממרק (see entry סַם).

• **הרפואה המכבסת** · **the cleansing medicine**: Arab. الدواء الغسال · Maimonides, *Medical Aphorisms* 23.100 · trans. Zeraḥyah Ḥen (BMMZ 230): הרפואה המכבסת והמטהרת היא אשר יסיר הלכלוך משטח הנקבים והפורי כמו הדבש וקמח הלופיני והשעורים והפולין והכרסנה והרבה מהזרעים (A cleansing and clearing medicine uproots sordidness from the outer layer of the pores and openings, such as honey, lupine flour, barley, beans, bitter vetch and a large number of seeds). Hebr. הרפואה המכבסת is not attested for in the current dictionaries. The *Pi'el* כִּבֵּס features in BM 2247 in the sense of 'cleansing the intestines with a clyster' in an attestation from the *Sefer ha-Kibbusim*. Nathan ha-Me'ati translates Arab. الدواء الغسال as הסם הרוחץ (see entry סַם).

• **הרפואה המעלה הבשר** · **the remedy that closes a wound with flesh**: Arab. الدواء الملحم (cf. DKT 245, s.v. الدواء الملحم: 'remedy making flesh grow, promoting cicatrization') · Maimonides, *Medical Aphorisms* 15.56 · trans. Zeraḥyah Ḥen (BMMZ 161): הרפואה המעלה הבשר ראוי שתהיה יותר מיבשת מהמצמיחה הבשר ולא יהיה בה ניקוי וריחוץ כמו שיצטרך לזה המצמיח הבשר אבל יהיה המעלה בשר מקבץ (A remedy that closes a wound with flesh should be more drying than a remedy that makes the flesh grow and does not need the same cleansing and purifying action as a remedy that makes the flesh grow. Rather, a remedy that makes the flesh grow should be astringent). Hebr. הרפואה המעלה הבשר does not feature in the current dictionaries. Nathan ha-Me'ati translates Arab. الدواء الملحم as הרפואה המדביקה (see entry above).

רְפָפוּת ‣ **twitching; palpitation:** Arab. اختلاج (Lane 783; cf. UWS 2:406, s.v. σφακελισμός (cf. LSG 1738: in gen.: 'spasm, convulsion')) · Shem Tov ben Isaac, *Sefer ha-Shimmush*, bk. 29, list 1 (SHS 1:485–486 (Resh 12)): רפפות ב"ה אכתלאג' (*refafut*; Arab. *ikhtilāj*). As an abstract noun, Hebr. רְפָפוּת features (for Arab. اختلاج) in BCD 266 (NM 1:188–189) in a later attestation from Zeraḥyah Ḥen's translation of Maimonides, *Medical Aphorisms* 7.40 (BMMZ 81). The regular term is Hebr. *Sing.* רְפָפָה, *Plur.* רְפָפוֹת (cf. BM 6689). The term רְפָפָה is particularly prevalent in medieval magical literature for the art of 'palmomancy,' i.e., the art of prognostication from twitchings in the limbs, called اختلاج in Arabic.

רֶפֶשׁ ‣ **humor:** Arab. خلط · Ibn al-Jazzār, *Zād al-musāfir wa-qūt al-ḥādir* · trans. Abraham ben Isaac, *Sefer Ṣedah la-Oreḥim*, bk. 1, ch. 9 (Ms Jerusalem, National Library of Israel, Fr. 95, fol. 88ᵇ): אם ירבו הכינים גם אל[309] ציבה שבראש ושאר הגוף ויהיה זה מחמת רפש רע מעופש תדחה אותו אל טביעה בין העור ובין הבשר (If lice and nits often appear on the head as well as on other parts of the body, and this happens because of a bad and putrid humor, which nature expels from [between] the skin and the flesh). Hebr. רֶפֶשׁ features in BM 6691 in the sense of 'mud, soiling' only. Moses ibn Tibbon translates Arab. خلط as ליחה.

• *Plur.* **רפשים** ‣ **superfluities:** Arab. فضول · Ibn al-Jazzār, *Zād al-musāfir wa-qūt al-ḥādir* · trans. Abraham ben Isaac, *Sefer Ṣedah la-Oreḥim*, bk. 1, ch. 5 (Ms Jerusalem, National Library of Israel, Fr. 95, fol. 86ᵃ–86ᵇ): והשני כאשר יעלה ההבל חד של רפשי[310] ארבע יסודות (The second [cause of dandruff is] a sharp vapor that arises from the superfluities of the four humors [to the brain]). In addition to רפשים, Abraham ben Isaac translates Arab. *Sing.* فضل as יְסוֹד (see entry). Moses ibn Tibbon translates Arab. فضول as מותרות.

רְקוּחַ ‣ **I. dye:** Arab. خضاب · Ibn al-Jazzār, *Zād al-musāfir wa-qūt al-ḥādir* · trans. Abraham ben Isaac, *Sefer Ṣedah la-Oreḥim*, bk. 1, ch. 4: ריקוח אחר להשחיר השיער ([Composition of] another dye for making the hair black). Hebr. רְקוּחַ is attested for in the Bible (BDB 955) and Piyyut literature (EM 1744) in the sense of 'perfumery, unguent,' in Rabbinic literature in the sense of 'perfume' (JD 1477), and in modern literature in the sense of 'fruit preserve, concoction' (EM 1744). Moses ibn Tibbon translates Arab. خضاب as צביעה.

‣ **II. liniment:** Arab. طلاء · Ibn al-Jazzār, *Zād al-musāfir wa-qūt al-ḥādir* · trans. Abraham ben Isaac, *Sefer Ṣedah la-Oreḥim*, bk. 1, ch. 6: וזה ריקוח אחר יועיל לחולי זה (Another liniment beneficial for this affliction). Moses ibn Tibbon translates Arab. طلاء as טיחה.

---

309 אל ציבה: الصئبان a.

310 רפשי: emendation editor רשפי Ms.

‣ III. **powder**: Arab. ذرور · Ibn al-Jazzār, *Zād al-musāfir wa-qūt al-ḥādir* · trans. Abraham ben Isaac, *Sefer Ṣedah la-Oreḥim*, bk. 1, ch. 8: וישקו לנער מריקות זה כי זה יועיל לאל סעפה (Or administer to the child the following powder beneficial for cradle cap ...). Moses ibn Tibbon translates Arab. ذرور as אבק.

‣ IV. **recipe**: Arab. نسخة · Ibn al-Jazzār, *Zād al-musāfir wa-qūt al-ḥādir* · trans. Abraham ben Isaac, *Sefer Ṣedah la-Oreḥim*, bk. 1, ch. 10: ואם תרצה לנקותך פעמיים בשנה בזה המשקה בניסן ובתשרי הוסף בריקוחם חלק אחד מסקמוניאה (If you want to cleanse [your head] with this potion twice a year, in Nisan and Tishri, add one part of scammony to the recipe ...). Moses ibn Tibbon translates Arab. نسخة as נסחה.

‣ V. **stomachic**: Arab. جوارش · Ibn al-Jazzār, *Zād al-musāfir wa-qūt al-ḥādir* · trans. Abraham ben Isaac, *Sefer Ṣedah la-Oreḥim*, bk. 1. ch. 14: ואם ישתה במים מן בושם הנקר׳ בלאדור יחיד חצי שקל 〈במים〉 יועיל לשכחה ויחזיק הגירסא ויאכל ריקוח הפלפלין (If one takes from the ingredient called 'marking nut' [*Semecarpus anacardium* L.] half a *shekel* with water, it is good for forgetfulness, it strengthens memory. One may also use the pepper stomachic). Moses ibn Tibbon translates Arab. جوارش as מרקחת; this term is also used by him for Arab. معجون ('electuary'); cf. BCD 163 (NM 4:107).

‣ VI. **recipe; composition**: Arab. صفة[311] · Ibn al-Jazzār, *Zād al-musāfir wa-qūt al-ḥādir* · trans. Abraham ben Isaac, *Sefer Ṣedah la-Oreḥim*, bk. 1, ch. 17: וזה ריקוח מרדים בשינה מעשה יצחק בן עמראן (This is the recipe [i.e., composition] of a soporific composed by Isḥāq ibn ʿImrān). Moses ibn Tibbon translates Arab. صفة as תואר. The term רִקּוּחַ is used by him for Arab. تأليف ('composition (of a remedy)'); cf. BCD 267 (NM 1:68).

‣ VII. **salve**: Arab. لطوخ · Ibn al-Jazzār, *Zād al-musāfir wa-qūt al-ḥādir* · trans. Abraham ben Isaac, *Sefer Ṣedah la-Oreḥim*, bk. 1, ch. 23: וזה מעשה ריקוח מספר יונס[312] יועיל למי שיבש חציו מן הקרירות והוא מנוסה (Recipe of a salve from the book by Paul,[313] beneficial for persons suffering from dryness of one side [of the body] resulting from coldness. It has been tested). Moses ibn Tibbon translates Arab. لطوخ as טיחה (cf. BCD 112 (NM 1:58)). Do'eg ha-Edomi translates Lat. *oleum* as משיחה.

• *Plur.* **ריקוחים** ‣ **medicines**: Lat. *antidotum* · Constantinus Africanus, *Viaticum* · trans. Do'eg ha-Edomi, *Sefer Ya'ir Netiv*, bk. 1, ch. 10 (Ms Oxford, Bodleian Library, Can. Or. 26, fol. 229b): אחרי זה נסדר הריקוחים הנאותים לזה (Later on I will make a list of the medicines that are good for this [i.e., headache caused by cold weather]).

[רקח] • *Part. Puʿal* **מְרֻקָּח** • **סיד מרוקח** → **סִיד**.

---

311 In addition to רִקּוּחַ, Abraham ben Isaac translates Arab. صفة as מַעֲשֶׂה (see entry).

312 יונס: بولس a.

313 Trans. after a; meant is Paul of Aegina.

ש

שׂאוֹר • מי שאור ← מַיִם

[שדל] • *Inf. Hitpaʿel* הִשְׁתַּדֵּל · **brooding:** Arab. إجالة · Isḥāq ibn ʿImrān, *Treatise on Melancholy* · trans. Anonymous, fol. 44ª (45ª): והם קרובים מן אלהוסואס אלסודאוי לרוב השתדלם וחשבם (They are close to [suffer from] melancholic delusion because of their constant [i.e., intense] brooding and thinking). Hebr. הִשְׁתַּדֵּל does not feature in this sense in the current dictionaries.

שׁוּם • שום מדברי · **water germander** [*Teucrium scordium* L.] · *Shinnui ha-Shemot ha-Niqra'im Synonimi*, Ms Florence, Bibliotheca Laurenziana, Or. 17, fol. 68ᵇ: איסקורדיאון הוא שום מדברי ובלשונם אסקורדיאו (ʾYSQWRDYʾWN [i.e., Arab. *išqurdiyūn*], i.e., ŠWM MDBRY [lit., wild garlic], and in their language [i.e., Rom.] ʾSQWRDYʾW). Hebr. שום מדברי is a non-attested loan translation of Arab. *thūm barrī* (ثوم برّي), a synonym of *išqurdiyūn* (إشقرديون); cf. SHS 1:515–516 (Shin 16); MIG 45.

שׁוֹק · **fibrous top of garlic:** Lat. *resta* (DMLBS 3158, s.v. 'restis') · Guillaume de Congenis, *Treatise on Surgery* · trans. Isaiah, fol. 56b: ולסרטן[314] ולפישטולא: קח זרניך ירוק הנחשת איירמן שליימא קרן איל שרוף עצם ארנבת שרוף צואת אדם שרופה שוק השומים שרוף (Against cancer and fistulas: Take orpiment,[315] verdigris, vitriol, rock salt, burnt horn of a ram, burnt bone of a hare, burnt human feces, burnt fibrous top of garlic …). Hebr. שׁוֹק does not feature in this sense in the current dictionaries.

שחורה ← שְׁחֹרָה.

שְׁחֹרָה • חלי השחורה ← חֳלִי.

שְׁחַרְחֹר • האדומה השחרחורת ← אֲדָמָה.

שִׂיחָה • שיחת הנפש · **affections of the soul (i.e., emotions):**[316] Arab. الأحداث النفسانية · Isḥāq ibn ʿImrān, *Treatise on Melancholy* · trans. Anonymous, fol. 41ᵇ–42ª (42ᵇ–43ª): ואלו הן הששה שהגוף צריך אליהם: השינה והתעורה התנועה וההשקט ההרקה והמלוי והמאכל והמשתה והאויר הסובב הנה בנשימה ושיחת הנפש (These are the six things [i.e., *sex res non naturales*] which the body needs: sleep and waking, movement and rest, evacuation and repletion, food and drink, the surrounding air that is inhaled, affections of the soul). Hebr. שיחת הנפש is not attested for in the current dictionaries. Constantine the African translates Arab. الأحداث النفسانية as *accidentia animae*.

[שים] • שם באפיו · **to apply a sternutatory:** Arab. سعّط · Ibn al-Jazzār, *Zād al-musāfir wa-qūt al-ḥāḍir*, trans. Abraham ben Isaac, *Sefer Ṣedah la-Oreḥim*, bk. 1, ch. 17: ואם הערות מיובש מרה שחורה אז נריק לו על ראשו מים מרותחין עם כמומילון ואכליל אל מלך הוא עשב סוריצילה וקליפת כשכאש ואניטו וזרע מלווא ודומ׳ ויגלח ראשו וימשחנו מחלב נשים או חלב

---

314 ולסרטן: Ms¹.

315 'orpiment': See entry זַרְנִיךְ.

316 In addition to שיחת הנפש, we find: חלאי הנפש for the Arabic synonym الألم النفسانية. See entry חֳלִי: חלאי הנפש.

אתון או חלב צאן וישים באפיו חלב אשה (If insomnia originates from dryness of the black bile, we pour water on [the head of the patient], in which camomile, melilot, i.e., the plant SWRYṢYLH, poppy calyces, dill, common marshmallow seeds, and the like have been cooked. After the head has been shaved, one should rub on it women's milk, milk of a she-ass, or milk of a goat. One should apply a sternutatory of women's milk). Hebr. שם באפיו is not attested for in the current dictionaries. Moses ibn Tibbon translates Arab. سعّط as שם בנחיריו (cf. BCD 274 (NM 4:204)) and Do'eg ha-Edomi translates Lat. *sternutationes facio* as היה העטוש.

שימור → שִׁמּוּר.

שינה → שֵׁנָה.

[שכך] • *Pi'el* שִׁכֵּךְ • **to repel**: Arab. ردع • Ibn al-Jazzār, *Zād al-musāfir wa-qūt al-ḥāḍir* • trans. Moses ibn Tibbon, *Sefer Ṣedat ha-Derakhim*, bk. 2, ch. 24: והרפואות אשר ישככו[317] המותרות אשר אמרנו שהם יעשו בתחלת החולי (The remedies that repel the superfluities and that we ordered to apply in the beginning of the illness). Hebr. שִׁכֵּךְ does not feature in this sense in the current dictionaries. Shem Tov ben Isaac, *Sefer ha-Shimmush*, bk. 30, translates Arab. ردع as הרתיע לאחור (cf. BCD 267 (NM 1:116)). Nathan ha-Me'ati translates the Arabic term as הרתיע in his translation of Maimonides' *Medical Aphorisms* 9.121 (BMMN 121), and Zeraḥyah Ḥen as הזיר (BMMZ 116). Hebr. הרתיע also features (instead of שִׁכֵּךְ) in *Sefer Ṣedat ha-Derakhim*, Ms Munich, Bayerische Staatsbibliothek, Cod. hebr. 19. See also entry סַם: סמים משככים.

• *Part. Pi'el* **מְשַׁכֵּךְ • סמים משככים** → סַם.

שֵׂכֶל • קל בשכל → קַל.

שָׁכֵן • שכנה • **(lit., neighbour); h.l., closely related to**: Lat. *vicina* (Arab. قريب) • Constantinus Africanus, *Viaticum* • trans. Do'eg ha-Edomi, *Sefer Ya'ir Netiv*, bk. 1, ch. 22: והאיפילימסיא שכינה אל אפופליקשיא כי המקום ההוא עצמו והטבע[318] מאשר נולדת הוא קר וגס (Epilepsy is closely related to apoplexy because [both originate from] that same place and the matter from which they originate is cold and coarse). Hebr. שכנה only features in the current dictionaries in the sense of 'neighbor' (cf. BM 7108–7109). Moses ibn Tibbon translates Arab. قريب as קרוב מן.

שלגיימה • **rock salt**: Lat. *salgemma* • Guillaume de Congenis, *Treatise on Surgery* • trans. Isaiah, fol. 49ª: משיחה לפישטולא: קח שלגיימה ומלח ושוגה בשוה וירקח עם חומץ ויפעל יותר ממשיחה ירוקה (A salve that is [good] for fistulas: Take equal amounts of rock salt, salt, and soot,[319] mix this with vinegar; it will have a stronger effect than an ointment made from verdigris). Hebr. שלגיימה is a non-attested loan word from Lat. *salgemma*.

---

317 ישככו: ירתיעו Ms Munich, Bayerische Staatsbibliothek, Cod. hebr. 19, fol. 50ᵇ.

318 והטבע: *et materia* L, cf. entry טֶבַע.

319 'soot' (ŠWGH) (O.Occ. *suia*, *sueia*, *suga*; cf. RL 5:288a): I thank Guido Mensching for this identification.

שַׁלְהֶבֶת · **fiery sensation in the body (i.e., inflammation):** Lat. *incensio* (Arab. التهاب) · Constantinus Africanus, *Viaticum* · trans. Do'eg ha-Edomi, *Sefer Ya'ir Netiv*, bk. 1, ch. 18 (Ms Oxford, Bodleian Library, Can. Or. 26, fols. 237ᵇ–238ᵃ): ונולד בשני ענינים או משלהבת האדומה עולה אל המוח או מרתיחת הדם בלב (It [i.e., phrenitis] may occur for two reasons, either from an inflammation of the yellow bile, which arises to the brain, or from a boiling of the blood of the heart). Hebr. שַׁלְהֶבֶת features in the current dictionaries in the sense of 'flame, flaming fire;' cf. BDB 529; JD 1587; BM 7123–7124. The term also features in the sense of 'heat' in the *Sefer Agur*, i.e., Do'eg ha-Edomi's translation of a Latin version of Hippocrates' *Aphorisms* (cf. BCD 275 (NM 3:227)). Moses ibn Tibbon translates Arab. التهاب as התלהבות (cf. BCD 76 (NM 3:73)) and Abraham ben Isaac as לְהִיבָה (see entry).

שְׁלִיקָה · **boiling:** Arab. سلاقة · Ibn al-Jazzār, *Zād al-musāfir wa-qūt al-ḥādir* · trans. Moses ibn Tibbon, *Sefer Ṣedat ha-Derakhim*, bk. 3, ch. 5: וכן יעשה בשליקת תאנים (The same should be done with boiled figs). Hebr. שְׁלִיקָה is only attested as a Rabbinic term in the current dictionaries; cf. JD 1584; BM 7163; EM 1839.

[שלך] • *Inf. Hif'il* • **הַשְׁלִיךְ** · **to expel; to expectorate; to spit out:** Arab. قذف · Ibn al-Jazzār, *Zād al-musāfir wa-qūt al-ḥādir* · trans. Moses ibn Tibbon, *Sefer Ṣedat ha-Derakhim*, bk. 3, ch. 7: ואם יקשה להשליך החומר מן הריאה נצוה החולה לשתות בשול איזוף עם סוכר ויאולד או יעשה הלחיכה הזאת (If the patient finds it difficult to expel the [superfluous] matter from the lungs, we tell him to take a hyssop potion with violet preserve or to use the following linctus …). In the sense of 'to expel,' Hebr. הַשְׁלִיךְ is a non-attested semantic borrowing from Arab. قذف. For *Part. Hif'il* משליך in the sense of 'expulsive,' see BCD 125 (NM 4:79), s.v. הכח המשליך ('the expulsive faculty'). Do'eg ha-Edomi translates the parallel Latin term *screo* as לרוק.

שְׁלֹמֹה • חוֹתָם שלמה ← חוֹתָם.

שָׁם • **משם** · **from that; therefrom:** Lat. *inde* (Arab. منه) · Constantinus Africanus, *Viaticum* · trans. Do'eg ha-Edomi, *Sefer Ya'ir Netiv*, bk. 1, ch. 23: גרגרישמי: פליטרי חרדל פלפל אשטאפישאגרא קלמנט זינזיבר דרכמ׳ וחצי ותשחוק לאבק ותמזוג בדבש ותעשה משם גרגרישמי עם אוקשימל למדת לוז ([Recipe of] a gargarism: Take two and a half *dirham* each of pellitory, mustard, pepper, stavesacre, water mint, and ginger. Pulverize this, mix it with honey and make therefrom a gargarism with oxymel similar to a hazelnut [in weight]). In the sense of 'therefrom,' Hebrew משם is a non-attested semantic borrowing from Lat. *inde*, which in addition to its regular meaning of 'from there,' can also mean 'from that, therefrom.' Moses ibn Tibbon translates Arab. منه as ממנו.

שִׁמּוּר · **abstention from food; diet:** Arab. حمية[320] · Ibn al-Jazzār, *Zād al-musāfir wa-qūt al-ḥādir* · trans. Abraham ben Isaac, *Sefer Ṣedah la-Oreḥim*, bk. 1, ch. 10 (Ms Florence, Biblioteca Medicina Laurenziana, Plut. 88.37, fol. 91ᵇ): ושיעור השתייה ב׳ שקלים במים

320 For *ḥimya*, cf. Lane 2:652a: 'The practising abstinence [especially the abstaining from things injurious in a case of sickness]; the abstaining, or desisting from eating.' In a med-

חמים[321] אחר שימור מאכל (Having abstained from food, one should take a measure of two *shekels*[322] with warm[323] water). Hebr. שִׁמּוּר features in Rabbinic literature in the sense of 'guarding, care' (cf. JD 1563; BM 7229–7230) and in modern literature in the sense of 'preservation [of foodstuff]' (cf. EM 1849). Moses ibn Tibbon translates Arab. حمية as שמירה (cf. BCD 278 (NM 1:69; 2:88)).

שִׁמָּמוֹן · anxiety; desolateness: Arab. توحّش · Isḥāq ibn ʿImrān, *Treatise on Melancholy* · trans. Anonymous, fol. 41[b] (42[b]): ונאמר שגבול המא⟨ל⟩נקוניאה הוא מחשבה ושממון שעוברין על הנפש (I say that the definition of melancholy is brooding and anxiety that affect the soul). Hebr. שִׁמָּמוֹן features in BCD 278 (NM 4:207) in an attestation from Jacob ibn Tibbon's translation of Ibn Zuhr's *Regimen of Health* in the sense of 'grief, affliction, distress, sadness' for Arabic كآبة or كرب.

שֶׁמֶן • שמן הדבש · (lit., honey oil); prob., a resin produced by injured olive trees [*Olea europaea* L.]: Arab. أومالي (cf. MIG 47) / Gr. ἐλαιόμελι (cf. Dioscorides, *De materia medica* 1.31) · *Shinnui ha-Shemot ha-Niqra'im Synonimis*, Ms Munich, Bayerische Staatsbibliothek, Cod. hebr. 8, fol. 193[a]: אומאלי הוא שמן חד נוזל מאילני סרק הגדלי' בישימון ובערבה ונקרא שמן הדבש ([Arab.] *ūmālī* is a heating oil [lit., sharp oil] that flows from trees that do not bear fruits and that grow in the desert and steppe. Its [i.e., *ūmālī*'s] [Hebr.] name is *shemen ha-devash*). Hebr. שמן הדבש does not feature in the current dictionaries.

שָׁמַע • *Part.* שׁוֹמֵעַ • הגיד השומע → גִּיד.

שֵׁמַע · listening to music: Arab. سماع[324] · Ibn al-Jazzār, *Zād al-musāfir wa-qūt al-ḥādir* · trans. Abraham ben Isaac, *Sefer Ṣedah la-Oreḥim*, bk. 1, ch. 20: וכבר אמר חכם אחד מן החכמים כי השמע הטוב כמו[325] הנפש והיין וכמו הגוף (A certain philosopher claimed that listening to music is like the soul[326] and wine is like the body). In the specific sense of 'listening to music,' Hebr. שֵׁמַע is a non-attested semantic borrowing from Arab. سماع. Moses ibn Tibbon translates Arab. سماع as שֵׁמַע as well. Do'eg ha-Edomi translates the parallel Latin term *sonitus* as קול.

• הברת השמע → הֲבָרָה.

• חסרון השמע → חֶסְרוֹן.

• כובד השמע → כֹּבֶד.

• כבדות השמע → כְּבֵדוּת.

ical context, the term features, e.g., in Maimonides, *Medical Aphorisms* 8.8, where it stands for Gr. ἀσιτία, 'abstinence from food' (cf. LSG 256).

321 חמים: فاتر a.

322 One *shekel* (Arab. *mithqāl*) is about 4.46 g.

323 'warm': 'lukewarm' a.

324 Arab. سماع in the meaning of 'listening to music' is common in Sufi literature.

325 כמו הנפש: كالروح a.

326 'soul': 'spirit' a.

[שמש] • *Part. Pi'el f.* **מְשַׁמֶּשֶׁת** · **scraper**: Rom./Lat. *rasta* (derived from Class. Lat. *raster*) · Guillaume de Congenis, *Treatise on Surgery* · trans. Isaiah, fol. 44^{b}: ובמשיחה[327] הזאת לא ימשח כי אם סביב המכה אך טוב הוא שיוסר עם המשמשת (This[328] ointment should only be used around the injury, but it is better to take it off with a scraper). Hebr. מְשַׁמֶּשֶׁת is not attested for in the current dictionaries.

שֶׁמֶשׁ • **מפסיד הראות בנטית השמש** → [פסד].

שֵׁן • *Dual* **שִׁנַּיִם** • **בשר השינים** → **בָּשָׂר**.

• **שינן השנים** → [שנן].

שֵׁנָה • **נדידת שינה** → **נְדִידָה**.

• **נידוד השינה** → **נִדּוּד**.

[שנן] • *Pi'el* **שִׁנֵּן** • **שינן השנים** · **to apply a dentifrice to the teeth**: Arab. استنّ / دلك الأسنان · Ibn al-Jazzār, *Zād al-musāfir wa-qūt al-ḥādir* · trans. Moses ibn Tibbon, *Sefer Ṣedat ha-Derakhim*, bk. 2, ch. 21: ממה שיועיל לזה שיקח חרס ולימסא וישחוק אותה יחד אחר שישרפם וישנן בהם השנים. או יקח חרס התנור קצף הים וישחקם יחד ויערב עמהם מעט מלח וישנן בהם שניו (Good for this [affliction] is to take potsherds and snails, to burn them and pound them together, and to apply this as a dentifrice to the teeth. Or take potsherds from the oven [and] sea[329] froth, pound them together, mix it with some salt and apply this as a dentifrice to the teeth). In the sense of 'to apply a dentifrice,' Hebr. שִׁנֵּן (coined from שֵׁן, 'tooth') is not attested for in the current dictionaries.

[שסע] *Pu'al* **שֻׁסַּע** · **to be cut; to be dissected**: Arab. شُقّ (Gr. ἐντέμνω; UWS 1:360–361) · Maimonides, *Medical Aphorisms* 15.31 · trans. Nathan ha-Me'ati (BMMN 158): כשתשוסע הכתנת הקרניית יהיה מה שיפגעך ראשונה הלחות הדקה הרקיקה ותשפך ותזול והיא הלחות אשר ברבים נראה אותה נוזלת ויוצאת מן הנקב אשר ינקב בעין אשר יוקדחו ממנה המים (If the horn-like tunic is dissected, the first thing you find is a fine and thin liquid streaming and pouring out. It is the moisture that you often see flowing out from the opening made in the eye that is being operated [on] for a cataract). In the sense of 'to be cut, to be dissected,' Hebrew שֻׁסַּע is a non-attested semantic borrowing from Arab. شُقّ. Zeraḥyah Ḥen translates the Arab. شقّ as קָרַע (see entry).

שְׁעִילָה · **cough**: Arab. سعلة · Ibn al-Jazzār, *Zād al-musāfir wa-qūt al-ḥādir* · trans. Moses ibn Tibbon, *Sefer Ṣedat ha-Derakhim*, bk. 3, ch. 12: ופעמים ירוק החולה בהתחלת החולי ר"ל ביום השלישי או ברביעי לדקות החומר ומהירות השמעו לפועל הטבע ויורה זה על קלות החולי ומהירות התכתו וכ"ש כשתהיה הרקיקה מעט לבנה מקובצת קלה לצאת ברקיקה אחת או בשתים (Sometimes the patient expectorates in the beginning of the illness [i.e., pleurisy], that is on the third or fourth day, because the [superfluous] matter is thin and reacts

---

327 ובמשיחה הזאת לא ימשח כי אם סביב המכה אך טוב הוא שיוסר עם המשמשת: *nec de isto unguento unguatur, nisi circa labia, sed melius est, ut remoueatur cum rasta* L.

328 Cf. L: 'Don't anoint it with this ointment, except around the lips, but it is better to take it off with a scraper.'

329 'sea froth': Cf. entry קֶצֶף: קצף הים.

quickly to the activity of nature [to expel it]. This indicates that the illness is mild, and quickly dissolved [i.e., healed], especially when the sputum is minimal, is white and concentrated and exits easily by coughing once or twice). In the sense of 'cough,' Hebr. שְׁעִילָה is a non-attested calque from Arab. سعلة. Do'eg ha-Edomi translates the parallel Latin term *tussis* as שעול.

שֵׂעָר • הלבנת השיער → הַלְבָּנָה.

שפא · **rob**: Lat. *sapa* (cf. DMLBS 3283: 'new wine boiled down to a fraction of its original volume; b) (other beverage); c) moisture, sap.') (Arab. ربّ) · Constantinus Africanus, *Viaticum* · trans. Do'eg ha-Edomi, *Sefer Ya'ir Netiv*, bk. 3, ch. 1: אחרי העשות כל אלה והליחות תכבינה נשוב אל הליחות שאינם נתרות ואשר נסגרות באברי החולה ונעשה גרגרישמי שפא מתותי העץ (Once we have done all these things and the [heat of the humors] has been extinguished, we turn to the humors that have not been dissolved and that are enclosed within the organs of the patient and prescribe gargles [prepared from] a rob of mulberries ...). Hebr. שפא is a non-attested loan word from Lat. *sapa*. Moses ibn Tibbon translates Arab. ربّ as בשול יין (see entry בִּשּׁוּל). See also entry: רֹב: רב ענבים.

שָׂפָה • *Dual* **שְׂפָתַיִם** · **edges (of a wound)**: Lat. *labia* (DMLBS 1870) · Guillaume de Congenis, *Treatise on Surgery* · trans. Isaiah, fol. 54[b]: כנגד חתוך הגידים קח תולעים מן האדמה ושחוק אותם ואחר שימם על שפתי המכה (When a nerve is cut, take earthworms, pulverize them and put them on the edges of the wound). Hebr. Sing. שָׂפָה, *Dual* שְׂפָתַיִם, does not feature in the sense of 'edges (of a wound)' in the current dictionaries.

• בקיעי השפתים → בְּקִיעַ.

• בקיעת השפתים → בְּקִיעָה.

שִׁפּוּי • שפוי הכובע · **larynx**: Lat. *guttur* (Arab. حنجرة) · Constantinus Africanus, *Viaticum* · trans. Do'eg ha-Edomi, *Sefer Ya'ir Netiv*, bk. 3, ch. 1: ואחרי ההקזה והכבוס יאות לשוב אל האברים באשר החולי מושל יותר ובתחלת הכאב נעזור באלה הענינים המפליגים אל הליחות היורדות אל הלהאה ומחזיקים עצם מהלהאה זהו גוטור שהוא שפוי הכובע (After the bleeding and purgation one should turn to the organ that is most affected by the illness and treat it in the beginning of the pain with medications that restrain the humors that descend to the larynx itself, i.e., GWṬWR [i.e., Lat. *guttur*], i.e., [Hebr.] *shippui hakova'*, and strengthen it). In the sense of 'larynx,' Hebr. שפוי הכובע features in BCD 282 (NM 4:210) in a later attestation from Nathan ha-Me'ati's *Sefer ha-Qanun*. Moses ibn Tibbon translates Arab. حنجرة as עליון הגרון (see entry עֶלְיוֹן).

שִׁפְלוּת • שפלות הקול · **hoarseness**: Lat. *raucitas* (Arab. بحوحة) · Constantinus Africanus, *Viaticum* · trans. Do'eg ha-Edomi, *Sefer Ya'ir Netiv*, bk. 3, ch. 4: משפלות הקול: שפלות הקול הוא מלחות מפריד[330] כלי הקול וזה הלחות מהלבנה או מהדם והוא ברדתו מן הראש יפריד[331] כלי הקול וישחית חלקות הדבור ולפעמים ממית מכל וכל הקול (On hoarseness:

330 מפריד: *infundens* L.

331 יפריד: *infundit* L.

Hoarseness originates from moisture, which soaks[332] the vocal organs. When this moisture—consisting of phlegm or of blood—descends from the head, it soaks[333] the vocal organs and harms clarity of speech. In some cases it causes a complete loss of voice). Hebr. שפלות הקול is attested for in BCD 283 (NM 4:211) in a later attestation from Moses ibn Tibbon's translation of the introductory title to ch. 4: השער הד׳ בשפלות הקול הוא בחוחה (see also BCD 25 (NM 3:28), s.v. אֲפִיסָה: אפיסת הקול).

שֶׁפַע · **superfluity; residu; superfluous matter**: Lat. *superfluitas* (Arab. مادّة) · Constantinus Africanus, *Viaticum* · trans. Do'eg ha-Edomi, *Sefer Ya'ir Netiv*, bk. 3, ch. 8: וכאשר נרפא אותו אשר ירוק דם יאות לתת לו מנוחה ושירגע מאד ושלא יוציא הנשימה בכח. ואם הוא חזק והעת מזוג וכפי שניו יוכל לסבול יאות לחסר המקור הבאשליקא ולהוציא הדם ב׳ פעמים או ג׳ עד שיכיר שיצא כל השפע גם יאות לחסר הדם מצד הכאב מן המקור אשר בין האצבע הקטן לאחיהו (If we want to cure someone who spits blood, we should [first of all] let him rest so that he becomes very calm and does not exhale forcefully. If he is strong and the weather is moderate and it fits his age, we should bleed from the basilic vein twice ot three times until it is clear that all the superfluous matter has come out. It is also fitting to bleed [the patient] from the saphenous vein that is on the same side as the pain). In the sense of 'superfluity, residu,' Hebr. שֶׁפַע features in BM 7405 in a later attestation from the *Sefer Almansur*, i.e., Shem Tov ben Isaac's translation of al-Rāzī's *K. al-Manṣūrī*. Moses ibn Tibbon translates Arab. مادّة as חומר.

שָׁקֵד • *Plur.* **שקדים** • **השקדים אשר בתוך הגרון** · **tonsils**: Lat. *glandes* (Arab. لوزتان) · Constantinus Africanus, *Viaticum* · trans. Do'eg ha-Edomi, *Sefer Ya'ir Netiv*, bk. 3, ch. 1: ואם השקדים אשר בתוך הגרון הם הגרנדולש (And if the tonsils, i.e., GRNDWLŠ ...). In the sense of 'tonsils,' Hebr. *Plur.* שקדים features on its own in BM 7419 in a later attestation from the *Sefer ha-Qanun*; cf. Nathan ha-Me'ati's glossary to the *Sefer ha-Qanun* (NM 2:120, 162 (Shin 5)): קראתי שקדים החטים שבגרגרת כי קראום כן הערביים (I called the tonsils (ḤTYM) in the throat ŠQDYM, because this is the name that the Arabs have given to them). Moses ibn Tibbon translates the parallel Arabic term لوزتان as שקדים הם החטי (cf. NM 2:162, n. 733, and BCD 93 (NM 4:65)).

שָׁקַט · **to be alleviated; to be eased; to abate**: Lat. *mitigor* (Arab. سكن) · Constantinus Africanus, *Viaticum* · trans. Do'eg ha-Edomi, *Sefer Ya'ir Netiv*, bk. 2, ch. 19: ואם לא ישקוט הכאב בכל אלה יאות להוציאם בברזל (If the pain [in the teeth] does not abate with any of the [remedies that I mentioned], one should extract the [tooth that causes the pain] with a surgical instrument). In the sense of 'to be alleviated (of pain),' Hebr. שָׁקַט is a non-attested semantic borrowing from Lat. *mitigor*. Moses ibn Tibbon translates Arab. سكن as נח.

---

332 'soaks': Trans. after L.

333 'soaks': Trans. after L.

• *Hif'il* הִשְׁקִיט · **to mitigate**: Lat. *mitigo* (Arab. سكّن) · Constantinus Africanus, *Viaticum* · trans. Do'eg ha-Edomi, *Sefer Ya'ir Netiv*, bk. 2, ch. 19: כל אלה ישקיטו הכאב ויגרשו התולעים (All these [ingredients] mitigate the pain and expel the worms). In a medical context, Hebr. הִשְׁקִיט features in BCD 284 (NM 3:126) in a later attestation from Nathan ha-Me'ati's translation of Hippocrates' *Aphorisms* 2.2. In the sense of 'to mitigate the pain' (השקיט את הכאבים), *Hif'il* הִשְׁקִיט features as a modern term in EM 1885. Moses ibn Tibbon translates Arab. سكّن as נח.

שֶׁקֶל · **weight**: Lat. *pondus* (Arab. جزء) · Constantinus Africanus, *Viaticum* · trans. Do'eg ha-Edomi, *Sefer Ya'ir Netiv*, bk. 1, ch. 17: ובבא התעורה ממאכל וממשקה חם נעזור אליו כפי הנראה אל הרופא הבקי עם דברים מישנים כמו אופי קשטור זעפרן גושקיאמי ליבור שחור מנדראגולא זרע פאפאבר בשקל שוה (If insomnia results from [the consumption of] hot foodstuffs or hot drinks, we treat it according to the opinion of an expert physician with a soporific, such as: opium, castoreum, saffron, poison hemlock, black hellebore, mandrake, and poppy seeds. [From each ingredient one should take] an equal weight). Hebr. שֶׁקֶל does not feature in this sense in the current dictionaries; cf. BM 7435–7437. Moses ibn Tibbon translates the parallel Arabic term جزء as חלק.

שְׂרָף • שרף רוטא מדברית · **(lit., resin of wild rue); thapsia** [*Thapsia garganica* L.]: Arab. السذاب البرّي (cf. M 380 (301): تافسيا هو الينتون وهو المثنان وهو السذاب البرّي نفسه وقيل أنه صمغ السذاب البري ('*Tāfsiyā*: It is *al-yantūn* and *al-maṯinān*. It is the wild rue itself, or it is said that it is the resin of wild rue')) · *Shinnui ha-Shemot ha-Niqra'im Synonimis*, Ms Munich, Bayerische Staatsbibliothek, Cod. hebr. 8, fol. 199a: ינתון הוא טפשיאה הוא שרף רוטא מדברית אך לפי דיאסקורידוס הוא עשב ואולי הוא העשב שהנוצרים יכנוהו בשם הזה ([Arab.] *yantūn*; i.e., thapsia; it is the resin of wild rue; but according to Dioscorides it is the plant itself; perhaps the Christians give it this name). Hebr. שרף רוטא מדברית is a non-attested calque of the Arab. السذاب البرّي.

שְׂרֵפָה • שרפת השתן · **burning urination; dysuria**: Arab.: حرقة البول (cf. SN 112) · Shem Tov ben Isaac, *Sefer ha-Shimmush*, bk. 29, list 1 (SHS 1:517 (Shin 39)): שרפת השתן ב"ה חרקה' אלבול (*serefat ha-sheten*; Arab. *ḥaraqat al-bawl*). Hebr. שרפת השתן is not attested for in the current dictionaries.

שרשפי · **epigastric**: Arab. شراسفي · Isḥāq ibn 'Imrān, *Treatise on Melancholy* · trans. Anonymous, fol. 50^{b} (51^{b}): ויגמע מעט מעט בכל עת במי כאשכאש עם קצת השמנים המרכבים שיש בטבעם למסס הרוחות והנפח השרשפי ([The patient] should regularly take small sips of poppy juice with some oils that by nature dissolve the winds and the epigastric flatus). Hebr. שרשפי is a non-attested loan word (or transcription)[334] of Arab. شراسفي. Constantine the African translates Arab. شراسفي as *hypochondriacus*.

שְׁתִי • בשתי וערב · **crosswise**: Lat. *in cruce* · Guillaume de Congenis, *Treatise on Surgery* · trans. Isaiah, fol. 45^{a}: [335]אם שבירת העצם גדולה ונכרת מגיד כי מן האזן ולמעלה ומן המצח

334 Cf. entry [מסס]: *Inf.* מְסוֹס.

335 המצח: emendation editor הצמח Ms *frons* L.

ולמעלה יאות לחתוך בשתי וערב (If the fracture of the bone is large and manifest, note that the incision above the ears and forehead should be crosswise). Hebr. בשתי וערב is not attested for in medieval medical literature.

שֶׁתֶן • שרפת השתן → שְׂרֵפָה.

תּוֹלֶדֶת/תּוֹלָדָה · **nature:** Lat. *natura* · Constantinus Africanus, *Viaticum* · trans. Do'eg ha-Edomi, *Sefer Ya'ir Netiv*, bk. 1, ch. 11: המוח נחלק באורך אל הימין ואל השמאל ושם קו אמצעי מפריד את מדוריו ובעלות עשן אחת הליחות ונדח בתולדתו אל הימין או אל השמאל שם כאב ונקרא מיקראניאה (The brain is divided lengthwise in a right and left [part], and there is a line [i.e., groove] that divides the ventricles; when vapors from one of the humors arise [to the head] and nature pushes them to the right or left, [head]ache called [in Lat.] MYQR'NY'H [i.e., migraine] occurs there). In the sense of 'nature,' Hebr. תּוֹלֶדֶת/תּוֹלָדָה is only attested for in medieval philosophical literature; cf. BM 7688; EM 1921; KM 4:182.[336]

• הרחבת התולדת → הַרְחָבָה.

תּוֹלָדִי · **natural:** Lat. *naturalis* (Arab. طبيعي) · Constantinus Africanus, *Viaticum* · trans. Do'eg ha-Edomi, *Sefer Ya'ir Netiv*, bk. 1, ch. 17: התעורה בשני ענינים תולדיים (Insomnia is natural in two ways). Hebr. תּוֹלָדִי features in BM 7689 in later attestations from Nachmanides' commentary on the Torah and from Me'ir Aldabi's *Shevilei Emunah*. Moses ibn Tibbon translates the parallel Arabic term طبيعي as טבעי.

תּוֹלֶדֶת → תּוֹלֶדֶת/תּוֹלָדָה.

תּוֹלָעִי • הדפק התולעי → דֹּפֶק.

תּוֹצָאָה • *Plur.* תוצאות · **emptying; purgation:** Lat. *egestio* (Arab. إسهال) · Constantinus Africanus, *Viaticum* · trans. Do'eg ha-Edomi, *Sefer Ya'ir Netiv*, bk. 3, ch. 1: וכאשר יכבה חדוד האדומה ויצא עם התוצאות אז יאות להקיז הספליקא עד צאת הדם הנלהב מן האדומה (When the heat of the yellow bile is extinguished and leaves [the body] with its purgation, one should bleed the cephalic vein until the blood heated by the yellow bile has been extracted). Hebr. *Plur.* תוצאות features in BCD 292 (NM 3:240–241) in an attestation from Do'eg ha-Edomi's *Sefer Agur* in the sense of 'evacuations, excrements, stool,' and in BCD 292 (NM 1:41) in a later attestation from Hillel ben Samuel's *Sefer Keritut* in the sense of 'emptying, voiding, excretion.' Moses ibn Tibbon translates the parallel Arabic term إسهال as שלשול.

תּוֹשֶׁבֶת · **anus:** Arab. مقعدة (cf. DKT 829) · Shem Tov ben Isaac, *Sefer ha-Shimmush*, bk. 29, list 1 (SHS 1:534 (Tav 12)): תושבת ב"ה מקעדה (*toshevet*; Arab. *maq'adah*). In the sense of 'anus,' Hebr. תּוֹשֶׁבֶת features in BCD 292 (NM 4:219–220) in a later attestation from Jacob ibn Tibbon's translation of the *Regimen of Health* by Ibn Zuhr.

תּוּת • *Plur.* תותים • תותי העץ · **mulberries** [*Morus nigra* L.]: Lat. *morus*, Plur. *mori* (Arab. توت) · Constantinus Africanus, *Viaticum* · trans. Do'eg ha-Edomi, *Sefer Ya'ir Netiv*,

---

336 In the sense of 'nature,' the term was actually coined by Abraham ibn Ezra, cf. Shl. Sela, *Abraham Ibn Ezra and the Rise of Medieval Hebrew Science* (Leiden 2003), 130–137 (following Freudenthal, McVaugh, and Mesler, 'Twelfth-Century Latin Medicine,' 244, n. 47).

bk. 2, ch. 24 (Ms Oxford, Bodleian Library, Can. Or. 26, fol. 275[a]): והרפואה המפליגה אל הליחות ראויה להיות כן: שפא[337] העשויה מתותי העץ (To restrain the humors, one should apply one of the following remedies: a rob composed from mulberries …). Hebr. *Sing.* תות העץ, *Plur.* תותי העץ, does not feature in the current dictionaries. The common term for 'mulberry' is תות (cf. BM 7710; LF 1:266 ff.). Moses ibn Tibbon translates Arab. توت as תותים.

תַּחְבּוֹשֶׁת › **poultice; plaster**: Lat. *cataplasma* (DMLBS 392) (Arab. طلاء) · Constantinus Africanus, *Viaticum* · trans. Do'eg ha-Edomi, *Sefer Ya'ir Netiv*, bk. 2, ch. 15: ותניח על המצח גרידא[338] מזוגה בחומץ ותחבושת מן שנדלש (And put on the forehead [of someone suffering from a nosebleed] chalk mixed with vinegar and a poultice from sandalwood …). In the sense of 'plaster, poultice,' Hebr. תַּחְבּוֹשֶׁת features in BCD 292 (NM 1:42) in a later attestation form Hillel ben Samuel's *Sefer Keritut*. Moses ibn Tibbon renders Arab. طلاء as טיחה.

תַּחְתּוֹן • הכניס בחור התחתון → [כנס].

תישית › **she-goat**: Lat. *capra* · Constantinus Africanus, *Viaticum* · trans. Do'eg ha-Edomi, *Sefer Ya'ir Netiv*, bk. 2, ch. 16: ואם יהיו הבקעים בעומק רב תמשח השפתים בשמן אווז או בשמן תישית (If the fissures [in the lips] are very deep, rub the lips with the fat of a goose or a she-goat). Hebr. תישית does not feature in the current dictionaries. The current feminine form of תַּיִשׁ is תֵּישָׁה (cf. BM 7741).

תָּכְנִית • חכמת התכנית → חָכְמָה.

תְּנוּעָה › **looseness (of teeth)**: Lat. *motus* (Arab. تحرّك) · Constantinus Africanus, *Viaticum* · trans. Do'eg ha-Edomi, *Sefer Ya'ir Netiv*, bk. 2, ch. 20: ואם תנועת השינים תהיה מהליחות הלבנות תקח ד' דרכמ' אלום מלח ב' דרכמ' ותשחוק לאבק ותשים על השינים (If looseness of the teeth is caused by phlegmatic moistures, take four *dirhams* of alum and two *dirhams* of salt. Pound these into a powder, and put this on the teeth). Hebr. תְּנוּעָה does not feature in a medical sense in the current dictionaries. Moses ibn Tibbon translates Arab. تحرّك as נוע.

• **תנועת החפץ** › **voluntary motion**: Lat. *voluntarius motus* · Constantinus Africanus, *Viaticum* · trans. Do'eg ha-Edomi, *Sefer Ya'ir Netiv*, bk. 1, ch. 18 (Ms Oxford, Bodleian Library, Can. Or. 26, fol. 240[b]): יאות אל השותים היין להרחיק הכמות היכול לשכר אותם. אם כן כל אדם יאות לחשוב איכויות גופו ואיבריו אשר להם תנועת החפץ וזכרנותם וטעמם (If someone drinks wine, he should avoid [drinking] a quantity that can make him drunk. For this reason, everyone should consider the qualities of his body and limbs that have voluntary motion [and also the strength of] his memory and reason). Hebr. תנועת החפץ does not feature in this sense in the current dicionaries. The standard term featuring in medieval philosophical literature is תנועה רצונית (cf. KTP 4:53, s.v. רצוני).

---

337 שפא: *sapa* L; cf. entry שפא.
338 גרידא: *creta* L.

A synonym for רצוני ('voluntary') on its own featuring in medieval philosophical literature is חפצי. (cf. KTP 1:320).

• *Plur.* תנועות • תנועות שלא מחפץ · **unvoluntary motions**: Lat. *non voluntarii motus* · Constantinus Africanus, *Viaticum* · trans. Do'eg ha-Edomi, *Sefer Ya'ir Netiv*, bk. 1, ch. 24 (Ms Oxford, Bodleian Library, Can. Or. 26, fol. 250^{b}): אלו הם תנועות שלא מחפץ (These are unvoluntary motions). Hebr. *Sing.* תנועה שלא מחפץ, *Plur.* תנועות שלא מחפץ does not feature in the current dictionaries. See previous entry.

תַּעֲרֹבֶת • *Plur.* **תערובות** · **humors (of the human body)**: Arab. خلط, *Plur.* أخلاط · Isḥāq ibn ʿImrān, *Treatise on Melancholy* · trans. Anonymous, fol. 49^{b} (50^{b}): אם כן התערובות הארבע והדם והמוח מפני לחות[339] כל אלה יוסיפו בתוספת הלבנה (For this reason the four humors [in the human body], and [especially] the blood and the brain increase during the waxing of the moon). Hebr. *Sing.* תַּעֲרֹבֶת features in the current dictionaries in the sense of 'mixture, intermixing,' not as one of the four humors of the body (cf. BM 7840). The standard medieval term for bodily 'humor' is לֵחָה. Constantine the African translates Arab. أخلاط as *humores*.

תְּפִישָׂה · **intake; ingestion**: Arab. شربة · Ibn al-Jazzār, *Zād al-musāfir wa-qūt al-ḥādir* · trans. Abraham ben Isaac, *Sefer Ṣedah la-Oreḥim*, Adaptation, bk. 1, ch. 10 (Ms Berlin, Staatsbibliothek Preußischer Kulturbesitz, Or. fol. 1058, fol. 94^{a}): וזהו מעשה הפילולי שתיקן גליאנו ... קח אלואי דאגרידיאו קולוקינטידה ... ועשה פילולי כעין אפונים ותפישתם ז׳ או ט׳ (A recipe for pills composed by Galen ...: Take aloe, diagridium [i.e., scammony], colocynth ... make pills resembling chickpeas, and take seven or nine [pills]). Hebr. תְּפִישָׂה, a variant reading of תְּפִסָה, does not feature in this sense in the current dictionaries, cf. BM 7851–7852. Do'eg ha-Edomi translates Lat. *dabis* as תתן. Moses ibn Tibbon translates Arab. شربة as לקיחה and Abraham ben Isaac as שיעור השתיה.

תָּפֵל · **raw; crude**: Arab. خام · Shem Tov ben Isaac, *Sefer ha-Shimmush*, bk. 29, list 1 (SHS 1:297 (Lamed 24)): לחה תפלה ב״ה ⟨כלט⟩ כ׳אם (*leḥah tefelah*; Arab. ⟨*khilt*⟩ *khām*). Hebr. תָּפֵל is not attested for in this sense in the current dictionaries.

תָּפַשׂ · **to take; to ingest** · Ibn al-Jazzār, *Zād al-musāfir wa-qūt al-ḥādir* · trans. Abraham ben Isaac, *Sefer Ṣedah la-Oreḥim*, Adaptation, bk. 1, ch. 10 (Ms Berlin, Staatsbibliothek Preußischer Kulturbesitz, Or. fol. 1058, fol. 94^{a}): וזהו מעשה הפילולי שתיקן גליאנו מה׳ מינין ויכולים לתפוש טרם האוכל ואחריו (Here follows a recipe for pills composed by Galen from five [different] kinds [of ingredients] and that can be taken before or after the meal). Hebr. תָּפַשׂ does not feature in this sense in the current dictionaries.

[תקן] • *Piʿel* תִּקֵּן · **to prepare**: Arab. دبّر · Ibn al-Jazzār, *Zād al-musāfir wa-qūt al-ḥādir* · trans. Abraham ben Isaac, *Sefer Ṣedah la-Oreḥim*, bk. 1, ch. 23: יתקן מהכל משיחה הנקר׳ בלשון ישמעאל מרהם ונקר׳ בלשון יון אליפי יתקן הכל עם דונג ויועיל לאשר אמרנו (Prepare a salve, called in Arab. *marham* and in Greek ʾLYPY [ἀλοιφή] from all [these

---

339 לחות: emendation editor לחותי Ms.

ingredients], with the help of wax and apply it. This will be beneficial for [the ailment] we mentioned). In the sense of 'to prepare,' Hebr. תִּקֵּן features in the Bible and Rabbinic literature (cf. BDB 1075; JD 1691–1692; BM 7880–7881; EM 1967). Moses ibn Tibbon translates Arab. دبّر as תִּקֵּן as well.

• *Part. Pu'al* מְתֻקָּן • מתוקן המלאכה · **well (properly) prepared:** Arab. المحكم الصنعة · Ibn al-Jazzār, *Zād al-musāfir wa-qūt al-ḥādir* · trans. Moses ibn Tibbon, *Sefer Ṣedat ha-Derakhim*, bk. 3, ch. 7: ואם היה הדם בתחלת החולי הזה רב והיה כחו חזק נקיזהו בתחלת החולי ויוציא מן הדם שעור הסיפוק ונזונהו במה שיקרר וידביק ויתבשל מהר כמו מי שעור מתוקן המלאכה (If in the beginning of this illness [i.e., pneumonia] there is a large quantity of blood and [the patient] is strong, we extract a sufficient amount of blood and then give him food that has a cooling and adhesive effect and is quickly digested, such as barley gruel that has been well prepared). In the sense of 'well prepared' in the context of food, Hebr. מְתֻקָּן is attested for in Rabbinic literature; cf. JD 1692. In medical literature, the term מתוקן המלאכה (for Arab. المحكم) recurs in Nathan ha-Me'ati's translation of Maimonides' *Medical Aphorisms* 17.14, 22, 30 (BMMN 172–174). The same Arabic term is translated by Zeraḥyah Ḥen as עשוי בחכמה (BMMZ 170, 172) or הנעשה בחכמה (BMMZ 171). Do'eg ha-Edomi translates the parallel Latin term *perfecta* as עשוי.

תַּרְדֵּמָה • תרדמת האיברים · **numbness:** Lat. *dormitatio membrorum* (Arab. خدر) · Constantinus Africanus, *Viaticum* · trans. Do'eg ha-Edomi, *Sefer Ya'ir Netiv*, bk. 1, ch. 25: ותרדמת האברים מחוברת בין התולדת והחולי והסבה היא קרירות שיקבוץ עצום הגידים ויקרר ויעצור שלא יוכל הכח המרגיש לנקוב שם (Numbness is a combination of nature and illness. Its cause is coldness, which coagulates the substance of the nerves, cools and restrains [them] so that the power of sensory perception cannot penetrate them). In the sense of 'numbness,' Hebr. תרדמת האיברים features in BCD 298 (NM 1:70–71; 2:94; 4:223) in later attestations, a.o. from Moses ibn Tibbon, *Sefer Ṣedat ha-Derakhim*. Moses ibn Tibbon translates Arab. خدر, featuring in the passage quoted here, as תרדמת איברים as well. Abraham ben Isaac renders the Arabic term as החולי הנק' אלכדר.

תַּרְנְגוֹל • תרנגול בחור · **young chickens:**[340] Arab. فرّوج · Ibn al-Jazzār, *Zād al-musāfir wa-qūt al-ḥādir* · trans. Abraham ben Isaac, *Sefer Ṣedah la-Oreḥim*, bk. 1, ch. 10 (Ms Jerusalem, National Library of Israel, Fr. 95, fol. 90ᵃ): וכך התרה עלינו גליאנוס לרפא ופרנס החולה כרושובלנא הוא אטרפיצי ופרפחינים ויירבוזין הם בליטין ואם אין לו חמימות אז האכילהו תרנגול בחור או עוף הנק' דראג' והקורא ודומיהן (For treating and feeding a patient [suffering from headache], Galen prescribed the following [ingredients]: garden orach, common purslane, and purple[341] amaranth, i.e., BLYṬYN. If he is not afflicted by

340 The same term features in the anonymous adaptation of *Sefer Ṣedah la-Oreḥim* (Ms Berlin, Staatsbibliothek Preußischer Kulturbesitz, Or. Fol. 1058, fol. 93ᵃ).

341 'purple amaranth, i.e., BLYṬYN': *Amaranthus blitum* L.

heat, he should eat young chickens, francolins, partridges, and the like). Hebr. בָּחוּר does not feature in this combination in the current dictionaries. Do'eg ha-Edomi translates the parallel Latin term *gallinarum pulli* as תרנוגלים קטנים. The same term features in the translation by Moses ibn Tibbon (for Arab. فرّوج). Hebr. *Sing.* תרנגול קטן features in the anonymous adaptation of Abraham ben Isaac's *Sefer Ṣedah la-Oreḥim* (Ms Moscow, Russian State Library, Guenzburg 165, fol. 100[a]).

תְּשׁוּמָה • תשומת כלי · **clyster**: Lat. *clystere* (Arab. حقنة) · Constantinus Africanus, *Viaticum* · trans. Do'eg ha-Edomi, *Sefer Ya'ir Netiv*, bk. 1, ch. 18: ואם לא יוכל לשתות משקה נעשה לו תשומת כלי הוא קלישטרי מן ויאולש שעור נקי גוגובש סובין (If he cannot drink the potion [we prescribed], we prepare for him a clyster, i.e., [Lat.] *clystere*, from violets, husked barley, common jujubes, [and] bran). Hebr. תשומת כלי does not feature in the current dictionaries. In addition to תשומת כלי, Do'eg ha-Edomi translates Lat. *clystere* with the Hebrew loan word קלישטרי. Moses ibn Tibbon translates Arab. حقنة as קלוח (cf. BCD 243 (NM 4:183)); Abraham ben Isaac renders the Arab. حقنة as חקנה הוא קרישטיר.

Bibliography

Adams, F. (ed.), *The Seven Books of Paulus Ægineta: Translated from the Greek with Commentary Embracing a Complete View of the Knowledge Possessed by the Greeks, Romans, and Arabians on all Subjects Connected with Medicine and Surgery*, 3 vols. (London 1844–1847).

Benedek, Th.C., 'Historical Background of Discoid and SLE,' in *Dubois' Lupus Erythematosus and Related Syndromes*, 8th ed., ed. by D.J. Wallace and B.H. Hahn, e1–e11 (Philadelphia 2013).

Bos, G., '*Balādhur* (Marking-nut): A Popular Medieval Drug for Strengthening Memory,' *Bulletin of the School of Oriental and African Studies* 59, no. 2 (1996): 229–236.

Bos, G., 'Two Comments on the Ben-Yehuda Dictionary' (in Hebr.), *Ha-'Ivrit* 65, nos. 3–4 (2018–2019): 106–108.

Bos, G., 'Jewish Traditions on Strengthening Memory and Leone Modena's Evaluation,' *Jewish Studies Quarterly* 2, no. 1 (1995): 39–58.

Bos, G., 'The *miswāk*, an Aspect of Dental Care in Islam,' *Medical History* 37 (1993): 68–79.

Bos, G., 'R. Moshe Narboni, Philosopher and Physician: A Critical Analysis of *Sefer Oraḥ Ḥayyim*,' *Medieval Encounters* 2, no. 1 (1995): 219–251.

Bos, G. and Kl.-D. Fischer (eds.), *A Glimpse into Medical Practice among Jews around 1500: Latin-German Pharmaceutical Glossaries in Hebrew Characters Extant in Ms Leiden, Universiteitsbibliotheek, Cod. Or. 4732/1* (*SCAL 15*), *fols. 1a–17b* (Leiden 2021).

Bos, G. and R. Fontaine, 'Medico-philosophical Controversies in Nathan b. Jo'el Falaquera's *Sefer Ṣori ha-Guf*,' *Jewish Quarterly Review* 90, nos. 1–2 (1999): 27–60.

Chauliac, Guy de, *Inventarium sive Chirurgia Magna*, 2 vols., ed. by M.R. McVaugh (vol. 1), commentary by M.R. McVaugh and M.S. Ogden (vol. 2) (Leiden 1997).

Dols, M.W., *Medieval Islamic Medicine* (Berkeley 1984).

Dugat, G. 'Études sur le traité de médicine d'Abou Djàfar Ah'mad, intitulé: زاد المسافر, *Zad al-mocafir*, 'La provision du voyageur',' *Journal asiatique* 5, no. 1 (1853): 289–353.

Ferre, L., *Práctica de Johannes de Parma: Un tratado farmacologico en sus versiones hebreas y catalana* (Granada 2002).

Freudenthal, G., 'The Father of the Latin-into-Hebrew Translations: 'Do'eg the Edomite,' the Twelfth-Century Repentant Convert,' in *Latin-into-Hebrew: Texts and Studies*, vol. 1: *Studies*, ed. by R. Fontaine and G. Freudenthal, 105–120 (Leiden 2013).

Freudenthal, G., M.R. McVaugh, and K. Mesler, 'Twelfth-Century Latin Medicine in Hebrew Garb: Do'eg the Edomite as a Cultural Intermediary,' *Medieval Encounters* 26 (2020): 226–284.

Galen, *Opera Omnia*, ed. by K.G. Kühn, 20 vols. (Repr., Hildesheim 1967).

Galen, *De usu partium corporis humani*, ed. by G. Helmreich, 2 vols. (Repr., Amsterdam 1968).

García González, A. (ed.), *Alphita: Edición crítica y comentario* (Florence 2007).

Hinz, W., *Islamische Maße und Gewichte umgerechnet ins metrische System*, photomechanischer Nachdruck mit Zusätzen und Berichtigungen, = *Handbuch der Orientalistik*, vol. 1, suppl. 1.1 (Leiden 1970).

Hippocrates, *Aphorisms*, in *Hippocrates*, vol. 4, ed. and trans. by W.H.S. Jones, 97–221, = *Loeb Classical Library*, vol. 150 (Cambridge, MA 1979).

Hippocrates, *Œuvres complètes d'Hippocrate*, ed. and trans. by É. Littré, 10 vols. (Repr., Amsterdam 1973–1982).

Ibn Ezra, Pseudo-, *Sefer Hanisyonot: The Book of Medical Experiences Attributed to Abraham ibn Ezra*, ed. and trans. by J.O. Leibowitz and S. Marcus (Jerusalem 1984).

Ibn ʿImrān, Isḥāq, *Maqāla fī l-Mālīḫūliyā (Abhandlung über die Melancholie) und Constantini Africani libri duo* De melancholia, ed. by K. Garbers (Hamburg 1977).

Ibn al-Jazzār, *Zād al-musāfir wa-qūt al-ḥāḍir (Provisions for the Traveller and Nourishment for the Sedentary): Books I and II—Diseases of the Head and the Face*, ed. and trans. by G. Bos and F. Käs, with Critical Editions of the Medieval Hebrew Translations by G. Bos and the Medieval Latin Translation by M.R. McVaugh (forthcoming).

Ibn Sahl, Sābūr, *Dispensatorium Parvum (Al-Aqrābādhīn al-ṣaghīr)*, ed. by O. Kahl (Leiden 1994).

Ineichen, G. (ed.), *El Libro Agregà de Serapiom*, vol. 2: *Volgarizzamento di frater Jacobus Philippus de Padua* (Florence 1966).

Kahl, O. (ed. and trans.), *Sābūr ibn Sahl's Dispensatory in the Recension of the ʿAḍudī Hospital* (Leiden 2009).

Karpp, G. and O. Riha, 'Aus der Geschichte der Rogerglossen: Ein bisher unbekanntes Wilhelm von Congenis-Fragment,' *Sudhoffs Archiv* 99, no. 1 (2015): 73–104.

Maimonides, *The Code of Maimonides*, bk. 5: *The Book of Holiness*, ed. by L. Nemoy, trans. by L.I. Rabinowitz and Ph. Grossman (Repr., New Haven 1965).

McVaugh, M.R., 'Medieval Paths to Surgical Practice: The Example of Montpellier' (forthcoming in *Micrologus*).

McVaugh, M.R., *The Rational Surgery of the Middle Ages* (Florence 2006).

McVaugh, M.R., Bos, G., and J. Shatzmiller (eds. and trans.), *The Regimen Sanitatis of "Avenzoar": Stages in the Production of a Medieval Translation* (Leiden 2019).

Penzig, O., *Flora Populare Italiana* (Genova 1924).

Richler, B., 'On the Existing Manuscripts of Marpé la-Ezem by ibn Waqar,' *Korot* 19 (2007–2008): 127–133.

Richler, B., *Hebrew Manuscripts in the Bibliotheca Palatina in Parma: Catalogue*. Palaeographical and codicological descriptions: M. Beit-Arié (Jerusalem 2001).

Richler, B., *Hebrew Manuscripts in the Vatican Library: Catalogue*. Compiled by the Staff of the Institute of Microfilmed Hebrew Manuscripts, Jewish National and University Library, Jerusalem. Palaeographical and Codicological Descriptions: M. Beit-Arié, in collaboration with N. Pasternak (Vatican City 2008).

Sela, Shl., 'The Fuzzy Borders between Astronomy and Astrology in the Thought and Work of Three Twelfth-Century Jewish Intellectuals,' *Aleph* 1 (2001): 59–100.

Sela, Shl., *Abraham Ibn Ezra and the Rise of Medieval Hebrew Science* (Leiden 2003).

Schönfeld, J. (ed. and trans.), *Über die Steine: Das 14. Kapitel aus dem* Kitāb al-Muršid *des Muḥammad ibn Aḥmad at-Tamīmī, nach dem Pariser Manuskript herausgegeben, übersetzt und kommentiert* (Freiburg 1976).

Shatzmiller, J., *Jews, Medicine, and Medieval Society* (Berkeley-Los Angeles-London 1994).

Steinschneider, M., *Catalogus Codicum Hebraeorum Bibliothecae Academiae Lugduno-Batavae* (Repr., Osnabrück 1977).

Steinschneider, M., *Verzeichniss der hebräischen Handschriften in Berlin* (Repr., 1 vol., Hildesheim 1980).

Sudhoff, K., 'Eine therapeutische Rogerglosse aus Montpellier', in: idem, *Beiträge zur Geschichte der Chirurgie im Mittelalter: Graphische und textliche Untersuchungen in mittelalterlichen Handschriften*, vol. 2, 265–297 (Leipzig 1918).

Tanḥum Yerushalmi, *Al-Murshid al-kafi*, ed. and trans. by H. Shy (Jerusalem 2005).

Ullmann, M. (ed. and trans.), *Rufus von Ephesos: Krankenjournale* (Wiesbaden 1978).

Zotenberg, H. (ed.), *Catalogues des manuscrits hébreux et samaritains de la Bibliothèque Impériale* (Paris 1866).

Corrections to NM 4 and BCD

Corrections to NM 4

210, entry **שפודיי**: The term features as a modern term in EM 1875.

Corrections to BCD

26, entry **אֹפֶל**: Gr. ἀμαύρωσις; correct: ἀμβλυωπία; cf. Ibn al-Jazzār, *Zād al-musāfir wa-qūt al-ḥāḍir*, bk. 2, ch. 6 (forthcoming, eds. Bos and Käs).

40, entry **בָּשָׂר: בשר נוסף**: Arab. بواسير; correct: نواسير; cf. MIG 480.

198, entry [**עור**]: *Piʿel* **עורר**; correct: *Polel*.

291, **תּוֹסֶפֶת: התוספות הדומות לשתי פטומות**: Arab. الزوائد الشبيهة بحملتي الثدى; correct: الزوائد الشبيهة بحلمتي الثدى.

ibid., **תּוֹסֶפֶת: התוספות הדומות לפיות השדים**: Arab. الزوائد الشبيهة بحملتي الثدى; correct: الزوائد الشبيهة بحلمتي الثدى.

292, **תּוֹסֶפֶת: התוספות הדומים בשני ראשי השדים**: Arab. الزوائد الشبيهة بحملتي الثدى; correct: الزوائد الشبيهة بحلمتي الثدى.

Index of Greek Terms

Index of Arabic Terms

Index of Latin Terms

Index of Romance Terms

www.ingramcontent.com/pod-product-compliance
Ingram Content Group UK Ltd.
Pitfield, Milton Keynes, MK11 3LW, UK
UKHW041844031026
15587UKWH00003B/999

9 789004 472792